4th Revised & Enlarged Edition

Indian Handbook of Hypnotherapy

ABOUT THE AUTHORS

Dr. Bhaskar Vyas (1937) and **Rajni Vyas** (1937) have distinguished themselves in their respective professions as plastic surgeon and obstretrician-gynecologist respectively. When they had initial exposure to hypnosis in 1976 from H. Jana, Modi and Athawale, they were excited to find some common ground between meditiation and hypnosis. They explored it further to learn hypnotherapy as a discipline from A.B. Khurana, Ratubhai Parikh, Kripa and Aruna Thakur, and Ernest Rossi. Vajrayana and Patanjali's Yoga Sutra gave further strategic support. They have conducted numerous workshops and trained several hypnotherapists. They initiated and are teaching hypnotherapy at M.S. University, Baroda, India. They have been Presidents of the apex hypnosis societies.

4th Revised & Enlarged Edition

INDIAN HANDBOOK OF HYPNOTHERAPY

FOUNDATIONS AND STRATEGIES

BHASKAR VYAS & RAJNI VYAS

Edited by

ULF SANDSTRÖM & SUSHEEL GUPTA

CONCEPT PUBLISHING COMPANY PVT. LTD.

NEW DELHI-110059

ISBN-13: 978-93-5125-195-8

First Published 2016

Published and Printed by

Concept
Since 1974

Concept Publishing Company Pvt. Ltd.
A/15-16, Commercial Block, Mohan Garden,
New Delhi-110059 (INDIA)
Phones : 25351460, 25351794, *Fax* : 091-11-25357109
E-mail : publishing@conceptpub.com
Website: www.conceptpub.com

Editorial Office: H-13, Bali Nagar, New Delhi-110 015, India.

Cataloging in Publication Data—DK Courtesy: D.K. Agencies (P) Ltd. <docinfo@dkagencies.com>

Vyas, Bhaskar, author.
Indian handbook of hypnotherapy : foundations and strategies / Bhaskar Vyas & Rajni Vyas; edited by Ulf Sandstrom & Susheel Gupta. — 4th revised & enlarged edition.
pages cm
Includes bibliographical references.
ISBN 9789351251958

1. Hypnotism—Therapeutic use—India. I. Vyas, Rajni, author. II. Sandström, Ulf, editor. III. Gupta, Susheel, editor. IV. Title.

RC495.V93 2016 DDC 615.85120954 23

Foreword

This scholarly volume of studies on Hypnosis by Drs. Vyas whom I call Indian Savants, introduces a new international standard of scientific excellence. Academicians, professionals in medical and psychological therapeutics, and their students will find each chapter in this book to be an authoritative source on the rich history and current status of the theory, research and practice of therapeutic hypnosis and mind-body healing in India. This is truly a scientific book on therapeutic hypnosis published by Indian savants as a major contribution to the psychotherapeutic art of the world.

India is one of the most unique nations of the globe in its ancient cultural heritage and rich practice of the creative arts of facilitating consciousness, spiritual states, and mind-body healing. The ancient religions of India, its gurus and teachers have long been a source of fascination and study by Western scholars. There has never been a single source of authoritative information about ancient and modern India that everyone could trust, however. This volume fulfils that need. Professor Vyas are at their creative best in this book.

Readers of this volume will find that therapeutic hypnosis, as it has developed and practiced over the past two centuries in the West since the time of Mesmer, is to a large extent a rediscovery of many of the mysteries of mind and behaviour that were first recorded, studied and practiced in India. Because consciousness and personal experiences are so subjective, however, there has always been a great deal of confusion about the philosophy, science, therapeutics or religion. Are studies of consciousness, spiritual experiences related to the body? If so, how is it possible? What are the integrative concepts and methods that bring mind, body, spirit, and therapeutics together?

One important and integrative concept of modern science that is consistent with and respectful of ancient studies of consciousness, spirituality, and healing as presented in this book is that which is now generally called information. Information is certainly communicated between guru and students of whatever art, science or philosophy as practiced in ancient and modern cultures. Information is rapidly becoming the central concept in the social, biological, physical, computer and mathematical sciences today. Since the monumental discovery of the molecular DNA code of life for which Watson and Crick received the Nobel Prize, information has become the central integrating concept for all studies of the art, science, and therapeutics. We now know and, as the book very lucidly portrays, information encoded in the molecular code of our genes functions as a space-time-energy-information transducer integrating our mind and body with our physical and psychosocial environment in a highly creative and adaptive manner.

It is preciously here in integrating information between scholarship in ancient and modern India—that this book serves a most important purpose for all academicians, students, and professionals in therapeutic practice. The authors of this impressive volume express a practical vision of how the subjective information of the mind can be integrated with scientific research to facilitate the art of healing the traumas and stresses of the modern world. This profoundly integrative book of therapeutic hypnosis is a new highway to the future of India's contributions to world of medicine, psychology, and philosophy.

Ernest Lawrence Rossi Ph.D.

Notes From the Editors

It is with joy I am part in bringing you this book about hypnotherapy by Doctors Rajni and Bhaskar Vyas. It reflects two lifetimes of vast experience in the field, and combines the science, the methods and the techniques with case studies, and the Indian perspective of a society with long traditions of spirituality, and an open mind to how the continuum of body, mind and soul affect each other.

The specific way Drs Vyas combine medical science with hypnosis and spirituality is the holistic view I believe will make the difference for stress related health issues in the future. I am a hypnotherapist, and my main interest is resolving symptoms of Emotional- and Post Traumatic Stress, based on how the neurology of trauma encodes in our amygdala and can evolve into phobias, allergies and even physical diseases. I am eternally thankful to Drs Vyas for their passion, sincerity and generosity in sharing their knowledge and skills.

Warm regards

Ulf Sandström,
Hypnotherapist, Sweden
Chairman International Hypnotists Guild, Peaceful Heart Network
ulf@ulfsandstrom.se

I am a medical doctor, working with cardiac patients as a resident (pre- and post-procedure care and emergency care) and I am practicing hypnotherapy. My skills in hypnosis took a sharp turn when I started working with Drs Vyas for the 3rd edition of this book. Whenever I see them, they teach me something new.

I know that current medical science is good for a lot of issues, and through working with hypnosis I have found that some of the diseases considered tricky in the psychosomatic realm of body and mind, can be cured. I want to serve this cure to the entire humanity and I hope for medical science to incorporate a lot more of the simple, yet efficient tools of hypnosis. This is the goal in my life.

Regards

Dr. Susheel Gupta, MBBS, DCAH,
Vadodara (Gujrat), India
susheelgupta25@gmail.com

The International Hypnotists Guild

IHG is a non-profit organization dedicated to collecting and distributing research, experiences and knowledge in all areas involving hypnosis. Please join.
If you have thought on how to improve this book please let us know, it is a living document under constant revisions. Mail ulf@ulfsandstrom.se

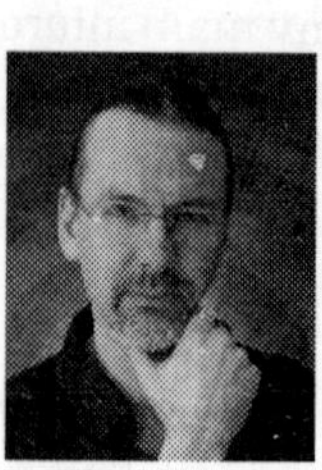

I'm a hypnotist. I've had the privilege to experience Drs Bhaskar and Rajni Vyas work live and they're truly effective and creative working in a way that is totally natural to them. In this book they generously share their knowledge and experience. Together with Ulf Sandström I am also on the board of directors of the International Hypnotists Guild. We believe in collaborating internationally to share the remarkable results that are possible with hypnosis.

Fredrik Praesto
General Master Trainer, IHG
NLP Master Practitioner, NLP-Trainer
Read more at www.internationalhypnotistsguild.com

Contents

Introduction

Hypnosis has global practice. However, clinical practice is culturally conditioned. The book relies heavily on Indian tradition. It has relevance to Indian society, culture and philosophy. We have therefore called it Indian Handbook.

The practice of hypnosis requires a wide range of fundamental understanding of physiology, psychology, philosophy (Western and Eastern) and psychotherapy. Attempt has been made in this direction. Because of this unique aspect of the book, it is relevant to all audiences. A lay person with scientific orientation may also find it interesting that hypnotherapy is a scientific discipline and the book should encourage him/her not to indulge in its unscrupulous practice. The book is meant for people who are legitimately entitled to practice hypnotherapy-medical doctors, psychologists, dentists, physiotherapists. It has to be emphasized that even this group needs practical training as much as a surgeon needs in his discipline. For the educationist and paraclinical personnel, there is scope to understand enough of hypnosis relevant to their interest and application.

Hypnosis is very easy to induce. However, that is only a change in the phase of consciousness. The subject has transgressed the ordinary awake state to merge into a distinctly different state with specific characteristics to it. Targeting a symptom, a syndrome, a disorder or a disease requires a strategy. The results can be demonstrated at workshops and be reproduced at the clinics. However, for an individual therapist, particularly a novice the situation is different. While dealing with unfamiliar cases, the most important question is how to proceed. What is the strategy?

This book gives some strategies as applicable to common conditions. It begins from the beginning as to how to structure the clinic/therapy rooms. It lays down a general format about what the ambience should be. Elementary protocols of courtesy, often forgotten particularly in the Indian context, are enunciated. Rapport building is formally illustrated.

Thus far it is common to all the situations. What most therapists want to know is how to structure a session for a particular condition. This is where the artistic ability of the therapist comes to be displayed. All surgeons perform operations; some of them do so more precise and deft. But every surgeon has a beginning and further evolution. Same applies to hypnotherapist. Regardless, therefore, of the status and length of practice, suggestions and formats for the design of the sessions are helpful. A Mona Lisa is painted only once: the inspiration so derived can cause innumerable replications.

A thorough mastery over the technique as well as complete familiarity with psychopathology is the prerequisite as a backdrop to successful therapy. Before venturing into therapeutics, the practitioner has to understand what is hypnosis and hypnotherapy. He has to be clear about what constitutes psyche and its compartments, howsoever hypothetical. There should be no confusion about consciousness and conscious, subconscious and unconscious mind. Philosophical collaterals of these concepts should be well versed. Most teaching is based on the Western concepts and, if the therapist is dealing with mainly Indian clients, he should be thoroughly conversed with cultural contradictions and predilections.

The strategies outlined in the book extend into several hours of work in clinical session. The tendency for stereotype copying will take away the joy of creation: still will succeed as much as command therapy also does. Taking a given instance as a model, the book aims to provide insights to the practitioners to design programmes for individual clients/patients. This will not only excel in the deliverance of the expected outcome but provide creative joy for therapist.

The singular distinguishing feature is a foreword by Ernest Rossi. He has painstakingly gone through the book and made detailed comments that led to further improvement of the text. This is one of the great strength of the book.

Prof. A.B. Khurana, Dr. Geeta Adwanenikar, Dr. Umakant Dave, Dr. Madhusudhan Jani, Dr. Bharat Kapadia, Prof. Sangeeta Chandawani, Prof. Uma Deshpande, Dr. Radha Mohan, Dr. Girish Vaishnav, Dr. Renu Sharma and Dr. Yogesh Chandarana made helpful comments regarding some of the chapters. Prof. Bimla Parimu inspired us.

The book is meant as a resource book for the course of Diploma in Clinical and Applied Hypnosis being offered at M.S. University, Vadodara: however, it will also serve as a handbook for anyone who is interested in hypnosis-at whatever stage.

Post Script to Introduction

The title of this book, The Indian Handbook of Hypnotherapy: foundations and strategies needs explanation.

Hypnosis is a universal attribute of mankind. Human beings any where, even those who have not been formally initiated to the subject would have experienced hypnosis at several occasions that are commonly associated with wonder, romance, awe, intense fear etc. So, it can be legitimately asked as to why the book should have an identity as Indian. The reason is clear and explicit.

While the experience is universal, its modulation so as to bring about a psychodynamic change is culturally conditioned. A mere view of anthropological situations among different cultures across the globe would ratify this: and yet, it is also pertinent that there can be several derivations to rich Indian tradition. This culture which is more than five thousand years old has flowed through the millennia by further enrichment with cultural and religious inputs of Buddhism, Jainism, Islam and Christianity. They all provide metaphors in the form of surrealistic images that impinge upon the archetype of the subject so as to bring about a radical transformation.

Recently there are two important publications[1,2]. Based on the postulates of these books hypnotherapy is for all those who believe that it brings about a radical metamorphosis. This book may therefore be called alternatively a global handbook.

However, as long as behaviour is culturally conditioned and values are formulated culturally, contortions of psychodynamics will manifest as disorders and diseases that way they are the symptoms of a troubled mind. The sure reversal of the order out of chaos of vitiated defenses of ego can be regained by utilizing high suggestibility of the hypnotic state. This is best translated by the idiomatic use of the axiom: we have to use the currency of the country. Earth is one; but geography makes the nations.

Preface to the Third Edition

Take this as a parody; take it really seriously: Fact of the matter is Hypnotherapy is a Science.

This may sound to be a platitude for those who are learned and practicing hypnotherapy with demonstrable results. However, for those who find them novice to the field, it does come as a surprise. Any idea that is novel, fascinating, luminous, dazzling or may be even, bizarre, —like a girl in the magic box being cut into two and jumping alive as one–produces a specific response from the observer. That also is common sense: One gets dazed and at times aghast! Hypnotic processes and magical demonstrations both appear extraordinary and yet, there is no magic about it: and, both are based on certain psychodynamic processes that are just being discovered – though such phenomena are a part of our every day life! Even noting certain details at a murder or terror scene and forgetting some is based on functioning of certain neurons and genes (!) at such times.

People mistakenly say; with the advent of quantum physics, Newtonian physics is outdated. They forget we are talking about an apple falling from a tree to the ground and the planets going round the solar system–even stock market functions as per the law of cause and effect! But did not Newton say that give me a long enough stick and make me stand in the solar system outside the earth and, I shall lift up the earth with my stick! For those who take a cue from this and try to use the law of gravitation for pulling money out of stock market through self-hypnosis–thinking themselves to be great telepathic programmers of the markets forget the elementary principle that in gravitational pull mass is the important factor. The gravitational pull of greed can be like a black hole so that huge finance institutions across the world also get sucked, shrunk and disappear. This is also science as the hypnotic process is: if you do not believe it, wake up some corpses that commit suicides following stock market crashes, and ask. They would tell you that stock market cast a hypnotic spell on them and, they likened themselves to Napolean Bonaparte – out to conquer the world.

So science is all about cause and effect, that cause causality to change the environment; results and variables, predictability and certainty. If physics and mathematics are such high precise sciences conforming to the principles of deductive logic, believe us when we say, hypnosis will also confirm to those principles. If you do not believe us, ask; but do not ask us; ask politicians. They will go a step further to prove that bluffing is also a science and, holding shares and not holding shares in IPL is all a make believe! Did not Sankaracharya say about the world being a mirage? *Brahma satyam*: *jagan mithya*! If all the world is a stage and we are but players in a drama, was Shakespeare not a great hypnotist to create such illusions that Romeo and Juliet still exist?

Some innocent genuinely nice people—to be innocent genuinely nice people is a hypnodrama being played most frequently by good, bad and ugly; all across the band–ask us: do you believe in the ghosts? We refer them to Dr. Jekyll and Mr. Hyde. It is pathetic to see that Mr. Hyde hides in most of us, most of the times–and some of us secretly love him too! and several expert psychiatric doctors Jekylls cannot exorcise him. Yet it may take a fresher in Clinical Psychology who has just walked out of the hypnosis workshop, a few sessions of cold fusion with hypnosis that the pathological ego states fuse into one forever.

Life is like that! Did not Meera Bai (a mad woman of god) sing about the fools being rewarded with kingdom and Pandits going a begging? Freshers will crack the psychodynamics of schizophrenics by just cataloguing the few years backwards of a young man to discover when was it that he was bit by a scorpion girl–*vishkanya* to be precise—that left him beaten, battered and perceptually blind so as to have disorientation in time and space. Most high profile psychiatrists will ravel in uncovering the schizophrenic gene and keep changing molecules after molecules for this young man. Yes, they are right in ridiculing psychoanalysis as the pursuit of lazy nineteenth century psychologists. Who has the time today to browse, read and mull over Romeo and Juliet! All the world is a stage, and we the doctors are just the actors in the melodrama that is played about: let us do our role to prescribe and change from one molecule to another. This may be an ordeal for most mentally wrecked, do not be surprised that naïve hypnotherapist age regresses empathetically to erase the traumatic memories by selective ablation of the past event. Of course, it is astonishing to see the post hypnotic suggestion work so that the boy passes his final examination with distinction. That should remind us of the fact that Jonathan Nash winning a Nobel Prize is a real life story.

Yet, if some credit is to be given to quantum physics as some kind of hypnodrama, it tells us about every particle changing its action with presence of an observer. Einstein refused to believe that a mouse looking at the Universe does change it. He said, God does not play dice. Neil Bohr's reply was: let God do his work and physicists their own. The hard core psycho-pharmocologists and psychiatrists would not believe that a tiny-mini clinical psychologist can look into the psychodynamics of a ravaged mind and, through the cyclic rotation of time dimension, can bring about a cure that would very soon be drugless.

The energy, which is unknowingly being provided by the consciousness of the observer in quantum physics, seems to be playing the same truant in the relationship between the subject and the therapist. The charisma of one influences reciprocally at times so great that one sees God when none exists. Poor hypnotherapist is trapped with the difficulty of studying the human behaviour which changes its route with presence of each different observer. There may be more interpretations of psychodynamics than the number of therapists and, none can be proved wrong! Knowing the real self, what lies deep within, what stirs up and stimulates within with every new experience; such questions are numerous! Like they say, knowing Shiva is enough for many, but for few it is the search of *Mahadeva* (a superior god), and for even fewer, it goes up to the search of *Mahakaala* (the god of time). As such, who would and who would not dare to discern the darkness which is lying deep with in the realms of Unconsciousness? Once again, hypnotherapist will answer such questions most humbly that he is just a poor scientist: for him the success of such probing lies in restoring his subject to functionality.

Humans are the most trainable species, and we train our minds with everything that we see or listen or just experience. Why would the *Panch Tantra* and Anderson tales be so effective in teaching a child about morals and discipline? Story telling being one of the oldest arts is enough to explain suggestibility and also to tell when someone is highly suggestible. We do not need to quote Milton Erikson—or for that matter our own Bhaskar Vyas for that. We can easily find the references of ill/well effects of the daily televison soap operas on the families following them. With the women having greater difficulty in finding peace and being content, and the men having trouble of searching the satisfaction with uncontrolled drive of ambition, we are talking about a society which is very high on indulgence. So, when a hypnotherapist cures a long history of infertility in just a few sessions, it is not miracle. It is a hundred per cent science, that restores the milleu interior to normal natural pulsatility that some one out there programmed the female since the times of Eve. It sounds incredible. So, let us take a simpler case: What happens when a woman is humiliated for her looks? Very simple, she develops twitching of face. Doctors call it a tic. It is wonderful to see hypnotherapeutic suggestions work and the woman being rid of her six years long abysmal trouble in just sixty days!

After all this persuasion, if the reader is now convinced that hypnotherapy is indeed a science as much is surgery, beware that we might just be fooling you as much as when we tell you we are sure that rebirth exists! Only a few centuries back, surgery was done by barbers: British respect that tradition even to-day! And if you respect British for all the imperial glory that they once had, how ingenuinely they are to carry on with the irrelevant tradition of Royalty? Ask Milton Erikson. He will carry on the tale till such times that you will end up convinced that any barber may become a surgeon but it requires a real creative genius to paint a Mona Lisa!

We agree. Milton Eriksons are not made: they happen as the flowering of the creative upsurge of a huge human potential. So, in the end, may be, we were just fooling you: hypnotherapy is not science: it is an art at its excellence: no Hadron Collider will ever produce a Leonardo da Vinci or a Milton Erikson!

Notes

1. Graham Burrows, Robb Stanley, Peter Bloom, *The International Handbook*, UK (2001).
2. Bruce Lipton, *Biology of Belief*, USA (2005).

Code of Ethics

To all participants of a course or workshop of hypnosis and/or hypnotherapy, the following pledge is compulsory for the continued participation to the course:

I solemnly pledge that:

I am privileged to undertake the course that exposes me to some aspects of Hypnosis. I now understand that the subject is vast and of immense potential.

I understand that just as a surgeon who wields a knife has to be highly skilled, so does a hypnotherapist who manipulates the mind, unskilled hypnotherapy can do harm as much or more than the knife of an unskilled surgeon.

I shall therefore not indulge in any act that shows hypnosis to be some kind of "magic" or "power" with me.

I shall undertake only as much of self-hypnosis as I understand that I understand.

I shall not undertake the treatment of psychological or "organic" diseases unless I am convinced that I have full training to do so and I have fairly mastered the technique for the same.

I shall refrain from treating my dear friends and near relatives form treating as far as possible.

I have understood the phenomenon of transference and counter-transference. With a view to save my clients/patients from transference, by and large, I shall not leave them with an obligation.

My motivation shall always be to help-honestly and transparently. In the process, when I derive any income, it is my rightful due.

I honestly and earnestly take a solemn pledge to abide by the above—both in letter and in spirit.

1
History of Hypnosis in India

At the onset, let us define hypnosis. The word is derived from Greek root *hypnos,* that means sleep. However, it is not a state of sleeping. The hypnotic trance does appear to resemble sleep, but the state is distinctly different from other states of consciousness–awake, sleep and dream states–that are ordinarily known to all of us.

Rishis of the ancient times knew different states of consciousness. *Mandukya Upanishad*[1] mentioned *Turya,* as Fourth State of consciousness. The Upanishad is tersely composed only in 12 verses. After elaborating on the initial three stages, *Turya* is described as thoughtless state where there is merging of self in the Supreme Self.

Patanjali's *Yoga Darshan-Yoga Sutras* of Patanjali (about 2500 B.C.) is unparalleled in its exposition of psyche and its dysfunctions. Yoga literally means to enjoin and, it lays down a royal road to spiritual enlightenment. Through a chiseled structured programme consisting of eight steps, it guides a beginner in practice of yoga to its highest advancement, to where that Alone is—*Kaivalya*. It postulates seven states of consciousness; well demarcated and yet, contiguous with each other.[2] Most commentaries interpret the *sutra* to connote seven states of intellect. However, further exposition of seven states is found in *Yoga Vashishtha.*[3]

States of consciousness beyond the ordinarily known three states are unfamiliar to most people. *Turya* and other states are not only experiential, but are a privilege of a few spiritually advanced meditators. They are not the subject of discussion here. But hypnosis, call it by whatever name of the state, is a fundamental attribute of all human beings. It is easily experienced by most. Though one need not be any way spiritually inclined to derive therapeutic benefits from it, it may prove a gateway to insights, leading to even enlightenment.

Hypnosis in Ancient India

The *Vedas* are the most ancient texts in Indian tradition. Savants like Tilak and Vivekanand date them to about 5000 B.C. *Atharva Veda* is the last of the four

Vedas. This is the most ancient source that mentions about psychotherapy. Certain of the therapeutic methods described here pertain to some of the techniques used in the present day hypnotherapy.[4] They are *mantra vidya*[5] in the form of *sankalpa* that is akin to auto-suggestion or self-hypnosis; and *sadesha,* that involves a therapist. To apply *sadesha,* refined application of symbolism, personification, metaphors and aversion are applied. The text does mention a specific word, *samvashikarana,* that translates as hypnosis and its use is described to enhance qualities of personality. It was used for diseases like epilepsy, hysteria and "consumption"[6].

Charak Samhita, magnum opus of Indian system (*Ayurveda*) was written about 2000 years back, mentions mantras and psychotherapy. Charak considered all the ailments to arise from the faulty functioning of discriminative wisdom. He makes a sweeping, all encompassing statement as

Pragyaparadha jayate sarva rogan!

That translates as; all the diseases arise from the faulty functioning of the intellect. But Charak does not seem to have mentioned hypnotherapy as such.

Patanjali mentions actually of several *siddhis* in *Vibhuti pada.* One of them is *vashita,* meaning ability to control the will of the others. Vagbhatta, who came after Patanjali, in *Ashtang Samhita* mentions meditation for psychosomatic disorders.

The Export of this Science to the West

Abbe Faria, who hailed from a Brahmin family from the South, was taught hypnosis by his father. After migrating to France in eighteenth century, he conducted shows with group hypnosis that involved as many as 5,000 people at one time and cured several of them. However, his impact on the Indian environment has been nil.

Before the discovery of drugs for anesthesia, James Esdaile, a Scottish surgeon operated on many patients under hypnosis at Calcutta (Kolkata now). His is a glorious chapter that has almost been lost. Let us retrieve it from a torn book.

James Esdaile, was born on February 6th, 1808 at Perth, Scotland. He graduated at Edinburgh in 1830 and then obtained an appointment in the East India Company. On April 4th, 1845, when in charge of the Native Hospital at Hooghly, Esdaile made his first experiment. He was operating on a convict with double hydrocele. As the usual injection had produced severe pain, Esdaile tried to hypnotise the patient; but did not expect to succeed,—as he knew nothing about mesmerism except what he had read. The man, however, fell into a deep trance, and became analgesic. Encouraged by this, Esdaile continued his experiments and soon reported seventy-five "mesmeric" operations to the

Company Board. His letter was not even acknowledged. When his operations amounted to over a 100, he placed the results before the Government The Governor of Bengal, Sir Herbert Haddock, at once appointed a committee mainly composed of medical men. Their report was an extremely favourable one. Esdaile operated over 375 patients before returning to U.K.

He failed to make any academic impact in U.K.: instead he faced ridicule.

And the glory ends there. On the contrary, *vashita,* if that meant to control the will of the others, went into serious disrepute, that lasts even today and the bias against hypnotherapy is widely prevalent.

Development of Hypnotherapy in Modern Times

On the other hand, the West, guided by the spirit of scientific inquiry and experimentation, has made great leaps in the understanding of this altered state of consciousness and its applications to psychotherapy that extend beyond the psychological domain. The British Medical Association took the cognition of this faculty as early as 1892. In 1955 it was accepted as a therapeutic modality by the same. Today, most of the European countries have done so and there are academic journals published by their Societies. American Medical Association recognized hypnosis as a treatment method in 1958. The Society for Clinical and Experimental Hypnosis was founded in 1949 and expanded into International Society in 1959. Prior to that, in 1957, American Society of Clinical Hypnosis was formed.

Today, a single *currency,* as body-mind, has already emerged. The recent understanding of molecular biological events, including the modalities of gene expression, link psyche and *soma.* This has brought the role of hypnosis in sharp focus. This is highlighted by the Nobel awards for the year 2004 in the field of physiology and chemistry.

Even though this is the case, modern medicine or clinical therapy has hardly any contribution to hypnotherapy from India. Its academic orientation and recent propagation is primarily due to the efforts of only a few individuals.

Dr. Hrishikesh Jana was the untiring pioneer. Dr. Jana was a physiologist. His detour to hypnosis began with an interesting event. One of his students at Manipal, South India, in 1959, demonstrated hypnosis in the class room. This started a journey for Dr. Jana to take up hypnosis as a mission for life. He is the first to have done a doctorate with hypnosis as a subject from Calcutta University. He was supported by Dr. Mody, an obstetrician and Dr. Athavale, a clinical psychologist, both from Mumbai. The authors gratefully acknowledge initial contribution by them to their learning. Dr. Mody was frowned upon by his peers. Dr. Athawale wrote a booklet on hypnosis. After some time, he gave up practice, founded Athawale Foundation and became a *'guru'*.

Dr. Jana is the Founder President of The Indian Society of Clinical and Experimental Hypnosis that was established in 1972. The Society is nearly extinct and we have initiated efforts to rejuvenate it. The Society so far has held four National Conferences. Dr. Anand Bhusan Khurana was the Chairperson and Dr. Bhupendra Palan was the organizing secretary for two of them that were held at Vadodara. Fifth conference is being organized at Vadodara in January 2009.

As of today, there is no formal recognition of hypnotherapy either as an adjunct or definitive therapy in academic circles in India except by some enlightened therapists. Obviously, therefore, there are no recognized courses for learning. It is being practiced at random. Bhaskar Vyas found great support from Bimla Parimu and Daftuar, at the Department of Psychology, M.S. University, Vadodara. He approached them with the syllabus from University College of London. A diploma course is now being offered at M.S. University, Vadodara. This is the only one of its kind, not only all over India but to the East of Suez. The course was initiated in 2001. By now about 90 students have qualified: some of them are already having post doctoral degrees and academic positions.

In 1987, Drs. Rajni and Bhaskar Vyas discussed hypnotherapy with a renowned philosopher, Dr. Rohit Mehta. Initially he was averse to it and deprecated the therapy. When presented with scientific advances, he regretted his bias and asked them to start an academic society. The Medical Hypnosis Society was formed in 1987 at Vadodara with Dr. Shivaji Udar as the Founder President and Dr. Ratubhai Parikh as Founder Secretary. Dr. Rohit Mehta inaugurated the Society. The Society was later converted into Indian Society of Clinical Hypnosis with Dr. Rajni Vyas as the President and Dr. Radha Mohan as the Secretary.

Prof. Ernest Rossi's interest in advancement of hypnosis in India was evident when he visited Bangalore for the conference organized by Prof. Ramachandran at the National Institute of Mental Health. He has been a pillar of strength behind us. The book is the culmination of collective knowledge and intelligence of the diplomats at the Psychology Department of M.S. University to whom the book is dedicated.

At the International Conference on Indian Psychology, Yoga and Consciousness, organized by the Indian Council of Philosophical Research in collaboration with the National Academy of Psychology and The Indian Academy of Applied Psychology in 2004 at Pondicherry, several members from the Indian Society for Clinical Hypnosis made presentations so as to impress the inclusion of hypnotherapy in the curricula for psychotherapy. The authors met Prof. Ram Krishna Rao there who has been an ardent exponent of Indian Psychology. With him as the Chairman of Indian Council of Philosophical Research, a seminar to explore hypnotherapy in Classical Indian tradition was sponsored in 2009.

The Society has also taken up the matter with Indian Medical Association, without any progress.

Post Script to History Chapter 1

Renaissance in Indian hypnosis and taking it to scientific foundation is due to three medical doctors. They are Shreedhar Sharma, Anand Bhushan Khurana and Hrishikesh Jana. Patronised by psychiatrist professors, Sharma and Khurana, Professor Jana organized initial six national conferences. The lead was followed by Bhupendra Palan.

Just when this is being written, Mehdi Fathi wrote from Iran as he is organizing a national conference there. "Facilitating hypnosis and hypnotherapists is not trouble for me. I feel it is my responsibility for expanding scientific hypnosis in my region. It may be wonderful if you know 20 years ago hypnosis was equal to magic, parapsychic and charlatanism in this region, I decided change it and begun presentations in universities and public societies. It was very difficult and boring. Now, we have trained more than 5000 medical staff, psychologists, nurses and. We have monthly demonstration in universities. We guide hypnosis researches in universities. Also people know hypnosis as science; not magic, and we have documented society for clinical hypnosis in health ministry. I have feeling about hypnosis like the feeling to my son, I have born it, grown it, try to secure it and, now enjoy from its expansion.

And from the other side of the globe, Sylvie Goldman is writing from Israel as "I use already the pledge from your book with my students-as is-and adapt the axioms. I thought to ask you: I want to propose to my students/colleagues your book as a Standard Book.... I began to study yoga, ayurveda and Sanskrit." Thus, there is a global spread and expansion of hypnosis; more, its synthesis with Indian traditions is also getting in vogue. Therefore it will make a highly readable, informative and entertaining book to write history of hypnosis. It will cut across eastern and western cultures. It will encompass various belief systems; even as they prevail in tribes of Africa, such as *Voodoo*[7].

At the same time it will reverberate to Dr. Larry Dossey performing "De-Hexing" at Brigham General Hospital at Boston; as an intern. It is well known that while de-hypnotizing an old man who believed in "Hexes", Dossey himself got converted into a different paradigm than his hard core scientific discipline.... It caused him to diverge from medical practice of today: that is based on Cartesian philosophy. This bifurcation created a different paradigm for health as well as medical practice for him; producing a wonderful book, Space, Time and Medicine.[8]

Most of such explorations were made unknow, proving a subtle point that hypnosis is all inclusive, pervasive phenomenon for human race. It further establishes the fact of its being a fundamental attribute of mankind. However, there is a moot point here. This kind of hypnotic experience is sub-luminal. It is indirect hypnosis.

The belief system routed in the deep alter state of consciousness pervades through the entire gamut of Tantric practices of Hinduism as well as Vajrayana of Buddhism. Viewed in this perspective the discovery of this phenomenon by Sharkot in nineteenth century appears relatively recent.

This suffices to convey that history of hypnosis covers the entire anthropological evolution of the mankind later so someday a historical genius will write this history that will cover several volumes.

Notes

1. *Mandukya Upanishad*, 12.
2. *Patanjali Yoga Sutra* II, 27.
3. *Yoga Vashishtha*, XXXI; 49-55.
4. Singh H.G., *Psychotherapy in India: From Vedic to Modern Times*, Agra, 1977 pp. 45-88.
5. Kapali Shastri T., *Further Lights, The Vedas and the Tantras*, Pondicherry, 1951, p. 108.
6. Arsh P., *Atharva Vediya Mantra Vidya*, Haridwar, 1991.
7. *Voodoo*–it is an occult practice. The tribes in Africa totally subscribe to a common belief. It is a mystic practice. It involves preparing a clay model of the enemy of the size of a doll. A word is scrumptiously passed to the victim that he/she is hexed. Everyday some clay is peeled off the clay model. The victim looses weight. When the clay doll finally collapses, the victim also dies.
8. Larry Dossey, *Space, Time and Medicine*.

2
States of Consciousness

While all of us are conscious, we may have hardly thought how consciousness arises, how does it transform and how and where does it vanish. The matter cannot manifest any thing that is not contained in it. If at some stage of biological evolution, the matter were to manifest consciousness as one of its properties, it must be intrinsically contained within it *ab initio.* If the implicate order of the matter is to incorporate consciousness, one has only to find the tools by which implicate, encoded order becomes explicit and unfolded. This epi-phenomenon, i.e. consciousness, that is evident in various forms of life is still a mystery though it manifests as self emergent quality of matter.

Expressing itself in the form of self-conscious, personal existence, the consciousness in man is in constant interplay with the phenomenal world. Awareness may be of ones surroundings, as inferred through the sensory inputs or it may be in terms of self-reference. Putting it another way, it involves the contact between the subject and object. And a step further, philosophers like Sri Aurobindo postulate that it is the fundamental attribute of all the matter. Theoretical physicist David Bohm defines consciousness as *an attribute that may be explicitly unfolded as seen in the life forms that are conscious or may be in the form of implicate order that remains unexpressed.*

The biophysics of consciousness[1] is still obscure; though the brain centers of its origin are well located. However, the play of consciousness seems physically a quantum electro-dynamic field, where the basic quantum currency is a single cell.[2] Applied to human beings, it leads to the possibility of infinite number of quantum fields in the process of being conscious.[3,4] This satisfies physical criteria that quantum theory stipulates–infinite degrees of freedom to systems, where quantum phenomena are taking place.

This kind of discussion is in the domain of philosophy. Philosophical reflections on the nature of consciousness have a bearing on the attitude of a hypnotherapist to therapeutic application. For instance, this is what Ernest Rossi commented on this chapter. *Consciousness is a novelty seeking modality of experiencing that turns on gene expression and brain plasticity.* An Indian philosopher would have never thought in such a manner: for him

Consciousness is primordial. On the other hand, hypnotherapist is primarily concerned with how vividly lived experiences in altered state of consciousness can reconstruct and heal the physical brain.

Since hypnosis is an altered state of consciousness, let us review what other states are. To be aware is to be conscious. Awareness may be perceptual of the external world, or it may be self-awareness. It is experienced by all of us in various states of consciousness. Ordinarily, they may be said to be, awake, sleep, and dreaming. Not familiar to all, there are other states of consciousness. In *Patanjali's Yoga Sutra*, it is said:

> *Saptadha prantabhumihi pragya.*[5]

That literally means that there are seven states of consciousness. They are demarcated and yet they are in continuity (as the demarcated geographical areas are). Having said that Patanjali leaves us to decipher what the seven states are.

As is common to philosophical interpretation of most classical Indian text, this statement also portends to be discursive with different semantics to word *pragya.* Most commentaries on Patanjali translate *pragya* as intellect here, though *pragya* is variously understood as intellect, discriminative wisdom and, it also means as intelligence in the life forms, i.e. consciousness. In support of such semantics, *rishi* of *Aitareya Upanishad* has this to say:

That which is known as the heart, the mind...that is consciousness or perception...all these indeed are names of consciousness (*pragyanam*[6]), consciousness is, indeed the cosmos (*Brahman*).

Summarising, there are seven states of consciousness, and the first three are:

- Awake
- Sleep
- Dream

During the experience of all of them, awareness that "I am there" persists.

The state of *Turya,* Fourth state is described as 'tranquil settlement in the state of liberation and the state of witness in action'. Indian tradition has varying concepts about *turya.* It is most poignantly narrated in *Mandukya Upanishad* as, *that which has no parts, soundless, the incomprehensible, beyond all the senses, the cessation of all phenomena, all blissful and non-dual AUM, is the Fourth, and verily it is the same as the Atman. He, who knows this, merges his self in the Supreme Self–the individual in the total.*[7]

This description stops short at Fourth State, describing *Turya* as a final submergence into the ocean of consciousness. It does not take the note of other states described in *Yogavashishtha.*

Since such classic descriptions of Turya go much beyond what is seen in hypnosis, it might be argued that later may not be called Fourth State: some say it is nearer the Fifth described in *Yogavasishtha* as, *Abiding in mere nonduality, with all distinction and division extinguished, he is seen as one asleep.*[8]

The Sixth state is described as, where he dwells "without knot", liberated while living and without conception or ideation. This is "*jivanmuktavibhavana*".[9] Having stayed in the Sixth state, he can reach Seventh state of enlightenment. This is the state of liberation without the body.[10]

Here, it is emphasized that narration of esoteric experiential states would differ from Pandit to Pandit. To quote from *Yogavashishtha* once again, *the sky of Pure Consciousness is only calm. This Supreme Spirit, some people ascertain as the state of Voidness, certain others, the state of mere knowledge and some others the state of the form of God, they quarrel mutually.*[11] However, to experience any of the states of consciousness is the fundamental attribute of all human beings and, is not culturally restricted or conditioned. William James said so in 1890-[12]1901-02[13]: Men involuntarily intellectualize their religious experience. They need formulas about the idea of 'fields of consciousness' with their centre or interest. Fields can vary in width and around what they are centered. These fields can experience incursions from beyond them, leading to sudden conversions marked by ecstatic feelings of happiness that need not be permanent to be critical to our lives. He describes various characteristics of mystical states such as their ineffability, noetic quality, transience, and involuntariness. He then gives some typical examples of mystical states and points out that while mystical experiences can occur naturally, certain religious traditions like Hindu yoga, Buddhist meditation, Islamic Sufi dance, and Christian prayer systematically cultivate them. Saint Francis and his disciples were, on the whole, of this company of spirits, of which there are of course infinite varieties.

In consonance, Patanjali describes different kinds of *Samadhi* (A state of communion where the presence of the observer is completely negated). They are:

- *Sampragyata Samadhi*[14]: Dialectic thinking, active mentation, abundance of interests and distinctive individuality are the factors constituting *sampragyata Samadhi* or an experience with thought-habit functioning as a center.
- *Asampragyata Samadhi*[15]: When consciousness retains only impressions of facts without their psychological associations, then is attained *asampragyata Samadhi*–an experience without any center of thought habit.
- *Savitarka Samadhi*[16]: In this state, there is an experience having thought modification as the center; there are variable interpretations due to the mind alternating between verbal and conceptual thinking. (Metaphors used in hypnotherapy illustrate this state).

- *Nirvitarka Samadhi*[17]: That is the experience in which the center of thought modification is non-existent—This state is attained when perception is clear so that subjective projections by the mind are dropped.
- *Sabijah Samadhi*[18]: This also centers round a thought seed.
- *Nirbijah Samadhi*[19]: When the very nucleus of identity is destroyed then there is a complete cessation of all reactive tendency, thus bringing into existence *Nirbijah Samadhi* or an experience in which there is not even a thought seed.
- *Dharma-Megha Samadhi*[20]: Here the state of meditation is an end in itself; not a means for the fulfillment of some motive (This is a stark contrast to hypnosis as well as *yoga-nidra*). There is pure and holistic awareness. It is a spiritual experience like benediction. There is infinity of wisdom and the psychological becoming through the functional activities of three *gunas* (all the defenses of ego) come to an end (so there is complete dissolution of ego). There is only That Alone—*Kaivalya*. The consciousness has regained its pristine, pure originality.

It will be of interest to most Indian hypnotherapist to know, understand and if possible to experience these esoteric, spiritual states. For successful practice of hypnotherapy it is not imperative to meditate and experience them. Therefore, we would rather describe as to what is the state of hypnosis, as it is well established by now through innumerable clinical and research observations.

Hypnosis: An Altered State of Consciousness

Since time immemorial, mankind has known a different state of consciousness. This altered/different state of consciousness is the attribute of entire mankind, but only a few are aware about it. This state is manifest in hypnosis (and meditation). But hypnotic state is widely researched through scientific tools by psychologists, physiologists and medical doctors. Therefore, the state of hypnosis is now widely documented. Objective criteria are now available for scientific validation about this subjective, experiential state.

The misconceptions about hypnosis are widely prevalent. This is because of its checkered history. It made its public debut in the West with stage shows by Mesmer in the later part of eighteenth century. Such stage shows, while claiming to bring about various cures, were motivated by craving for personal power. They indeed resulted in so much myth and mysticism being associated with hypnosis. This caused fear, distaste and dislike.

Mesmer did another mistake. The age of reason had just arrived then. The philosophy of Descartes' and Newtonian discoveries had established the relationship between causality and change. The whole universe was seen as a huge clock and every event was connected to some causative agent like the wheels of a clock. Going by the scientific spirit that was just dawning upon his time, Mesmer tried to postulate a scientific hypothesis. He claimed that the phenomenon of hypnosis and associated cures were because of a field that he called Animal Magnetism. When the Charcot commission in 1784 failed to find any such field[21], the baby was thrown with the bath water. The hypnosis was discredited and the stigma still sticks in the minds of the lay people. There was enormous empirical data to suggest the existence of a hypnotic state but the misconceived rationalization caused the damage. It attached a further stigma about hypothetical imposition of one's will on the other. No body can be hypnotized against his/her will or be made to do actions against his/her will. It put fear and disgust in the minds of people: so much so that subsequent clarification by Abbe Faria that hypnotic phenomena are entirely dependent upon the expectancy and co-operation of the subject; and are therefore in the nature of self-hypnosis, was also given a go-bye.

Hypnosis begins by transforming our ordinary consciousness to an altered state of consciousness. It is indeed a different state of consciousness, as much as sleep and dream states are. A sense of differing awareness about the experience is common to all the four states; even in sleep and dreams; the feeling of awareness is there. Hypnosis is not a delusion. It is not anything extraordinary either. Like awareness, sleep and dream state, this is a natural attribute of entire mankind. It is easily accessible by all, may be with a little help initially. Even when not formally told about it, most of us are familiar with it. In ordinary experiences, childhood fairy tales, a beautiful landscape, a piece of fine poetry, an absorbing novel, a magnificent painting, or simply a creative thought has given us a glimpse of this natural attribute. A good glimpse of this not so unfamiliar dimension is obtained in mystic verses from various traditions.

Such intuitive connection remains only a glimpse for most of us, because, caught as we are in the cross traffic of the profit and loss in our worldly trade accounts, we are immediately drawn away from this almost 'other worldly' experience; only to remember it as some precious moments. The memory of the precious moments can and do turn into "ever present now". For this to happen repeatedly, we have the doorway of the altered state of consciousness that is easily provided through hypnosis.

Phenomena in Hypnosis

Hypnosis and all kind of meditative states begin with the Fourth State of consciousness (Based on the description of *Turya* in *Mandukya Upanishad,* many *gurus* will not agree to hypnosis being called Fourth state; call it by whatever number, and accepting that hypnosis, *yoga-nidra* and meditation are not the same, there is much common to hypnotic and meditative states as we shall soon see). For the generation of the Fourth State of consciousness, most of the traditions rely on reflection, or self-absorption or simple relaxation along with deep breathing. There are sophisticated techniques for each of these, but one need not be familiar with them to begin. As the process goes forward, within a few minutes there is spontaneous onset of Fourth State of consciousness.

The characteristics of this state are that the mind is quiet, calm and peaceful. A general sense of well-being prevails. The person is awake but the state is more like sleep than awake. It is a state of alert restfulness. In this state there is focalization on the subject, be it an image or a *mantra* and, the marginal inputs fade. The focal point becomes symbolic, i.e. it gathers content that goes on expanding in its abstract meaning. There is attention on the focalized idea, but it is not accompanied by any kind of tension. There may be distraction by the surroundings, but there is no disturbance. There is choiceless extensive awareness but it is not exclusive of any thing in particular. Surreal metaphors translate into real.

The subjective time moves slowly and an hour may appear to have been only a few minutes. But if so programmed, the time shall pass very slowly. Or the time many so undulate that the distinction between the past, present and future is lost. There is shift of space location and one can experience oneself at several different locations in space. This is trance. It may be mild, moderate and intense in depth. And in the state of trance, one may experience the space-time dimension to shift. It is possible to regress in time and be at places at times in the past, which may have been forgotten. There can be time progression too. This is utilized in therapy for setting up a goal.

The state has been studied physiologically by Herbert Benson.[22] And there are extensive studies on the physiology of meditative state.[23, 24, 25, 26] Initially the pulse rate and the blood pressure rise; but soon go below the resting levels. The respiratory rate rises first, but soon falls below the resting level and, as the trance progresses, it may be accompanied by small periods of apnea. The metabolic rate falls steeply and it may fall below the level of sleep. The peripheral flow of blood increases and the body and the face may be flushed. Plasma cortisol levels decline. There is increased coherence of functions of both the hemispheres of the brain. In the electroencephalogram there is preponderance of *alpha* waves. There is increase of the galvanic skin resistance.

For the regular practitioners of self-hypnosis, there are lasting psychological benefits. Overall the stress levels decline. There are better interpersonal relationships. There is realistic goal setting and achievement. There is increase in productivity and creativity. Probably the most important outcome of the process is clarity of perception and the generation of intuitive insight.

Altered states of consciousness are useful tools to clarify perception. In every day living, one is led to several fallacies about perception. What is seen is coloured by various projections of mind. We shall discuss later about this as defenses of ego in terms of Freudian psychology. Before they become diseases of mind, they persist and perpetuate themselves as neurotic compensation thus acting as coping mechanisms in the service of the ego. Such a conditioned mind refuses to accept perceptual clarity. There is a constant striving by the mind to weigh each and every matter in its own favour. In the process, the perception of reality is tilted.

The mind is a mirror that has a tendency to gather dust through stress and strife of every day life. And this dust must not be allowed to remain. Better still the dust should not generate and if there is any, it must constantly be wiped out. Meditation is the remedy. J. Krishnamurthy[27] has explained it thus:

How is a mind that has so many problems, to meet new problems? There is problem of time, the problem of space, the problem of relationships, and the problem of living, of earning a livelihood, the problem of disease, health and old age. How is the mind to meet all these problems all at once, not one by one but the whole of them all at once, without effort? The way we meet them now, our problems are all fragmentary. There is the problem of fear, the problem of boredom, the problem of enjoyment—a multitude of problems one after the other. Is there a way of meeting all these problems not separately, but totally? For the mind to be totally free from pressure, pleasant or unpleasant, all motives, however subtle or noble, must wither away.

In contrast, hypnosis is goal oriented and therefore, circumscribed. What happens to the mind following the experience of meditation is a kind of transformation. It has been variously described as metamorphosis of the self and, mutation of the mind. There is awakening of intelligence[28] so that the very ground from where the intelligence arises undergoes a multifold transformation.

This kind of the awareness is different from the ordinary awareness. In this profound state of awareness, one is a participant and a witness too. Of course, on the way further, the participant and the witness both cease to be. Observer and observed also merge[29] to disappear altogether. One can say this is self actualization or the peak experience of Abraham Maslow. It is a state of self-realization in the timeless moment!

In this state there is steadiness of perception without any object to hold on and there is total stillness of mind without dependence on any image. It is this new mind that has come out of a radical transformation that can comprehend true nature of time.[30] There is a clear understanding about the perception of time being dependent on the moment of consciousness. While the past and future turn out to be mental constructs, the ever present *now* is just a moment dependent on the consciousness.[31] Since consciousness itself is modulated, the experience of *now* also subjects itself to change. Time dilatation and constriction as well as stoppage of time are the natural outcome.

Anatomy of Consciousness: Physiological Basis

So consciousness seems to be more than a mere function of brain: no matter that we have identified the reticular formation in the mid brain extending down to medulla oblongata as the seat of consciousness. Firing of the cells from the cells located in this region upward to the cerebrum causes the subject to be

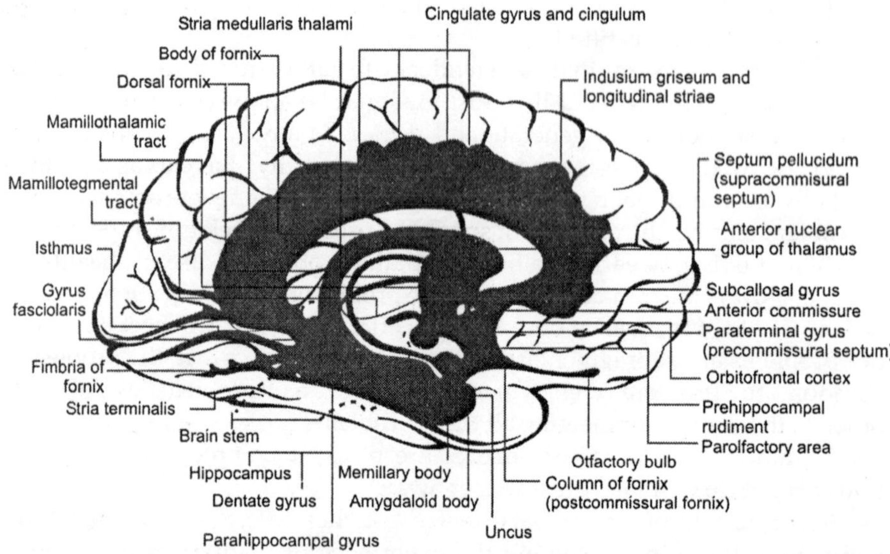

Fig. 2.1: Cross Section of the Cerebrum

conscious. However, such an activity does not happen in isolation and the role of genes is being recognized in psychobiology of consciousness. According to Rossi[32], consciousness can be understood as a series of continuously emerging experiential states that focus attention to evoke activity-dependent gene expression and neurogenesis in the dynamics of self reflection and co-creation of the self. It should not be long before there is conclusive evidence that the state of hypnosis is gene activity dependent. And we believe the physics of consciousness shall soon be understood in terms of quantum mechanics.

Hypnosis and Meditation

Though there are several features common to both as seen above, meditation is not the same as hypnosis. Meditation, when practiced, begins as self-hypnosis. It happens spontaneously too. And it may extend along an uncharted path to lands without boundaries. Hypnosis is restricted and much circumscribed. Both have been subjected to scientific research but it is difficult to standardize the results since the experience is subjective and input qualitative. On EEG, both the experiential states generate alpha waves and cannot be distinguished by it. Both are royal roads to unconscious mind and can lead to the experience that "a moment reveals what the ages toiled to express." "*Siddhis*" accrue to the meditator. Hypnosis generates creativity. Hypnotherapy alleviates or cures.

Let us compare them in a nut shell.

Hypnosis	Meditation
1. Scientific and therapeutic	Spiritual
2. Subject of scientific scrutiny	Philosophical
3. Studied scientifically since last two centuries	Spiritual experience since ages Difficult to quantify
4. Fertile ground for research; difficult to quantify the experience	A moral and ethical code of living is a prerequisite before initiation; esoteric
5. Any one can learn 6. Goal oriented	There are many kinds of *Samadhi*: goal oriented; goalless; and Nameless experience.
7. Relaxation and deep breathing are utilized as induction tools	Stillness of body and mind is essential; esoteric breathing exercises, pranayam, facilitates the experience.
8. Utilized for therapeutic healing and for personality development	Health giving, disease preventing and helps spiritual growth.
9. Self hypnosis is easy to learn and practice and can be taught individually and in group by academicians	Requires a *guru*. Difficult to find a *bona fide guru*.
10. Archetypal symbols and meaningful images may be utilized	Focalization on a form of sound, *mantra* or visual symbol of a deity.
11. Insight generation and creativity is a step by step process	It is a pathless land where there is no destination, no goal. Enlightenment "happens".
12. Guided hypnosis is unlikely to do any harm	Meditation has driven people crazy when not practiced under the supervision of a *guru* or a guide.
13. Freedom from affliction by hypnotherapy	Attainment of *kaivalya* – Journey alone to Alone.

Psychedelic State of Consciousness

The altered state arising out of drug ingestion, habit, dependence, abuse is pathological. The damage to self and the civilization are devastating that the use is criminal. Drug abuse is most difficult to treat; in a willing subject, hypnosis promises to be a good adjunct in combination with professional psychiatric help.

The following is only for the sake of academic interest. If this were to be the universal experience, *nirvana* seems to be only a pill away! No wonder, Arthur Koesler[33] dreamt of a substance that can be mixed with the drinking water so that it heightened creativity and sense of peace for the general population!

The highly aesthetic experience is given a poetical description by Aldous Huxley.[34] Huxley was drawn to experiments with altered states of consciousness and was in close contact with Milton Erickson. They closeted themselves for some time and did several experiments to study consciousness at Huxley's home. The home caught fire and the records were destroyed.

Huxley studied Buddhism and had practiced meditation. His description of what happens in the State (induced by ingestion of mescaline) is immaculate. Huxley states, "I was seeing what Adam had seen on the morning of his creation—the miracle, moment by moment, of naked existence. In an instant I experienced in things around me a transience that was yet an eternal life, perpetual perishing, that was at the same moment, pure being. In this state, a simple look at the flower in the vase was to provide the beatific vision of *sat, chit, ananda*, viz. Being, Consciousness and Bliss". He saw the *dharma* body of the Buddha in the flowers. The doors to a new way of perception seemed to be open. Spatial relationships ceased to matter. Instead there was intensity of existence, profundity of significance and relationships within a pattern. He instantaneously realized the experience of Van Gogh in the painting of the Chair. While Huxley gazed at the legs of the Chair, he experienced, "Being my Non-self in the Non-self that was the Chair."

Huxley's description is following his personal experience with ingestion of mescaline. Hypnosis, meditation and the drug-induced state are not identical. However, one may note many similarities to the experiences.

Summarizing, States of consciousness beyond the ordinarily well known three, are experiential states of esoteric people. The Rishi of *Mandukya Upanishad* was perfect in being brief and not explicit. Patanjali after defining *pragya* having seven states knew well to leave exposition. Vashishtha[35] after describing *Turya* elucidates seven steps to reach the pinnacle of *yoga*. In a broad sweep, he clubs initial three stages as one and describes four advanced stages with enlightenment as the ultimate.

So, call it by any name, or label it as you have experienced. Even to hypnosis, we assign three well documented stages; light, moderate and deep trance. Let us leave philosophic dissection and experience the whole. Sugar and honey by any name will taste same sweet: the sweetness of each is different. And yet, a rose is a rose is a rose.

Post Script to Chapter 2: States of Consciousness

The focus of hypnotherapist is to bring about a change in the health status for better. Towards this aim he utilizes various phenomenon as they occur during what we may classically called a hypnotic state: however, we come across different levels of hypnosis during trance. The subject does experience numerous variations of the altered state of consciousness. Their descriptions we come across in an ancient scripts as well as on treatises on meditation.

It will be in fructuous to discuss more about the differences between hypnosis and meditations. *Pandits* and *Gurus*, practising their own style of meditation assert their meditation is not self-hypnosis. This cannot be proved wrong.

"A rose by any other name will smell same sweet", says Shakespeare.

Meditation, *de facto* begins as self hypnosis except the phenomenon of spontaneous hypnosis. The experience of spontaneous hypnosis is ubiquitous but rare. Spontaneous hypnosis is confined to a selected few esoteric sages like Socrates, Ramakrishna Paramhans and J. Krishnamurti, who describes the experience of meditation as pathless land.

Today the value of any discipline, is determined by the number of people it is likely to help, at the minimum cost. Therefore, the therapist aims to bring about a change, a radical cure or transformation by utilising the altered state of consciousness that can be easily and certainly induced with a time frame.

Hypnotherapy by name of fourth state of consciousness—*yoga nidra*—or by utilisation of the phenomena attributed to 5th, 6th, 7th states of consciousness, is finding validation, acceptance and spread primarily because it helps.

Notes

1. Amit Goswami, *Physics of the Soul*, New York, 2002.
2. Bhaskar Vyas and Rajni Vyas, *Space Time Consciousness: The Fifth Dimension*, Delhi, 2004.
3. Ernest Rossi, *Dream, Consciousness, Spirit: The quantum experience of self-reflection and co-creation*, Arizona, 2002.
4. Schwartz J. and Begley S., *The Mind and The Brain*, London, 2002.
5. *Patanjali Yoga Sutra II*, 27.
6. Swami Chinmayananda, *Aitareya Upanishad*, III, 2,3.
7. *Mandukya Upanishad*, 12.
8. Sri Jnanananda Bharti, tr. by Samvid, *The Essence of Yogavashishtha*, XXXI, 50.
9. *Ibid.*, XXXI, 51.
10. *Ibid.*, XXXI, 53.
11. *Ibid.*, XXXI; 21.
12. William James, *Exceptional Mental States Lectures in Principles*, London, 1890.
13. *Ibid.*, *Varieties of Religious Experiences*, London, 1901-02.
14. *Patanjali Yoga Sutra*, I, 17.
15. *Ibid.*, I, 18.
16. *Ibid.*, I, 42.
17. *Ibid.*, I, 43.
18. *Ibid.*, I, 46.
19. *Ibid.*, I, 51.
20. *Ibid.*, IV, 29, 32, 34.
21. It is important to note that after that, there has not been any scientific investigation about the physical nature of hypnosis. Such an inquiry with refined modern tools is overdue.
22. Herbert Benson, *The Relaxation Response*, Boston, 1980.
23. Maharshi Mahesh Yogi, *Creating an Ideal Society*, Salisberg, 1977.
24. Wallace Robert Keith, *The Physiological Effects of Transcendental Meditation*, A Proposed Fourth Major State of Consciousness, Los Angeles, 1970.
25. Orme-Johnson D.W. and Farrow J.T. Scientific Research on the Transcendental Meditation programme: Collected papers. Meru, Switzerland, 1976.
26. Charles Tart, Altered States of Consciousness and the Spiritual Traditions: The Proposal for the Creation of State Specific Sciences, in K. Ramkrishna Rao *et al.*, *Handbook of Indian Psychology*, Delhi, 2008, pp. 577-605.
27. Rohit Mehta, J. Krishnamurty and *The Nameless Experience*, Delhi, 1979, pp. 128-153.
28. J. Krishnamurty, *Awakening of Intelligence*, Madras 1970.

29. *Patanjali's Yoga Sutra,* Section III, 3.
30. *Patanjali's Yoga Sutra,* Section III, 16.
31. Dwarakanath Reddy, *The Dicey Problem of New Age Science: Einstein, Hawking and God at the Casino,* Chittor, 2003.
32. Ernest Rossi, *The Psychobiology of Gene Expression,* New York, 2002.
33. Arthur Koesler, *The Ghost in the Machine,* London, 1955.
34. Huxley Aldous, *The Doors of Perception,* London, 1956.
35. *Yogavashishtha,* XXXI.

3
Phenomena in Hypnosis

Since time immemorial, mankind has known a different state of consciousness. This altered/different state of consciousness is the attribute of entire mankind, but only a few are aware about it. As discussed in the previous chapter, this state is manifest in hypnosis (and meditation). But hypnotic state is widely researched through scientific tools by psychologists, physiologists and medical doctors. Therefore, the state of hypnosis has now been widely documented. Objective criteria are now available for scientific validation about this subjective, experiential state.

Hypnosis begins by transforming our ordinary consciousness to an altered state of consciousness. It is indeed a different state of consciousness, as much as sleep and dream states are. A sense of differing awareness about the experience is common to all the four states; as experienced even in sleep and dreams, awareness is there. Hypnosis is not a delusion. It is not anything extraordinary either. Like awareness, sleep and dream state, this is a natural attribute of entire mankind. It is easily accessible by all, may be with a little help initially. Even when not formally told about it, most of us are familiar with this altered state of consciousness. In ordinary experiences, childhood fairy tales, a beautiful landscape, a piece of fine poetry, an absorbing novel, a magnificent painting, or simply a creative thought has given us a glimpse of this natural attribute that all humans possess. A good glimpse of this not so unfamiliar dimension is obtained in mystic verses from various traditions.

Such intuitive connection remains only a fond memory for most of us because, caught as we are in the cross traffic of the profit and loss in our worldly trade accounts, we are immediately drawn away from this almost 'other worldly' experience; only to remember it as some precious moments. The memory of the precious moments can and do turn into "ever present now". For this to happen, we have the doorway of the fourth state of consciousness.

Characteristics of the Hypnotic State

The lyrical/philosophical description in the previous chapter applies in common to both, hypnosis and meditation. It may be summarized qualitatively and objectively as follows:

Paradigm Shift in Consciousness

There is a total shift of perception of the external world and internal environment. The characteristics of this state are that the mind is quiet, calm and peaceful. A general sense of well-being prevails. The person is awake, but the state is more like sleep than awake. It is a state of alert restfulness. Self awareness persists except in deep trance. In this state there is focalization on the subject, be it an image or a *mantra* and the marginal inputs fade. The focal point becomes symbolic, i.e. it gathers content that goes on expanding in its abstract meaning. Surreal is perceived as real. There is attention on the focalized idea, but it is not accompanied by any kind of tension. Focalized awareness is accompanied with fading of marginal sensory inputs. There may be distraction by the surroundings, but there is no disturbance. There is choiceless extensive awareness that accepts the suggestions by the therapist uncritically, but it is not exclusive of any thing in particular. Control is passed over to the therapist so that most suggestions (except unethical, immoral or those that are repulsive to the subject's unconscious mind) take the form of command.

As per *Rig Veda,* there are 28 characteristics to consciousness. All of them undergo a change and the change is available for therapeutic utilization. Let us enumerate them before we take the discussion in psycho-physiological parameters. They are: Five kinds of *prana* (Western translation is impossible since the concept is alien to Western thought; at best they may be equated with metabolic processes); five elements viz. earth, water, fire, air and space; five senses viz. sound, touch, vision, taste and smell; mind, speech, body (form) and (organs of) action; five sheaths to the self viz. *annamaya* (physical), *pranamaya* (vital), *manomaya* (mental), *vigyanamaya* (intuitional) and *anandamaya* (blissful); *atma* (self), *antaratma* (inner self), and *paramatma* (self beyond self).

Hypnosis and all kind of meditative states begin with the Fourth State of consciousness. For the generation of the Fourth State of consciousness, most of the traditions rely on reflection, or self-absorption or simple relaxation along with deep breathing. There are sophisticated techniques for each of these but one need not be familiar with them to begin. For induction of hypnosis also there are numerous standard techniques and one has to master only a few. As the process goes forward, within a few minutes there is spontaneous onset of the Fourth State of consciousness.

Psychological Phenomena in Hypnosis

- ***Time Perception and Location in Space***

The subjective time moves slowly and an hour may appear to have been only a few minutes. But if so programmed, the time shall pass very slowly. Or the time many so undulate that the distinction between the past, present and future is lost. On the other hand, perception of time may be made very sharp. A subject when suggested to wake up after one hour does so nearly in time. There is shift of space location and one can experience oneself at several different locations in space during this state. This is trance. And in the state of trance, one may experience the space-time dimension to shift. It is possible to regress in time and be at places at times in the past, which may have been forgotten. There can be time progression too. This is utilized in therapy for setting up a goal.

For the regular practitioners of self-hypnosis, there are lasting psychological benefits. Overall the stress levels decline. There are better interpersonal relationships. There is realistic goal setting and achievement. There is increase in productivity and creativity. Probably the most important outcome of the process is clarity of perception and the generation of intuitive insight.

Altered states of consciousness are useful tools to clarify perception. In every day living, one is led to several fallacies about perception. What is seen is coloured by various projections of mind. We shall discuss later about this as defenses of ego in terms of Freudian psychology. However, before they become diseases of mind, they persist and perpetuate themselves as neurotic compensation thus acting as coping mechanisms in the service of the ego. Such a conditioned mind refuses to accept perceptual clarity. There is a constant striving by the mind to weigh each and every matter in its own favour. In the process, the perception of reality (in the ordinary every day sense of the meaning) is tilted.

The mind is a mirror that has a tendency to gather dust through stress and strife of every day life. And this dust must not be allowed to remain. Better still the dust should not generate and if there is any, it must constantly be wiped out. J. Krishnamurty[1] has explained it thus:

How is a mind that has so many problems, to meet new problems? There is problem of time, the problem of space, the problem of relationship, and the problem of living, of earning a livelihood, the problem of disease, health and old age. How is the mind to meet all these problems all at once, not one by one, but the whole of them all at once, without effort? The way we meet them now, our problems are all fragmentary. There is the problem of fear, the problem of boredom, the problem of enjoyment—a multitude of problems one after the other. Is there a way of meeting all these problems not separately, but totally? For the mind to be totally free from pressure, pleasant or unpleasant, all motives, however subtle or noble, must wither away.

Hypnosis is goal oriented and therefore, circumscribed. What happens to the mind following the experience of meditation is a kind of transformation. It has been variously described as metamorphosis of the self and mutation of the mind. There is awakening of intelligence[2] so that, the very ground from where the intelligence arises undergoes a multifold transformation.

In this profound state of awareness, one is a participant and a witness too. Of course, on the way further, the participant and the witness both cease to be. Observer and observed also merge[3] to disappear altogether. The consciousness then assumes whatever form is presented to it, knower, known or the act of knowledge. One can say this is self actualization or the peak experience of Abraham Maslow. It is a state of self-realization in the timeless moment!

In this state there is steadiness of perception without any object to hold on and there is total stillness of mind without dependence on any image. It is this new mind that has come out of a radical transformation that can comprehend true nature of time.[4] There is a clear understanding about the perception of time being dependent on the moment of consciousness. While the past and future turn out to be mental constructs, the ever present *now* is just a moment dependent on the consciousness.[5] Since consciousness itself is modulated, the experience of *now* also subjects itself to change. Time dilatation and constriction as well as stoppage of time are the natural outcome.

- ***Rapport in Hypnosis***

Rapport is fundamental to therapeutic efficacy. In most clinical situations, its importance cannot be overemphasized. One of the causes of superior therapeutic efficacy of hypnotherapy is easy establishment of rapport. Therefore, hypnosis maybe considered as communion in consciousness.

Particularly in the deep state, the *rapport* generally intensifies. The subject responds to the operator alone; and, while the latter's slightest gesture or softest whisper is instantly obeyed, he remains inert though others may stimulate him by speaking loudly or acting roughly.

- ***Memory in Hypnosis***

Memory in relation to hypnotic states varies widely arid is influenced by the depth of the hypnosis.

It may be unchanged and the subject can recall the events of normal life, and on awaking remember all that has passed during the session. Such memory may be increased, diminished or circumscribed. The subjects can recall during hypnosis the events of waking life and those of previous sessions with a clearness corresponding to their memory in the normal state, but, on awakening, the incidents of hypnosis are more or less forgotten. The subjects usually assert that they are able to remember all that has passed during hypnosis. Questioning, however, reveals the fact that their memory is not nearly so perfect as they believe it to be. Further, what they do recall soon fades, resembling ordinary dreams, which, although vivid on awakening, are often quickly forgotten.

The memory during the sessions and of the sessions at times surpasses the normal one. The improvement shows itself: (a) in an increased power of recalling impressions received during hypnosis, and (b) in reviving the lost impressions of normal life, so that what is told during hypnosis is better memorized.

The recollection during hypnosis of the events of waking life, and of those of previous hypnoses, rarely occurs spontaneously in the untrained subject. The suggestions of the therapist, however, readily evoke these memories, and his indirect suggestions produce the same result. Thus, when a disagreeable suggestion is given, the subject is able to recall, despite the wishes of the therapist, the feelings, sentiments or prejudices of his waking life and, may reject the suggestion. The subject, on the other hand, who has been frequently hypnotized and taught to revive lost memories by suggestion, soon comes to do so spontaneously. When hypnosis is induced, the subject takes up his hypnotic life at the point at which he left it when he was last hypnotized; and the memories of past hypnoses and of waking life are at once restored. Events reappear, just as ordinary memories would, with every association of ideas that is brought about by his surroundings. Cases are said to have occurred in which the forgotten dreams have been spontaneously recalled in hypnosis.

Sometimes the events of profound hypnosis cannot be recalled by suggestion. If the subject is told to sleep deeply, and to be unconscious of everything until awakened by the operator, two widely differing conditions may be observed: (1) Despite the commands of the operator, the subject at once manifests consciousness if any experiment, of which the subject disapproves, is attempted. (2) If, however, he is neither questioned nor touched, he generally takes no notice of anything said or done around him. On awaking, he frequently has no recollection of what has passed, and suggestion in hypnosis may fail to revive the lost memory.

A hypnotized individual cannot recall events that occurred during the period of his normal sleep. This is obviously so. So is the case with non-hypnotic double personality. What happened during an "attack" is not recalled in hypnosis.

- ***Echolalia***

Hypnotised subjects are capable of repeating like phonographs. This has utility in school studies.

- ***Memories of Long Past: Age Regression***

Memory of remote events is the basis of age regression. Memories of even intrauterine events have been explored. So is the case with memories that are repressed into unconscious mind. Some of the subjects can be time regressed so that they relate what had happened at the age of two or three, and one girl has described a children's party given on the first anniversary of her birthday. When the samples of handwriting are obtained, they alter in character with the age that was suggested: the subjects are unable to produce these in normal state. The increase in hypnotic memory is closely related to the depth of the hypnosis, and reaches its fullest development in somnambulism.

- ***Revivification***

Apart from a simple recall, the subject can be made to relive an event up to any age. There is at least one case report of age regression up to intra uterine life. A subject with phobia for sharp object regressed up to three months of fetal age. He saw a sharp object approaching him then. The mother confirmed an attempt at abortion that had failed. The memory was selectively ablated and phobia was cured. Thus, reliving can be very usefully utilized, particularly of emotional traumatic events.

- ***Past Life Regression***

Belief in past life can never be proved wrong: so far there is only one scientific investigation by Ian Stevenson. After a life time of work, he claims to have accounted over 2000 authentic cases. What matters is that apart from being a fundamental tenet of Hinduism and Buddhism, it is also a matter of faith for so many in other parts of the world.

Considering that the hypnotherapist uses the currency of country concept, he does not challenge the belief of his client. If the client ascribes his present ailment to some unfinished agenda of his previous life, it is possible to make that client experience his past life. In furtherance to age regression, he will further go back to his previous life(s), and will come across people with whom he had left agenda unfinished.

It is not to be offered by the therapist; but when asked by the client for a specific ailment, it does work. One of our client was dysfunctional since she had unfinished agenda with Lord Krishna. After regressing to several thousand years and meeting and dancing with him then, she came back to sleep for two days continuously: fully functional thereafter.

- ***Catharsis***

Reliving particularly of emotional traumatic events can produce a sudden letting off the repressed feelings. The subject may burst out crying or sobbing or even run about furiously.

Some times a novice of a therapist may get alarmed and think of terminating the session. It is better is to see that the subject does not harm herself, and wait till the outburst subsides. Invariably there is relief/cure after this. Therapeutic benefit is ascribed to state dependent memory that after reliving is replaced by another positive emotion.

- ***Memories of Future! Age Progression***

Paradoxical as it may sound, there is no suggestion of a design argument for the future here. What is implied is that suggestions so given that the subject is likely to pursue a particular goal and achieve it in foreseeable future, is followed by the subject. This works when the goals suggested are realistic. Subjects have been experimented with commands to execute after weeks up to an year successfully.

- ***Post-Hypnotic Suggestions***

This is a condition in which the subject, who has been previously deeply hypnotized, will accept suggestions similar to hypnotic ones, without having been subjected to any further hypnotic process, or having passed through any state resembling sleep or trance. The suggestions may have as powerful an effect as given during trance or even more

Under ordinary circumstances, the instant hypnosis is terminated all the phenomena which have characterized it may not disappear. In response to suggestion, one or more of these phenomena may manifest themselves in the subject's waking life. This is brought about in two ways: (1) Where the operator suggests that one or more of the phenomena shall persist after waking. For example, the analgesia successfully suggested in operative cases. (2) As a consequence of post-hypnotic suggestions, the appearance of the phenomena can also be delayed until some remote time after the termination of hypnosis. The production of sleep at night, the prevention of the return of periodic pain, the excitation of the action of the bowels, or of the menstrual flow, are examples of this from the therapeutic side. Sometimes the suggestions are forgotten almost immediately, at others they are remembered for a longer period, and in some cases are recalled after the lapse of weeks.

- ***Post-Hypnotic Amnesia***

Most hypnotic sessions are characterized by a decrease of memory of the events during session, on awakening, which usually corresponds to the depth of the hypnosis. Sometimes the subject recalls and retains a certain proportion of the incidents of his hypnotic life; at others he remembers everything on waking, but forgets it all a few minutes after. Finally, he may have absolutely no recollection of anything he has said or done during hypnosis.

It is difficult to determine whether post-hypnotic amnesia ever appears without either direct or indirect suggestion. Moreover, the lost memories of hypnosis cannot be revived by chance association of ideas and, therefore are fundamentally different from those of the waking state.

- *Selective Ablation of the Past*

The amnesia may be limited by suggestion. Here the subject cannot remember selected events and ideas of his past life. For example, he may be made unable to recall certain traumatic events after reliving them. This kind of post-hypnotic amnesia is of therapeutic value in post traumatic stress disorder and several other conditions.

- *Automatic Actions*

The hypnotic subject can be trained to perform/not perform automatic acts under hypnosis. If some simple movement is suggested, of which volition does not disapprove, it may after a time becomes *automatic,* i.e. after having been frequently voluntarily and consciously performed, it may be executed unconsciously as a genuine automatic act in response to the habitual stimulus, which has excited it. This is the basis of correction of tics and habits as well as sports hypnosis.

Physiological Phenomena in Hypnosis

- *Changes in the Voluntary Muscular System*

The first muscular change observed in hypnosis is usually a sudden or gradual closing of the eyes and muscular relaxation all over the body.

The appearance of the lids varies; sometimes they are closed more tightly than natural by muscular spasm, at others they are not quite shut, and a portion of the eyeball remains visible. When closed, the eyelids either remain motionless, or quiver as long as the hypnosis lasts. In some instances, just before or immediately after the closure of the lids, the eyeballs roll upwards, usually, however, quickly returning to the normal position. During induction, quite often nystagmus is noticed. Occasionally, the eyeballs turn inwards as well as upwards. In many cases of deep hypnosis, however, the eyes remain open, not only in the state itself, but also while it is being induced.

Eye movement desensitization and reprocessing (EMDR) is a new technique for induction. It is effective therapeutically too. It is an information processing psychotherapy that was developed to resolve symptoms resulting from disturbing and unresolved life experiences. It uses a structured approach to address past, present, and future aspects of disturbing memories. The approach was developed to resolve the development of trauma-related disorders such as rape. Clinical trials have demonstrated EMDR's efficacy in the treatment of post-traumatic stress disorder (PTSD).

The limbs can be bent at the joints easily at times like soft wax, and maintain any position in which they are placed. There is absence of muscular tiredness, so that, when uncomfortable positions are suggested or assumed during hypnosis, the fatigue and pain, which usually follow excessive muscular exertion in a fixed position, are apparently absent. This is useful to the plastic surgeon.

- ***Catalepsy and Arm Levitation***

Conversely, tonic contraction of all the muscles of a particular part or limb can be suggested. This is catalepsy. Catalepsy can be induced in all subjects who have passed the first stage. The amount of muscular contraction varies widely, sometimes being barely sufficient to maintain an upraised limb in position, at others passing into a tonic contracture of nearly all the voluntary muscles. An arm made rigid by suggestion drops slowly arid gently.

The subject must thoroughly understand what the therapist wishes. Common and most natural way of affecting this is by telling the subject what he should do, i.e. verbal suggestion. Verbal suggestion is made more effectual by means of the operator's assistance. Catalepsy cannot always be excited by mere verbal suggestion, and then gentle help may be necessary.

- ***Increase of Muscular Power***

During hypnosis, suggested increase in power of selected group of muscles happens. It can be further suggested that this increase strength is maintained after the session as post-hypnotic suggestion. This is utilized in therapy following recovery of paresis or paralysis.

- ***Paralysis***

A single muscle, or a group or a limb, may be selectively suggested to be paralyzed. However, this has hardly any clinical utility.

- ***Kinesthetic***

A subject so suggested that he is moving fast, may see himself doing so. From there he can be suggested to run. While he visualizes himself doing so, he may even start movements of the limbs. So suggested that his muscles are now tired because of a fast run, he slows down, but may persist with increased pulse and respiratory rate. Visualizing himself on a sea shore, he may withdraw his toes when suggested that now the sea water is touching him.

- ***Muscular Features Independent of Suggestion***

Certain muscular features arise independently of suggestion as a part of hypnotic process.

Lethargy—The limbs are relaxed and fall by their own weight; the tendon reflex is increased. There is neuro-muscular hyperexcitability, i.e. the muscles tend to contract under the influence of mechanical stimuli, whether applied to a tendon, or nerves of supply, or the muscles themselves.

Catalepsy—Any position given to the limbs is maintained for some time; there is no tendon reflex.

Gentle stimulation of the skin causes rigid contraction of the underlying muscles, which does not cease when the antagonistic ones are excited, but disappears when the original stimulation is repeated.

- ***Miscellaneous***

Ideation in hypnotic state does transform into predetermined movement before starting the session. This is called ideomotor signals. These changes such as ideomotor response from yes and no fingers, such other motor changes like wriggling the toes as a sign of throwing of the tension; 'yes', 'no' and 'I do not know' movements of the pendulum are useful for therapy. Movements of a pendulum, classically associated with hypnotherapist, as is the stethoscope with the medical doctors, may be utilized as a good method for induction. They can also be interpreted as answers in the above mentioned format. Wonder, one of the most efficient component for producing good results is inbuilt here. Nothing can ever happen in contravention of principles governing the Universe: a body that is at rest will and must remain at rest unless some force is applied to it. Of course, there is no cheating and no external force is applied to the pendulum and yet it moves. This is because all the muscles of the body, as of the hand holding pendulum, are constantly undergoing minor twitching. These are not perceptible but are enough to impart movement to the pendulum.

Therapeutic relevance comes in when the movements are given a direction to answer in the form of yes, no and I do not know. It happens as ideomotor signals; just as yes and no answers by moving the previously determined fingers. Here, the difference is that each individual has a different way of movements of the pendulum to answer yes, no and I do not know. This is most useful in hypnoanalysis.

Summary regarding the phenomena about voluntary muscles.

There are few, if any, changes in the voluntary muscles which are absolutely characteristic of hypnosis; and none which arise independently of direct or indirect suggestion. The most noticeable phenomenon is the long maintenance of an uncomfortable posture, associated with extreme muscular rigidity, and the subsequent absence of fatigue.

Changes in the Involuntary Muscular and Vasomotor Systems

- ***Pulse***

The induction of hypnosis is sometimes accompanied by an acceleration of the pulse initially. This, although regarded as a characteristic phenomenon by some authorities, appears to be due to emotional causes; for, although it frequently appears the first time hypnosis is induced, it rarely occurs afterwards. During deep hypnosis, when the subject is allowed to rest undisturbed by suggestions of any kind, the pulse falls spontaneously.

The frequency of the pulse can be altered by suggestion. It may be only necessary to state quietly that the pulse should beat faster or slower. At times. the suggestion may not be successful unless it is associated with an emotion. Thus, to quicken the pulse, the subject may be told that he is hurrying to catch a train. Slowing may be more difficult to produce, but occurs spontaneously in deep hypnosis.

- ***Respiration***

Most methods of induction include some kind of suggested breathing, like "deep breath in; deep breath out". Left to himself, a hypnotized subject shows some slowing of the respiratory rate in deep trance. The respiration can be accelerated, slowed or temporarily arrested by suggestion.

- ***Bleeding***

Before the availability of blood components, hypnosis was the only tool for the arrest of bleeding in bleeding diathesis like purpura. Rasputin probably used hypnosis to arrest bleeding in Russian princess and, in the process came to occupy powerful position around Russian royalty.

- ***Local Redness of the Skin; Blistering***

Local redness of the skin by suggestion can be induced as well as reduced or even, effaced. Blisters may also be so produced and, cases with superficial burns can be suggested to cool and not produce burns. They do not if suggested immediately after the occurrence of burns.

- ***Changes in the Temperature***

With the suggestion that there is increase in circulation of blood in a particular part, it can be made to warm up. Parts showing ischemia can be made to increase circulation. With the suggestion that ice is being applied to a part, it actually cools down by several degrees and, this is an easy method of producing analgesia/anesthesia.

- *Menstruation*

It is possible to initiate or arrest menstruation by suggestion. It may be made to appear at a given moment by post-hypnotic suggestion and, regulate its duration and intensity. This can have wide applications in menstrual disorders.

- *Action of the Bowels*

The action of the bowels can be excited or arrested by suggestion. Since, the autonomic control is easily accessible to the therapist, subjects with irritable bowel syndrome are most benefited by hypnosis.

- *Micturition*

Suggestion not only removes difficulty in micturition, but may also augment the amount of urine secreted. More over, a tighter control of the sphincter may be suggested and, unless there is organic cause, incontinence, say due to old age, may be improved or controlled altogether.

- *Lachrymal Secretion*

While a person is undergoing hypnosis and before he closes the eyes, they become slightly watery. It is postulated that before formal suggestions are made, there is increase in the parasympathetic tone by itself. This leads to increased lacrimation and, at the end of the session some tears may indeed roll out.

This is to be differentiated from catharsis where the subject actually cries reliving a painful or traumatic situation.

- *Perspiration*

Perspiration is regulated by autonomic control. Since this is easily accessed in hypnosis, patients with hyperhydrosis can be assured a sure help. At times, even a single session with only command suggestion to stop perspiring that much, has benefited the subjects permanently.

- *Secretion of Milk*

Secretion of milk cab be increased or arrested by suggestion. As an exception, two notable historical cases are being reproduced here because of great relevance. One of the earliest is cited by Esdaile. His sister-in-law, when weaning a child, suffered from the accumulation of milk in her breasts, which rendered them painful and swollen. Esdaile hypnotized her and in half an hour she was free from pain. Next morning the breasts were soft and comfortable and, there was no further secretion of milk.

An experiment, the reverse of this, is related by Braid. He hypnotized a patient who was nursing, and suggested an increased secretion of milk in one breast. On awaking she had no recollection of what had been done, but complained of a feeling of tightness and tension in the breast. Her husband then told her that Braid had been trying to increase the secretion of milk. She was skeptical as to the result, as her child was fourteen months old and the milk had almost disappeared. Her breast, however, almost immediately became distended with milk, and a few days later she complained that her figure was deformed in consequence. Braid again hypnotized her and successfully repeated the experiment with the other breast. The patient suckled her child for six months longer, the supply of milk being more abundant than it had been at any time since her confinement.

- ***Miscellaneous***

Physiological changes extend lowering of the metabolic rate and decrease in the lactic acid levels in blood; lowering of stress as evidenced by the serum cortisol levels; increased galvanic resistance of skin; appropriate homeostatic hormonal changes as per the built in suggestions in the session; changes in immune status. Dominance of α waves in electroencephalogram.

Ideosensory Changes

Such as visual, touch and pain perception; analgesia and anesthesia.

- ***Hearing***

In deep hypnosis, the hearing could be rendered more acute by suggestion. On the other hand, there can be selective shutting off some sounds or all the sounds except the therapist's voice. This can also be shut off with the command that "you will not hear even my voice till I call you by your name after sometime".

At a mental asylum, Forel had conducted an interesting experiment in 1890. This is narrated as it is of historical interest.

The warders were hypnotized, trained to sleep by the bedside of dangerous patients, and to awake the instant the latter attempted to get out of bed. Sounds which had no reference to the warder's duties were inhibited by suggestion, while those they should hear were rendered more acute. In addition to their ordinary routine of hard work, these warders performed night duty for six months at a stretch, without being unduly fatigued. The results, as far as the patients were concerned, were uniformly successful and no accident of any kind occurred.

- ***Alterations in Olfactory Sensation***

Subjects can be made to experience a particular sense of smell as well as shut of any or all sensations of smell. While so many phenomena in hypnosis remain unexplained scientifically, this is one area where some progress is made.

Nobel prize for physiology and medicine for the year 2004 narrows the gap between the genetic arousal and sense perception as well as memory of an experience. American researchers Richard Axel and Linda Buck have explained how people can smell a lilac flower on one fine spring morning and recall the smell years later. They discovered that about 1000 genes were responsible for this. The genes give rise to a huge variety of proteins in the cells of the nasal mucosa that are responsible for a particular smell to be sensed by the brain. What remains to be proved is that at the time of recall of a given smell, the arousal of the specific genes was produced through a process akin to hypnosis. We have incorporated the suggestion of a pleasant fragrance in the initial few minutes of every session. This is perceived by most subjects and, has significant reinforcement value.

And with this pointer, it is difficult not to narrate a spectacular case of anosmia that we have successfully treated. In brief, the story is:

A professional lady, aged about 40, with two children was brought for therapy as she had lost the sense of small since past seven years. She was teaching biochemistry at a college. The loss occurred around the time that she was working towards her Ph.D. and, it was a severe professional handicap.

In history taking it was soon evident that the period around her Ph.D. work was highly stressful with the demands of the teaching job, care of the young children as well as running the house. In giving up her sense of smell, she seemed to have "genetically engineered" a coping mechanism to offload some thing special.

After putting her in deep trance, she was age regressed to the period prior to the stress times. By eliciting the ideomotor signaling, it was confirmed that now she was at a period when her sense of smell was intact, by making her "sense the smell" of some of the common aromatic compounds she worked with as well as the smell of flowers of her choice. She was then age progressed to the present time, but with selective ablation of the stressful time.

Following the session, when she reached her sister's home, she suddenly told her, Oh I never knew you had *parijat* (A flower occurring in India with delicate fragrance) in your garden!

- ***Anesthesia***

Hypnosis can be remarkably effective in controlling pain whether of psychogenic or non-psychogenic origin. Although hypnosis has been used successfully as the sole anesthesia in major surgery, very few medical indications are found for performing major surgery with hypnosis as the sole anesthesia. Rather, hypnosis should be considered an adjunct that permits comfort with lower doses of anesthetic agents and that may speed recovery and diminish intraoperative blood loss, especially if those expectations are established preoperatively.

In nineteenth century, Esdaile reported better than 80 per cent surgical anesthesia with hypnosis. Esdaile's series of 3,000 patient also showed a 10-fold decline in operative mortality from 50 per cent to 5 per cent, that presumably resulted from avoiding the effects of shock. Highly hypnotizable subject often can achieve full anesthesia: persons with a lower responsiveness can learn to transform their perceptions or to divert their attention from the pain.

The familiar example is the inhibition of pain for operative purposes. Anesthesia may be suggested, when the patient can revive neither painful nor tactile sensations; or analgesia alone may be induced, when the patient can recall the steps of the operation, but has no memory of pain. That this inhibition of pain is a real, not an apparent one, is proved by the fact that the patients remain passive during operation and the physiological signs of pain are absent, *i.e.* there is neither dilatation of pupil, nor increase of pulse. Even corneal reflex may be absent. The nose and' throat also can be rendered insensible, and subjected to careful examination without pain or discomfort to the subject. There may be persistence of analgesia after awaking. Pain on awaking can be prevented by post-hypnotic suggestion. It is also potentially useful for the relief of preoperative anxiety that will augment post-operative pain. Furthermore, the patients with post surgical or trauma induced pain, as well as some with chronic distress, may be taught to hypnotize themselves to cope with pain better. The healing process is said to be unusually rapid.

- ***Childbirth***

Hypnosis may be under recognized as a helpful technique in natural child birth. During antenatal period, expectant mothers are taught relaxation, particularly of pelvic diaphragm. They are also taught self hypnosis with emphasis on pain relief. Such measures taken with the presence of the hypnotherapist during labour can lead to a painless delivery.

- ***Cutaneous Sensibility***

This can be enhanced, diminished or eliminated as in case of pain sensation. Thermo-sensibility can be manipulated the same way, so much so that changes of the burns may either be minimized to a great extent if the suggestion is given so immediately after the burns. Healing is also acclerated.

- ***Appetites, Hunger and Thirst***

Suggestion can induce hunger in patients suffering from anorexia. Reverse is also true, subjects with obesity, when so suggested, lose appetite and are less hungry.

- ***Vision***

Illusions in the form of visual imagery are the common therapeutic mode to replace negative events with positive. Most subjects use vision acutely all the time and to that extent, programmes are generally formatted with imagery. The subject is made to visualize objects, scenes of landscape, mountains, sea beach as per his/her sensibility.

The visualization can be so intense that the subject may see an object that does not exist in front of open eyes: the visualized object may even block other objects as if they were real in preventing the view of other objects. An object can disappear in response to the suggestion. Visualization takes place with eyes open or eyes closed too.

- ***Gustatory***

Any taste may be simulated by suggestions. Combining with other sensory inputs, an anorexic person can be made to smell, see, and hear various kinds of foods being cooked and served. This produces even salivation and, healthy appetite. On the contrary, person can be so suggested that having eaten all such goodies, he/she is fully satiated and has no more any hunger left to eat.

- ***Somnambulism***

Subject in deep trance can perform several actions like walking out of chair, coming back to the chair, write, calculate, draw etc. They may engage in conversation on command. Such a state can last till such time as there is reinforcement by the therapist. Usually, the memory is lost of what happened during the trance; but it can be recalled at a subsequent session of hypnosis.

While this is generally true, it cannot be said that the subject can be robbed or raped in hypnosis. Instances, particularly abound when somebody makes such charges, mainly in lay hypnosis and matter goes before a court. The attitude of the court is not guided by belief in what may happen in hypnosis but by hard evidence.

It is on this count that an attendant must always be present during a therapeutic session. And, we work with half open door all the time.

Miscellaneous Ideosensory Phenomena

- ***Dissociation***

A subject may separate himself from what is going about himself and the surroundings. This is achieved in deep trance and may persist for a long time. This is useful with subjects faced with incurable diseases like terminal cancer, persistent pain or when the surroundings are intractable.

- ***Depersonalization***

A person may lose his identity and may identify himself as someone else. This is rarely useful in therapy. We have never employed it.

The meditative state is studied physiologically by Maharshi Mahesh Yogi, Herbert Benson and others.[6] There are extensive studies on the physiology of this state of consciousness.[7, 8, 9] Initially, the pulse rate and the blood pressure rise; but soon go below the resting levels. The respiratory rate rises first but soon falls below the resting level and as the trance progresses, it may be accompanied by small periods of apnoea. The metabolic rate falls steeply and it may fall below the level of sleep. The peripheral flow of blood increases and the body and the face may be flushed. Plasma cortisol levels decline. There is increased coherence of functions of both the hemispheres of the brain. In the electroencephalogram there is preponderance of alpha waves. There is increase of the galvanic skin resistance.

In this age of reason, we should be able to delve deep into the depth of what happens to various body functions during different states of consciousness. Quantum jumps in technology say, PET and fMRI scanning of brain can reveal illuminating data about therapeutic mechanisms and experience of spirituality. Some how, the fascination about the ghost in the machine[10] seems to have vaned, in spite of huge funds liberated from shackles of cold war. Utilitarian research is in the forefront and, till such time that mankind is once again riddied with fundamentals about the nature of Being, as it happened with Genome project, such answers will have to wait. However, different states are there for experiencing and flying high in spirits: as a rose is a rose is a rose; and, it will smell the same sweet with no understanding of its biochemistry.

Post Script to Phenomena in Hypnosis

The physiological, psychodynamic as well as somatic changes (inclusive of changes in the hormone and other molecular biological substances) have been well defined for meditation.[11, 12]

Suffice it to say that hypnosis and meditation are conducive to relaxation and distressing. The stress mediators will therefore diminish and such molecular substances and gene expression that are conducive to regeneration and rejuvenation will flow all over the body, through the blood stream, through the lymph and interstitial spaces and, within the cell too. A radical change in the blood chemistry comes about that is fundamental to the change in health paradigm. To illustrate the above point the reader may refer to the chapter on genomics of the hypnosis process. However, some of the potent molecular substances that are affected by the hypnotic process are discussed in brief here to emphasize the vast ranging effects that hypnosis can modulate.

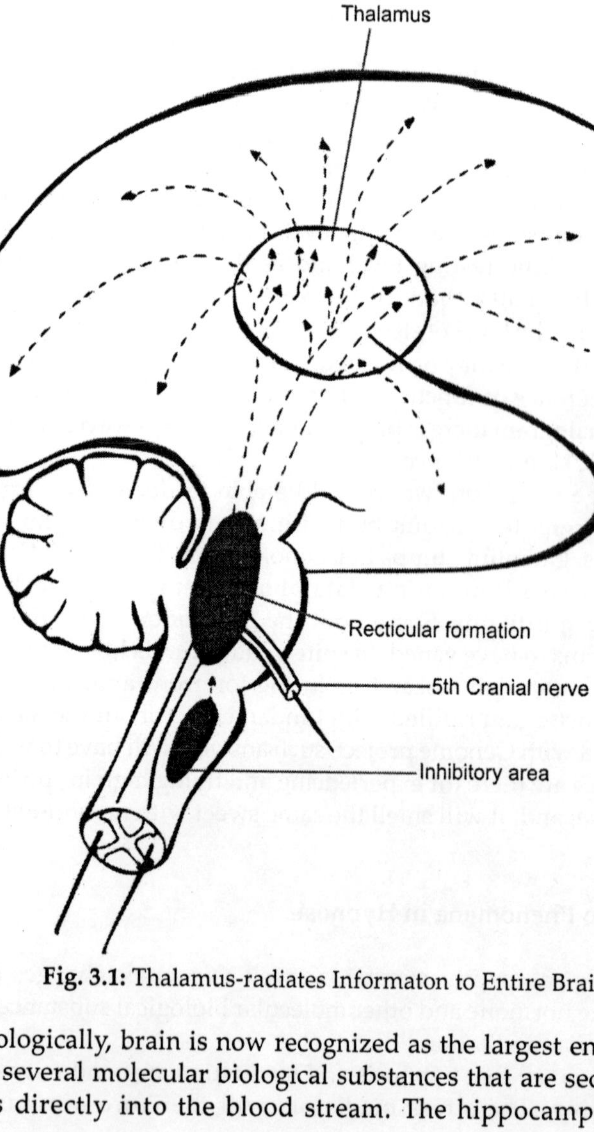

Fig. 3.1: Thalamus-radiates Informaton to Entire Brain

Physiologically, brain is now recognized as the largest endocrine gland. There are several molecular biological substances that are secreted by brain structures directly into the blood stream. The hippocampus, amygdala, pituitary, hypothalamus, and the limbic system secrete information substances in response to stimuli from environment, as well as thought processes. The neurotransmitters convey information. And there are substances that cause arousal that releases energy.

Endorphin produces "euphoria' similar to the effect of exogenous morphine; since it is endogenous to body, therefore the name, endorphin. Endorphin was the first of these substance that was discovered by Candace Pert. While it is secreted by physical pain, it is responsible for causing a sense of pleasure and joy in various situations including love and sex. Masochistic, narcissistic and sadistic traits have their roots with the association of pleasurable experiences that would have been derived through endorphin levels earlier. Endorphin secretion gets triggered and, an unfortunate connection in the brain is established in the Pavlovian model. Catharsis and crying helps since it stimulates endorphin secretion. Painful relationships get tolerated or even sustained because the brain has learned to expect good feelings.

Following case history illustrates the role of endorphin release related memory encoding leading to a stereotype behaviour.

A newly married couple came for therapy. The woman was depressed after marriage though marriage was with her explicit consent. She will burst out into sobs after love making. The husband and his family were caring and, concerned. Yet, the depression would not abate.

Psychodynamic exploration revealed a premarital relationship which the women had taken seriously: her paramour was just flirting. They had slept together and, woman had experienced ecstasy at the climax. When the boy plainly told about his casual attitude and moved away to Australia, she accepted the situation and, got married.

However, the boy continued to flirt. He would call her from Australia and make love talk. She will derail. The therapist called up the boy and suggested to the boy that if he really loved the girl, he must not now call her.

This change, along with a strategy for selective ablation of past, substitution of euphoria with pain and time progression to happy family building almost restored her; till the boy returned to the city to get married and, invited her to the marriage. In spite of desistance and warning from the therapist, she attended the marriage and, crashed once again.

Wise learn from the mistakes of others, fools from their own; but idiots who have experienced euphoria of a bygone endorphin release situation would not learn ever. Then a psychodrama of confrontational therapy was enacted and, it worked. So, of course, with help even idiots do learn to re-modulate their endorphins.

Dopamine

Dopamine is a neurohormone. It is responsible for the awake state. It can enhance the joy of finding—the "eureka"! It is also released by the hypothalamus. It has many functions in behaviour and cognition such as voluntary movements, motivation, punishment and reward and prolactin production inhibition. It is rated to play a role in pain processing in multiple levels of the central nervous system. Dopamine increases general arousal and goal directed behaviour and, decreases latent inhibition; all three effects increase the creative drive of idea generation.

Melatonin

Melatonin is secreted into the blood by the pineal gland in the brain. It is best secreted in darkness. It may also be produced by a variety of peripheral cells such as bone marrow cells, lymphocytes, and epithelial cells.

Melatonin is a geroprotector. Melatonin receptors appear to be important in mechanisms of learning and memory such as long-term potentiation (LTP). In perimenopausal women it produces an improvement in thyroid function and gonadotropin levels, as well as restoring fertility and menstruation and preventing the depression associated with themenopause. Melatonin is an effective preventive treatment for migraine and, since itaeliorates circadian misalignment, it is the only drug for jet lag after travel. It is an anti-oxidant and suppressant of tumour development. Melatonin acts as a mild hypnotic. Melatonin is effective in treating depression and seasonal affective disorder.

A team lead by Bhaskar Vyas and Renu Sharma, comprising of various disciplines is engaged at M.S. University in fundamental research (2013-2014) in the role of melatonin in hypnosis. There are 2 genes that regulate the production of the hormone by pineal gland. It is postulated that these genes get up-regulated during hypnosis. It will be ideal to study the activation of melatonin genes; before and after hypnosis. However, the research on gene expression is highly expensive. Therefore, with limited funding from the surplus of 9th National Conference of Indian Society of Clinical and Experimental Hypnosis at Vadodara, the current research is likely to provide path breaking findings for melatonin metabolism.

A clear message has already emerged from the results under analysis: there is a pulsatile production of melatonin under/after hypnosis. This will explain several regenerative and rejuvenating outcomes following hypnotherapy.

Oxytocin

Oxytocin causes the feeling of being safe and bonded in social situations. It acts as a neuro-modulator in the brain. In lactating mothers it causes flow of milk. It is important for cervical dilation before birth and causes contractions during the second and third stages of labour. This explains the facilitation of labour with hypnosis. There is correlation of oxytocin with human bonding; increase in trust, and decrease in fear are attributed to the hormone. Certain learning and memory functions are impaired by centrally administered oxytocin. Oxytocin is involved in the initiation of maternal behaviour. Oxytocin inhibits the development of tolerance to various addictive drugs (opiates, cocaine, alcohol) and reduces withdrawal symptoms.

Serotonin

Serotonin produces the feeling of being respected and is responsible for feeling proud.

Cortisol is the stress hormone. It triggers different survival behaviours depending on whether it is paired with low blood sugar, or the scent of a predator, or social exclusion. The actions of cortisol are best summarized as fight or flight response. Hypnosis converse the response to flow.

Survival builds without effort or intent because neurochemicals pave pathways. The ability of a therapist lies in elucidating a particular phenomenon as a strategic tool in a correcting disorder/disease of a particular client/patient. Almost all client's coming to a therapist are under stress therefore it is prudent/ proven to structure initial session of the therapy for all client's, thereafter different phenomenon may be utilize so as to negate/alleviate a particular disorder. Say a patient with claustrophobia–fear with close spaces may be met to experience expansion of spaces. This is further buttress by giving a cue during hypnosis that by following the given cue, whenever the phobia is likely to occur, there will be expansion of space, there will be expansion of space, this results in a permanent cure.

A patient with irritable bowl syndrome has his sympathetic system in overdrive. When the metaphor that following heavy rain now the flood are subsiding so that the river is no more in spite (illustration of a rare use of No) and the flow is slowing down will permanently cure IBS. The ingenuity and talent of therapist lies in utilization of heighten suggestibility of hypnotize subject together with an appropriate illustration of a certain phenomenon together with surrealistic metaphors that results in excellent therapy.

Notes

1. Rohit Mehta, J. *Krishnamurty and The Nameless Experience,* Delhi, 1979, pp. 128-153.
2. J. Krishnamurty, *Awakening of Intelligence,* Madras 1970.
3. *Patanjali's Yoga Sutra,* Section III, 3.
4. *Patanjali's Yoga Sutra,* Section III, 16.
5. Dwarakanath Reddy, *The Dicey Problem of New Age Science: Einstein, Hawking and God at the Casino,* Chittor, 2003.
6. Herbert Benson, *The Relaxation Response,* Boston, 1980.
7. Maharshi Mahesh Yogi, *Creating an Ideal Society,* Salisberg, 1977.
8. Wallace Robert Keith, *The Physiological Effects of Transcendental Meditation: A Proposed Fourth Major State of Consciousness,* Los Angeles, 1970.

9. Orme–Johnson D.W. and Farrow J.T. Scientific Research on the Transcendental Meditation programme: Collected papers. Meru, Switzerland, 1976.
10. Arthur Koestler, *The Ghost in the Machine*, London, 1958.
11. Jeffery A. Dusek, Jeffery A. Dusek1,2,3,6#, Hasan H. Otu3,4#, Ann L. Wohlhueter1, Manoj Bhasin3,4, Luiz F. Zerbini3,4, Marie G. Joseph4, Herbert Benson1,3,5*, Towia A. Libermann3,4*, *Genomic Counter-Stress Changes Induced by the Relaxation Response*, PLoS ONE v.3(7); 2008.
12. Davidson, R.; Lutz, A. (2008). "Buddha's Brain: Neuroplasticity and Meditation [In the Spotlight"]. *IEEE Signal Processing Magazine* **25** (1): 176-174.
13. Davidson, R.J. (2004). "Well-being and affective style: Neural substrates and biobehavioural correlates". *Philosophical Transactions of the Royal Society B: Biological Sciences* **359** (1449): 1395-1411.12.

4
Mind and Matter

Mind has no matter; and yet, it is only the mind that matters.

Various definitions and structures about the mind fall in the realm of psychology, philosophy and neurosciences. Religions also have a view on it. The authors subscribe to the psychodynamic theory of behaviour that can cause disorders, diseases and derangements. It is restated for emphasis that faulty functioning of the discriminating mind is the fundamental etiological factor for most diseases. This apparent exaggeration will find simplification when we wonder as to how even the accidents happen because of the faulty functioning of intellect. Did not the princess Diana and her paramour die in an accident that was caused by the derange perceptions of the two and the chauffer?

Philosophers had the first say about the mind. Plato said idea is the first reality. De Cartes brought about the age of renaissaince by proclaiming, I think; so I am (*Cogito ergo sum*). In the nineteenth century, there was no difference between philosophy and psychology. Freud initiated psychological studies and elevated the study of mind to the level of a science through a systemic study of nature of mind.

The concept of the mind as given by Freud, to begin with was a philosophical one. Its scientific relevance as of today lies in being practicable, as a scientific construct for about hundred years. His postulations of mind being structured in three layers viz. conscious, subconscious and unconscious layers are fully functionally applicable for understanding psychodynamics of health, neurosis, disorders, psychiatric diseases and psychosomatic illnesses.

Freud's emphasis of the childhood environment in conditioning the mind is so vital that it is applicable to all cultures. Several personality theories have subsequently emerged with Karl Jung, Erik Erikson, Abraham Maslow, Carl Roger and Ken Wilber etc. The genius of Freud stands tall among them. The common factor shared among all psychologists is that most of the theories are philosophical and are being propagated with the label of science.

By comparison the construct about the mind in eastern traditions have some distinct differences. However, the fact that mind is conditioned by environment is basic to east and west, both.[1]

With the above discussion as the background let us now reflect on certain facts of science, and eastern philosophy that will provide better understanding.

A de-cerebrated subject does not have any perception of the world around; thus brain is the materialistic base for the sensorium and the mind. (Yet the brain has no sensation by itself!) Poetically speaking matter does not know what the mind knows; mind does not know what is beyond mind.

How is the mind structured is still an unresolved debate; but it is surely true that both the seed –genetics- and the soil – environment are both important. Though genetics have a large say in the in structuring the personality, so that, some say we are the product of our genes. That is only partly true. Beginning with Pavlov's experiments on conditioned reflexes, we are led to Watson and the successive behavioural psychologists, who proposed that man is a conditioned animal. Subscribing to such a view will negate the acceptance of a fundamental creative attribute of human mind and personality. Human creativity is an undisputed fact. It is rooted in the capacity of the mind to generate a perception of external reality through sensory inputs.

Mind synthesizes our perceptions of the external reality into concepts (heightened sensibility of hypnoidal state enhances this capability). This provides the knowledge base for the individual, from this raw data mind can further generate an endless number of algorithms so as to provide fountain heads of the creativity that range from poetry, arts, mathematics and other scientific inventions to common place neurosis, neurotic defences of ego and a certain psychosis.

Thus creativity, though arising from some hidden corners of the mind takes the mind beyond mind. Mind in such a state is beyond its usual habit of understanding by definition, comprehension by successive steps, understanding with sprinkling of past experiences and future projections and their subjective interpretations.

Uncultured mind is a poor slave of brute; id. Id surreptitiously creeps up to assert its assertion through heightened ego. It Is through the cultural conditioning of the civilized society that the brutal dominance by id of the ego-self, is brought down within the definition of Freudian concept that ego strives to maintain a balance between the irrational drive of the id and restrictive, constrictive commands of superego. Twentyfirst century has inherited this unstable equilibrium of the mind from the consumerist, affluent Western culture. Mind was driven to the verge of being a mercenary when I for myself emerged with a capital I in the past century.

But simultaneous, concurrent divergent forms of behaviour are clearly evident. Though ego is generally accepted as the motivating driving force for the mind, there has been a consistent emphasis on negation of self-assertion in Indian and Buddhist psychology. Here the mind is credited with the faculty with the creation of chimerical world. It is driven by the insatiable demands of irrational self to persistently strive and struggle for the attainments of wants that have no relevance to the real needs. The situation is the genesis of the neurosis.

The eastern traditions emphasize on even the minimization of the needs. Self-esteem is accepted as a need for purposeful and fruitful functioning. This is to be practiced with constant appreciation of the diminutive role of an individual, so as humility and regards for the others are emphasized in social behaviour.[2]

The discussion has so far has taken us to the formation of perception, generation of concepts and formative cultural conditions that would decide the virtues and vices, Buddhism has several illustrative metaphors to illustrate this, and one of them begins by postulating the mind as a pale full of clear oil. Various thoughts in the mind are equated with the images that the oil reflects (see the chapter on group hypnosis). Another metaphor equates the mind as a mirror; here the emphasis is on the emptiness of the glass itself, it simply reflex the light and, Tibetan Buddhism takes the metaphor a step further by including the effect of stress on the quality of reflection by the mirror. Classically it says, a mirror does not reflect well when it gathers dust. Only a clear perception of a situation, devoid of all the kind of ego defences (dust particles) will lead to right action.

Hindu and Buddhism tradition both lay tremendous emphasis on what they call *samskara*. These are deeply in grain-what one might call deep unconscious-values. These systems are carried over as subtle mind even to the next birth. There is an obvious paradox here. The essential nature of the mind is to be totally empty on itself. But it derives its existence by its contents, some of these can be forgotten or wished away or washed out by meditative practice[3] even if the therapist does not wish to be dwelling deep in mysticism of meditative practice, mindfulness is a simpler and easy to understand way of keeping the mind healthy, here the emphasis is on, here and now. Living in the present moment and at the present location reads the mind of a tremendous burden of futile memories and jettisoning of the garbage of ego defences.[4]

While the perceptual contents of the mind are primarily derived from sensory inputs, its ability to synthesize concept and, make them progress algorithmically makes it one of the sense organ by itself and the algorithm may proceed with a freedom of 359 degree. This is the basis of creative genius. On the other hand it will also explain compulsive obsessive behaviour and schizophrenia. Therapist's understanding of algorithms in the psychodynamics of the patients of these disorders will provide him with cues for restoration to the algorithm for here and now.

For those who computer savvy it might be appropriate to understand mind in computer language, here we will say that brain is a computer and mind is the software, that is stored in it. This software has the capacity for auto renewal as well as corruption as we understand in computer language. To illustrate succinctly say a terrorist mind is infested with viruses. Almost all the characteristic of hardware for the computer apply to the brain. Its function is also by comprehending successively; how so ever small, the electronic pause may be between two successive processes. Some individuals develop comprehension in a simultaneous fashion. This kind of faculties will provide them with what one might call a holistic perception.

Akin to the computer, the brain has the faculty to running several programmes simultaneously. This is what we call the ability to have multiple intelligences. But simultaneous running of several programmes slows down the computer; when the dust of stress gathers on the mirror of the mind, it reflects poorly. Perception, memory, conceptualization and intelligence all dim. Most important, insight generation wanes. This is evident in stress, and such a functioning for a prolonged period causes mental exhaustion or a break down similar to hanging of a computer. Analogy to the computer repeated for the recovery of the health: close all programmes by shutting the computer. Have a pause and restart. Functioning of the mind is analogues to the mathematics of the computer languages; it is didactic, dialectic, analytic, as well as synthetic. However fast, these processes are successive and continuous. There is a possibility of simultaneous functioning of multiple, numerous (? All) the programmes that is describes by various connotations as *Samadhi, satori, sunyata, zen,* etc.

Other analogies are ROM—read only memory of the computer is the analogues to the conscious mind as the ROM of a computer may be enhance so as to make the computer faster, the awareness of the mind can also broaden, however increase in the awareness of the mind through meditative practices can create problematic situation, intense and extensive awareness, apart from producing stress can also produce jarring in the data processing so that a person may land up in a mental disorder.

Central data processing unit of the mind is difficult to locate. Even in a simple perception like a flower, there is a simultaneous parallel firing of the neurons from various sensory and the motor areas so as to retrieve the memory of a flower called rose. Neurologically, one fact is clearly evident. Almost all that passes through the sensorium is recorded in the brain. This is categorized in short term and long term memory. Short term memories get completely erased; such as what one might have eaten as a dinner few days back. Long term memories are very important for over all functioning of an individual. Encoding pathways are different. Repeation, revision, recapitulation, recitation and recollection enhance the long term memory.

Association, how ever logical or illogical helps in retrieval. This is exemplified by the usage of acronyms. Emotional bonding of the content goes a long way such as parental fondling, school teacher's punishments, peer ridicule, first gold medal and first love. The joyful bonding overrides the painful experiences. Application of Neuro linguistic programming is useful. For students, it is important to identify their personal trait in NLP. After focalising on one, say, visual, the student may learn to "photograph" the pages in the mind's eye, with the preference for music may associate a particular memory with a tune etc. What is associated with incorporation of all senses and emotional content will be remembered as a whole. The faculty of the mind as the sixth sense, in deriving analysis, such as subheadings and meaning contributes to retention with understanding. Understanding by the mind is greatly enhanced by a pause (does the mind ever pause?[5]) and juxtaposing with analogy and metaphor contributes constructively. Reinforcement after a pause and, review with reinforcement again after a gap of sometime would seal the memory. A simple computation of all the strategies above would mean three revisions should be ordinarily enough.

Philosophers have postulated that even a cell has memory. The concept of state related memory, physiologically envisages a hologram of the body in a particular state. A given state has x number of physiological number of constituents in xyz quantities. Recollection to the extent of coming alive of the experience—reliving in a hypnotic state would hypothetically reconstruct the same physiological state. This is a far reaching hypothesis but the proofs are visible in the work of Candace Pert, where we have come to decipher the molecules of emotions.

Such a memory is further encoded with various fast experiences that would have caused different kind of association; this is relevance in hypnotherapy and in NLP (Neuro Linguistic Programme), such strategies that cause the arousal of a large sensory-motor input so as to make the experience come alive —reliving make the therapy better.

Putting a programme on the computer screen is like putting in subconscious mind, shutting down a programme and yet keeping it on the computer keeping it of the software of computer, though not entirely analogues may be compared to putting it in the unconscious mind. In order to retrieve it, a fresh reprogramming is necessary. This is easily done on a computer: requires deftness and expertise for the therapist. Disk cleaning as well as defragmentation of the data on the disk are so analogues between the computer and mind that the metaphor may be quickly grasp for a computer literate in the therapy.

In personality disorder depression and person suffering from severe stress, there is indeed a vast catering of the data in their mind so as to create dissociation. The metaphor is utilised in therapy as follows. "You know when a computer is fan fresh information; it throws in information a random where the empty space is. With accumulation of such larger data the fragmentation becomes more disperse retrieval of a particular file in a compact form, therefore takes a longer time, as a computer literate person you are familiar with the defragmentation programme, here the fragmented beets are taken from diverse location and compacted so as to format uniformly.

Let us start the computer, go to defragmentation programme and double click the switch... on the screen see the play of the different colour bricks.

They are compacting living so much of an empty space on the hard disc... as the hard disc gets the defragmented so does your mind and the brain, the speed and the clarity of your thinking and perception is now so much better.

A similar computer programme is disc cleaner; the programme cleans the files of the viruses. It will permanently delete the infested files.

A comparable metaphor in therapy is visualization of a black board randomly scribbled with corrupted data and the client visualizes the cleaning of the black board with the repeated swipes.

At the bottom line a fact emerges clear and explicit. Fast computing capability might be a property for those who practice self-hypnosis. Hypnosis deals with consciousness, that can be modulated, expanded and even be transformed. May be, therefore, there is a possibility to develop super-intelligence as the art is practiced. And they must be developing fast computing capability without knowing! That is how, perhaps, hypnotherapists understand the depth of other's mind.

Ordinarily, the speed at which we can compute is not adequate to predict events of the past and the future. There certainly is such ingredients of elevating the computing capacity ingrained within the scope of hypnotic realities. But it is certainly amazing to harness collective wisdom from different fields to move towards the ultimate, where during the journey, the preliminaries of expertise in hypnotherapy come and disappear as one moves higher up in the journey.

One thing is clear. The power of ideas from multi-sources and to grasp them, shall accelerate the development process to move towards the ultimate. However, what is the ultimate is difficult to fathom.

Our strategies in hypnotherapy are based on psychodynamics. But we donot do and donot advocate, classical psychoanalysis. We understand psychodynamics by our hunch; when we fail, we rely on the subject's innate attribute to generate it through passive, permissive hypnotherapy.

It will be simplistic to assume that passive, permissive hypnotherapy will always generate insight for the client/patient. The aim and the goal is restoration to normative functioning of the individual. This is generally achievable.

Some of the useful books for understanding the psychodynamics:[6]

Michael E. Kerr and Murray Bowen, *Family Evaluation*, 1988, New York, London.

Nancy Mc Williams, *Psychoanalytic Diagnosis: Understanding Personality Structure in the Clinical Process*, Second Edition, 2011, New York.

Frank James Fish, Patricia R. Casey, Brendan D. Kelly, *Fish's Clinical Psychopathology: Signs and Symptoms in Psychiatry*, Third Edition, 2008, London.

Notes

1. The materialistic concept of mind is that it is derived from functioning of the

nervous system; some even exaggerate that as the stomach secretes gastric juice, the brain secrets mind. Though the existence of the mind without brain is a matter of discussion between theologist and parapsychologist. We should limit this possibility only as far as it may have relevance to therapeutics; see the chapter on past life regression.

2. Bangladesh is one of the poorest nations in the world; the paradox is that it has the highest happiness index also.
3. *Vipassyana* meditation may be a reflection on *kayanupassana,* where the flow of the breath and the memory of the body are the objects of contempletation in two different forms called *anapana sati* and *kayagati sati* respectively. *Vedana anupassana* observes the flow of feelings leading to subtle sharp mind. *Chitta anupassana* passively reflects on the contents of the mind. *Dhammanupassyana,* a contemplation on the philosophical aspects of religious experience like nature, inherent quality, void, merit, and *Samadhi* is the final stage of *vipassyana* meditation.
4. For further study of this method, the readers are referred to the literature of J. Krishnamurthy, as well as to the life he live, described in the biography by Marry Lutens.
5. When the mind pauses, may be or a fraction of second, it is *Samadhi.*
6. Michael E. Kerr and Murray Bowen, *Family Evaluation,* 1988, New York, London. Nancy McWilliams, *Psychoanalytic Diagnosis: Understanding Personality Structure in the Clinical Process,* 2011, New York.
   Frank James Fish, Patricia R. Casey, Brendan D. Kelly, *Fish's Clinical Psychopathology: Signs and Symptoms in Psychiatry,* 2008, London.

5
Body-Mind Continuum

French philosopher Descartes propounded the foundation of one's being as, "I think, so I am." He was also to link causality and change. In so doing, he ushered in the age of reason and laid the foundation of present day Western civilization. He postulated body as a separate entity from mind. Body worked like a clock that operated through a set of interconnected wheels. The duality propounded by him propagates to a great extent even today but much evidence is gathering to efface it and, affirm scientifically that bodymind is one: so that, there is no interface but there is constant and perpetual exchange.

A hypnotherapist work rests on the fundamental basis that body-mind is one single entity. About a quarter century ago such a statement may have been interpreted as make belief.

The continuum is in the following manner. There are ideas and thoughts. There are emotions. Thoughts are in the form of suprathalamic *stimuli* that are conveyed in the form electrical impulses to the centers lower down. There may as well be another mode of transport in the form of molecular substances secreted by the brain cells at hypothalamus, limbic system and several other areas all over the body. Our understanding of these kind of interplay between the electrical impulses, secretion of neurotransmitters, neurohormones, neuropeptides and several other chemical substances like endorphins, opiates, valium and others, in the pipeline of discovery, have established a scientific link between emotions and their chemical equivalence. There are molecules of emotions.[1] They are floating as particles in the blood stream and also in extra cellular fluid. Putting it other way, cerebral *stimuli* in the form of thoughts and emotions have their molecular equivalents.

We have now come to understand that the target organs for these substances can be many and in wide locations. The magnitude of the effect of a substance would be determined not only by the concentration of substances, but also by the number of receptors for the same on a particular cell or an organ. More over the different target organs have different mechanisms to increases the action within the cell by a specifically driven action.

Let us visualize what is happening to the emotional brain in a given emotional state. Following the arousal of these centers, there will be an instantaneous release of some molecules that trigger a response in several organs and in some genes too. These will set up a cascade of molecular biological events all over the body across the systems. In terms of biochemistry, in such a moment the biochemical composition of the organism is changed. It is a different kind of human body than what was just a few moments before. And it seems the body has a built in mechanism to encode these biochemical states as state dependent memory.

Additionally, there is constant recording in the brain of what has been perceived through the sensorium. While operating on awake subjects, Canadian neurosurgeon Penfield evoked memories of long forgotten events by stimulating certain areas of brain with microelectrodes. His successor, Pribram postulated that events are stored as holograms in a large area of cerebral cortex. This data is likely to provide clues as to how hypnosis works. What we can prove scientifically for sure today is the fact that bodymind is one.

Therefore, as a simplistic statement it may be said that a particular emotional state has its biochemical equivalent. The hypnotherapist attempts to produce a cascade of molecular biological events, may be through the activation of genes, manipulating the ideation and reliving the emotions. The transformation brought about through hypnotherapy is because of subtle strategic psychocybernetics. And the information substances are the keys.

Brain and Neural Network

Let us first understand the basics of brain function.

From a functional standpoint, the brain and its two hemispheres may be divided into five major components:

- Prefrontal Cortex,
- Frontal Cortex,
- Primary Sensory and Motor Cortex,
- Secondary Sensory and Motor Cortex,
- Tertiary or Association Cortex

And

- Limbic Cortex.

The upper levels of the nervous system operate not by sending signals directly to the periphery of the body but instead by sending signals to the control centers of the spinal cord, simply commanding the cord centers to perform their functions. This is based on neurological circuitry. However, brain has now been identified to secrete more than 150 substances called information substances. They are directly secreted into the blood stream and, therefore, their effects to bring about changes by transferring information are radically in a different mode than neurotransmission.

The limbic cortex is composed of the brain structures that lie in the border region between the hypothalamus and its related structures on one hand, and the cerebral cortex. Major structures of this system include the hippocampus (sea horse), amygdala, septum (partition), mammillary bodies, olfactory bulbs, fornix, and caudate nucleus. We shall discuss mainly amygdala and hippocampus. They are particularly relevant to hypnotherapy. Let us see how.

Each component of the limbic system has some involvement in the modulation of mood and effect. The amygdala and related cortical-limbic areas are associated not so much with the generation of emotion itself as this is most probably coordinated chiefly by the hypothalamus, but rather with directing emotions to their proper object and perhaps to the proper mental content. Input could enter this circuit from other structures to be elaborated as emotional. Hence, the term limbic system means this entire basal system of the brain that mainly controls a person's emotional behaviour and drives; falling under psychological dominion of the primary process thinking by the id.

In general, the intricate limbic circuitry can be divided into the amygdaloidal and hippocampal spheres of influence. The hippocampus and its connections seem to be more closely associated with memory functions. Whereas the amygdala and its pathways are more closely related to the affective (or emotional) components of the human experience, it is the limbic cortex and the association cortex that provides the neural networks that mediate between those inner urges of an individual and the contingencies of his extra personal environment.

The limbic cortex participates in the regulation of autonomic tone; stimulation tends to produce gastrointestinal responses, cardiovascular and respiratory changes, inducing inhibition of gastric peristalsis, respiratory rate changes, and marked blood pressure changes (as much as 100 mm Hg) depending upon the specific area of stimulation. Stimulation of different areas of the hippocampus can cause almost any one of different behavioural patterns, such as rage, passivity, excess sex drive, and so on.

Cells in the caudate are known as tonically active neurons (TANs). They process information from an emotion-processing part of the brain, the amygdala. Through another set of cells, information from the thinking, reasoning cerebral cortex reaches the caudate. Thus by virtue of their position, TANs can integrate emotion and thought. They fire in a characteristic pattern when the brain senses something with positive or negative emotional meaning. Cognitive-behavioural therapy in hypnotherapy mode may change how TANs respond to various triggers.

TANs respond dramatically to visual and auditory stimuli that are linked through behavioural conditioning to a reward. TANs conceivably play a central role in behavioural responses to hints (or cues) of an upcoming reward. Studies have demonstrated that TAN firing rates changed when a once-neutral cue became associated with a reward. Consider, for example, that a visual cue such as a flashing light means that a monkey will get a reward (juice) if that monkey performs a simple behavioural response (licking a spoon). But TANs do not respond to the light cue if that monkey has not learned to associate it with a reward. As the monkey's brain learns to recognize a reward, TANs fire in that characteristic pattern. When TANs detect a potential reward, they pause at first and then fire faster.

The Reticular Formation

The Reticular Formation extends in widely scattered area of brain stem. The consciousness seems to originate by the firing of the neurons in reticular formation to the higher centers. The location of respiratory center is in the medulla oblongata in the vicinity of the reticular formation. It is hypothesized by us that crossover of the impulses from the respiratory center to reticular formation may be involved in bringing about the altered state of consciousness.

Limbic System and Behaviour

- *Feeding Behaviour*: Amygdale regulates not only the food intake, but movements associated with eating. The ability to discriminate edible and inedible objects is also vested in amygdale.
- *Sexual Behaviour*: Human sexual functions are extensively encephalized and conditioned by social and psychic factors. They are regulated through limbic system and hypothalamus. This involves the entire range from courtship to copulation to pregnancy and lactation.
- *Maternal Behaviour*: Home making, caring and child raring functions are regulated by the limbic system.

Thus, the entire range of the emotions is controlled by the limbic system including the social behaviour like propriety, protocol, attire, etiquette and decorum. They are instinctively dictated by the emotional brain. The control is through potent molecular biological substances that provide matrix to the emotional state. Such a matrix can be redesigned through hypnotic manipulation.

Having understood the transduction of information in various locations of the brain, let us now have an overview of the various information substances that bring the change.

Information Substances

Neurotransmitters such as acetylcholine (ACh) and dopamine (DA), act upon the specialized proteins, which are located on the post-synaptic membrane of the recipient neuron. Receptors, as these specialized proteins are called, bind the neurotransmitter substances. Three neurotransmitters in the brain are believed to be important in emotional behaviour : dopamine (DA), norepinephrine (NE), and serotonin (5-HT). Each of these substances are manufactured in various areas of brain and sent *via* long axons to various places, especially to one in the forebrain. Norepinephrine (NE), triggers the *beta*-2 (β-2) receptors of the sympathetic nervous system, as well as receptors involved in long-term memory. Epinephrine (Epi), acts as a catalyst, locking memories of exciting, shocking, or stimulating events in the brain. Serotonin (5-HT) is yet another neurotransmitter which is actively involved in many activities of the brain from its perception of pain to the prevention of depression and even the production of sleep.

The loss of dopaminergic cells results in Parkinson's disease. Loss of axons of certain neurons that project to the limbic system is believed to occur in schizophrenia. Abnormalities in norepinephrine (NE), and serotonin (5-HT) secreting neurons are suspect in some symptoms of depression.

All the above biochemical active substances are secreted to a varying degree during emotional states. Thus, emotions are the heart of therapeutic change in hypnotherapy. Changes in emotion will ideally be accompanied by corresponding changes in attitude, behaviour, self-image, family structure, discipline and enjoyment. The symptoms should be thought of as unconscious metaphors for the patient. Just as symptoms are the symbols or metaphors of experience, they too are the coping or defense mechanisms that may have made a great deal of sense to the patient in the context from which they arose. Taking the point further, *diseases are the metaphors that the mind creates to give vent to its unresolved conflicts.*

Table 4.1: Influence of Cytokines on the Hypothalamic—Pituitary-Thyroid Axis

Cytokine	*Effect*
On the Hypothalamus	
E. coli endotoxin, interleukin-1	Inhibits synthesis of thyrotropin-releasing hormone; stimulates somatostatin secretion (which inhibits thyrotropin secretion)
Glucocorticoid	Excess inhibits secretion of thyrotropin-releasing hormone
TNF-α	Lowers hypothalamic mRNA content of thyrotropin-releasing hormone
On Anterior Pituitary	
E. coil endotoxin	Stimulates pituitary production of interleukion-1 (mainly by the thyrotroph cells); stimulates production of interleukin-6 by folliculostellate cells
TNF-α	Reduces glycosylation of thyrotropin, decreasing its biologic potency
On the Thyroid Gland	
Interleukin-1	Decreases iodide uptake, accumulation of cyclic AMP, thyroglobulin synthesis and secretion, expression of peroxides gene; stimulates growth
TNF-α	Inhibits iodide uptake, inhibits response to thyrotropin
Interferon-γ	Increases expression of HLA class I and II molecules; increases iodide uptake and accumulation of cyclic AMP; reduces thyroid peroxidase levels; blocks stimulation of triiodothyronine release induced by thyrotropin; inhibits growth

Other mediators of inflammation that influence the hypothalamic-pituitary-adrenal axis are:

1. *Growth Factors*

- Epidermal growth factor
- Transforming growth factor β

2. *Lipid Mediators*

Prostanoids: In short the message as follows: there is a molecular basis to thinking and emotions. Therefore when a subject under hypnosis is strategically manipulated to experience the positive feelings of joy, happiness and a particular desired change in the behaviour, the hypnotized person, de facto, is experiencing at molecular biological level a renewal and rejuvenation in the brain and the related systems.

3. *Psyche, Information Substances and Immune Function*

Since last few years a possibility has emerged that the course and occurrence of some diseases known to be due to abnormalities in the immune function, can be modulated by some aspects of personality, behaviour, emotional state, stress and coping style. This integration of behaviour, brain and immune reactions is known as psychoneuroimmunology. The three important homeostatic mechanisms namely nervous, endocrine and immune system are well connected with each other and they communicate *via* various chemical substances like neuropeptides and neurotransmitters. These information substances and their receptors are part of all three systems mentioned.

Psychoneuroimmunology consists in study and relationships of component parts; psyche comprising of the cognitive and emotional processes involving conscious, subconscious and unconscious mind and how they collate with the neurological connections that bring about neurotransmitter and neuroendocrine secretions. And, how the immune system, e.g. the cellular and humoral components is impacted by psyche.

Thus, psychoneuroimmunology is the study of the interaction of behavioural, neural, and endocrine factors and the functioning of the immune system. The study involves bidirectional communication occurring between behaviour, brain, immune and endocrine systems.[2] So, it is an interdisciplinary science that studies the interrelationships between psychological, behavioural, neuroendocrine processes and immunology.[3]

Neuroimmunomodulation is the influence of the nervous system on immune responses. Neuroendocrinoimmunology is the study of neuroendocrine influence on the functions of immune system and cybernetic influence of immune system on neural and endocrinal activity. Suffice it to say that there is enough scientific evidence about the interconnectedness of these systems.

Research on Psychoneuroimmunology

In 1936 Hans Selye noticed that in rats exposed to stressors, adrenal glands were enlarged and thymus and lymph nodes shrunken. Subsequently cortisone was found to possess anti-inflammatory activity. The first systematic investigation in Psychoneuroimmunology (PNI) was by Ader and Cohen in 1975 of studies of conditioning and immunity. It was based on learned taste aversion requiring only one pairing of neutral taste and unconditional *stimuli.* These researchers in 1981 and 1986 found that a single taste stimulus and cyclophosphamide—a immunosuppressant drug that can eventually kill, produced association between taste and the immune system. The experiment was feeding mice with saccharin and simultaneously injecting a drug that caused suppression of the immune system. The mice died. When the experiment was repeated without cyclophosphamide, even then a high proportion of the mice died when receiving saccharin alone. The conditioning had been so successful that saccharin alone suppressed the immune system enough to kill the mice.[4] This study showed that it is possible to classically condition the immune system. Some evidence of conditioning of immune responses in humans has been reported too.

Conditioned immuno-suppresion reduces the graft versus host rejection response. The use of conditioning in bone marrow transplants, to help suppress the immune system rejection of the graft, has been described by Storb in1994.[5] Recently it is shown that antitumor functions of some lymphocytes can also be conditioned. Animals were exposed to pairing of a camphor odor with injection of an immunomodulator and responded to the odor alone by showing increases in cytotoxic T and NK cell activity. These findings provide new information about how conditioning of autonomic responses may occur.

What is of importance is not whether we have our emotional ups and downs, but rather that lingering unresolved emotions and inflexible ways of coping, can become the source of chronic low grade stress, which can undermine immune system functioning. This may not necessarily cause disease; however, given the right genetics, a weakened physical condition, or an existing illness and one may be sitting on a time bomb. Robert Ader, one of the foremost researchers in the field of PNI says "we are not talking about causation of disease, but the interaction between psychosocial events, coping and pre-existing biologic conditions."[6]

Clinical Studies

Norman Cousins who achieved remission of his ankylosing spondylitis by psychological means was the one who popularized the idea that there is a possibility that some aspects of personality, behaviour, coping style or emotional state influence the course of diseases due to abnormalities in immune functions. Simonton and Simonton[7] in 1975 treated cancer patients with the use of guided imagery with astonishing results and postulated psychoneurogenic basis. These results remain non-replicated as of today.

There are reports about some new discovery of a drug that caused many cancer patients to regress till they read the reports that the initial reports were found not true. This establishes at least psychobiological linkage. The cancer cells are produced in the body all the time at all ages. The normal immune resistance is able to destroy the abnormal cells. A break down in the immune level thus may be contributory to the appearance of cancer.

Whether these psychological and emotional factors can influence the course of autoimmune disease, cancer and infectious diseases in humans in evidence based manner is a subject which is yet to be resolved satisfactorily. The crux of the entire matter is to demonstrate that psycho cybernetics can reverse it; *via* hypnotherapy or any other kind of psychotherapy. However, we shall examine two areas where the research and clinical findings correlate.

Neuroimmunology

- *Brain*

The activation of cytokines in the central nervous system can lead to profound changes ranging from mild behavioural changes to destruction of neurons. A number of cytokines are synthesized in glia. This is activated to local tissue injury brought about once again by cytokines such tumor necrosis factor, interleukins etc. The damage can extend to the necrosis of brain cells in a scattered manner leading to Alzheimer's disease.

- *Joints*

Experimental destruction of the sensory innervation of joints that will destroy neurons containing substance P, somatostatin and other tachykinins, reduces the intensity of inflammatory arthritis. The so called osteoarthritis, ascribed to wear and tear due to aging, appears to have an auto immune component too, as inferred from the Lewis and Fischer rat models.

The expression of auto antibodies in the form of IgA, IgG and IgM appears to be time related. By the time IgM antibodies are found, the immune process may have gone on for 5-10 years. Reversal of such a slow, continuous damage through reversal of psychodynamics, at the moment is not clinically proven and appears a distant vision.

However, some idea of this complex psychoneurohormonal immune modulation can be visualized by a review of Tables 4.1-4.3. Table 4.4 further deals with cytokines.

Table 4.2: Immunoregulatory Effects of Hormones and Peptides

Hormone or Peptide	*Immune Function Affected*
Inhibitory	
Glucocorticoids	Lymphokine synthesis, inflammation
Corticotrophin	Macrophage activation, synthesis of IgG and interferon-γ
	Activity of T cells and natural killer cells
Chorionic gonadotrophin	IgG synthesis, T-cell proliferation
α-Endorphin somatostatin	T-cell proliferation, inflammatory cascade
vasoactive intestinal peptide	T-cell proliferation and migration in Peyer's patches
α-Melanocyte-stimulating hormone	Fever, prostaglandin synthesis, secretion of interleukin-2
Stimulatory	
Estrogens	Lymphocyte proliferation and secretion
Growth hormone	Thymic growth, lymphocyte reactivity
Prolactin	Thymic activity, lymphocyte proliferation
Thyrotropin	IgG synthesis
β-Endorphin	Activity of T, B, and natural killer cells
Substance P	Proliferation T cells and macrophages, inflammatory cascade
Corticotrophin-releasing hormone	Lymphocyte and monocyte proliferation and activation

Table 4.3: Hormones and Neuropeptides found in Immune competent cells

Hormones	*Source*	*Comments*
Corticotrophin	B lymphocytes	Stimulated by corticotrophin—Releasing hormone; inhibited by cortisol
Growth hormone	T lymphocytes	Stimulated by growth hormone
Thyrotropin	T cells	Stimulated by thyrotropin—releasing hormone; inhibited by somatostatin
Prolactin	Mononuclear cells	
Chorionic gonadotrophin	T cells	
Enkephalines	B lymphocytes	
Vasoactive intestinal peptide	Mononuclear leukocytes, mast cells	
Somatostatin	Mononuclear leukocytes, mast cells, poly morphonuclear leukocytes	
Vasopressin	Thymus	
Oxytocin	Thymus	
Neurophysin	Thymus	

Table 4.4: States Potentially Associated with Suppression or Activation of Immune-Mediated Inflammation through Defects in the Hypothalamic-Pituitary-Adrenal Axis (HPA), or its Target Tissues

Suppression of Immune-Mediated Inflammatory Reaction:	*Activation of Immune-Mediated Inflammatory Reaction:*
Increased HPA- axis activity	Decreased HPA- axis activity
Cushing's syndrome Melancholic depression Chronic alcoholism	Adrenal insufficiency Rheumatoid arthritis Atypical or seasonal depression
Chronic stress	Chronic fatigue or fibromyalgia
Long-term excessive exercise Pregnancy (last trimester) Fischer-rat model	Hypothyroidism Post-traumatic stress disorder Nicotine withdrawal After successful treatment for Cushing's syndrome After glucocorticoid therapy Postpartum period After chronic stress Lewis-rat model Obese-chicken model of autoimmune thyroiditis
	Conditions resistant to glucocorticoids are: Rheumatoid arthritis Steroid-resistant asthma AIDS Degenerative osteoarthritis Systemic lupus erythematosus*

*Due to increased catabolism of cortisol in target tissues.

Enormous data has accumulated about the information substances and their complex interactions. What triggers the secretion/activation of a particular substance or a molecular biological event? Psyche and soma being one, we hypothesize the trigger switch in the psychodynamics. While narration of such evidence in brief may provide the basis for a hypothesis, hypnotherapists will have to provide hard core laboratory/clinical evidence to prove the effectiveness of hypnotherapy.

- ***Consciousness, Brain Plasticity and Neurogenesis***

It is platitude to say that neurons do not regenerate nor do they multiply. However, their synaptic connections do grow and multiply[8] in response to genetic expression of behaviour state related genes as well as late activated genes. This expands the horizons of learning a fresh. It also provides us with a clue that how we can create ourselves a new as per the programme that we desire. This is the basis of NLP-neurolinguistic programmes that revolve around hypnotherapy. This explains how fresh learning through hobbies can generate psycho-cybernetic replays that delay ageing. That also explains how hypnotherapy works. To quote, Eric Kandel[9], Nobel Laureate in medicine for 2000:

Table 4.5: A summary of the main classes of neuromediators or putative neuromediators found in the nervous system

Cytokines and their effects

Cytokines	*Sources*	*Targets*	*Primary effects*
Mediators of natural Immunity:			
Type 1 interferon (alpha IFN, beta IFN)	Monocytes, macrophages, others	All NK cells	Antiviral, anti proliferative, increased class 1 MHC expression Activation
Tumor necrosis factor (TNF)	Monocytes, macro-Phages, T cells	Neutrophils liver T cells, B cells Hypothalamus	Activation (inflammation) Acute phase reactants Co-stimulator Fever
Interleukin-1 (Il-1)	Monocytes, macrophages, others	T cells, B cells Hypothalamus	Co-stimulator Fever
Interleukin-6 (IL-6)	Monocytes, macrophages, others	T cells, B cells Mature B cells	Co-stimulator Growth
Mediators of lymphocyte activation			
Interleukin-2 (IL-2)	T cells	T cells NK cells B cells	Growth, cytokine production Growth, activation Growth, antibody production
Interleukin-4 (IL-4)	CD4+ T cells	T cells B cells	Growth Activation, isotype switching to IgE
Transforming growth factor-beta (TCF-beta)	T cells, others	T cells Monocytes, macrophages	Inhibit activation and proliferation Inhibit activation
Mediators of effecter Cell activation:			
Interferon gamma (IFN-gamma)	T cells, NK cells	Monocytes, macrophages, NK cells	Activation
Interleukin-5 (IL-5)	T cells	Eosinophils B cells	Activation Growth and activation
Mediators of effecter cell growth and differentiation:			
Interleukin-3 (IL-3)	T cells	Immature progenitors	Growth and differentiation to all cell lines
Granulocyte-macrophage colony stimulating factor (G-M CSF	T cells, monocytes, macrophages, others	Immature progenitors Committed progenitors	Differentiation to granulocytes, monocytes, and macrophages
Macrophage CSF	Monocytes macrophages, others	Committed progenitors	Differentiation to monocytes, macrophages
Granulocyte CSF	Monocytes, macrophages, others	Committed progenitors	Differentiation to neutrophils, eosinophils, basophils
Interleukin-7	Fibroblasts, bone marrow stromal cells	Immature progenitors	Growth and differentiation to B cells

Abbreviations: CD-clusters of differentiation; CSF-cerebro-spinal fluid; MHC-major histocompatibility complex; NK-natural killer.

It presumably does so by producing changes in gene expression, that alters the strength of synaptic connections and structural changes that alters the anatomical pattern of interconnections between nerve cells of the brain.

Further research was needed to convert the philosophical vision of Rossi into a probability. How does an order by the brain in terms of an idea to requite a particular behaviour undergoes transduction into molecular biological events of intricate subtlety and, return is granted in the form of explicit behaviour (ideodynamic transformation)? And how is the genetic play for the same brought about? Let us see this most fascinating evolution of the (w)holistic scientific paradigm step by step.

Carew *et al.* (1983)[10], Hawkins *et al.* (1983)[11] and Walters and Byrne[12] described the information transduction within cells as activity dependent neuromodulation. This was brought about by secondary messenger systems such as camp, Ca^{++} and diacylglycerol. Kandel[13] in 1983 in a seminal work, described the passage from metapsychology to molecular biology.

Rossi, independently of his own, in 1983, 1985 and 1986[14], hypothesized mind gene connection and postulated that as molecular basis of therapeutic hypnosis. This was indeed a giant leap forward based on logical positivism. It still needed to be buttressed by empirical evidence.

Glaser *et al.*,[15, 16] deriving from the experimental results, documented the path of information transduction in 1990 as: primary messengers from neuroendocrine system → trigger cell receptors → initiate a cascade of secondary messengers → mediation of gene transcription → mRNA production → protein synthesis and other information substances that act on their specific receptors.

During the concluding decade of the last millennium, there has been a torrential cascade of path breaking research. There have been Nobel[17] prize winning contributions. Rather than cataloging them here, reference is made to the monograms.[18, 19, 20, 21, 22]

So consciousness seems to be more than a mere function of brain: no matter that we have identified the reticular formation in the mid brain extending down to medulla oblongata as the seat of consciousness. Firing of the cells from the cells located in this region upward to the cerebrum causes the subject to be conscious. However, such an activity does not happen in isolation and the role of genes is being recognized in psychobiology of consciousness. It should not be long before there is conclusive evidence that the state of hypnosis is gene activity dependent. And we believe the physics of consciousness shall soon be understood in terms of quantum mechanics.

Post Script to Chapter 5: Body-Mind Continuum

A given behaviour is the sum total of the effects of several neurotransmitters, hormones and hormone like substances secreted from the brain down to the cells. Symptoms of any particular disorder or disease therefore, are only metaphors displayed by the body of discomfort of the mind.

The following cases are examples.

- *Case 1*

A Muslim girl, aged 25 years came with the complaint of severe migraine. She started having headaches around the age of 18. The intensity and frequency increased with passage of time.

She was a super-intelligent girl. She came from lower socio-economic status. Though the family was a conservative Muslim family, they were not orthodox, They encouraged the child for higher education from very childhood. She topped the ranks and by choice took physics for higher studies. At bachelor level she was first ranker in the state. She was called for a national fellowship. The frequency and intensity of migraine forced her to abandon her fellowship.

The psychodynamics of migraine was written in bold letters in this scenario.

Hypnotherapeutic strategies aimed at generating the insight about the conflict. She was made to visualize a meeting with Late Dr. A.P.J. Kalam (former President of India), who also is a Muslim coming from a poor family. As a physicist he developed missiles with nuclear capability. Then he was to become the President of India.

Though her situation abated and she could verbalize her situation, her protest was that Dr. Kalam, after all was a man. In a subsequent session, she was made to visualize herself as Malala Yousafzai (The Pakistani girl, victimized by Taliban). In hypnosis, she saw Malala walking bravely and defiantly; through crippled.

A few months after she called to say that her migraine has almost gone. She asked for some cosmetic advice, since she wants to be prettier to get married.

A point is to be made here about the goal setting in therapy. The goal was to get rid of her migraine and, not aimed at making another Dr. Kalam or Malala.

- *Case 2*

An infertile couple approached Dr. Rajni Vyas. Physiologically, they were normal. Following previous treatment the woman had an ectopic pregnancy and, abortion at about six weeks. Exploration about psychodynamics revealed that the couple, prior to marriage was in a triangular relationship with another man in the triangle. The woman preferred to marry her husband out of material considerations. However, she had considered the other man a soul mate. While she was taciturn about the premarital physical proximity to the men, it was fair to assume that she was close to both. The reproductive behaviour of this woman can be exemplified as the expression of Bruce Effect.

Bruce Effect is well established in rodents. Whenever a pregnant female mouse comes in contact with another male, she aborts. It is likely that it extends to all mammals. This phenomenon is mediated through pheromones (volatile aromatic compounds that emanate from mammals).

To take the proof of body-mind continuum further we may document Whitten effect here as well. It was initially observed in mice as synchronization of estrous in a group of females in presence of a male. This extends to humans as well. It is observed that girls living in a dormitory with good empathy synchronize their menstrual cycles.

The above scientific data was presented as story telling through indirect hypnosis to the above mentioned couple across a few sessions. They seem to have understood when they adopted two children and lived happily far away from "soul mate".

We hypothesize that mind can block reproduction at any one or all of the following ways:

1. Erectile dysfunction in man and frigidity in female.
2. Oligospermia, azospermia in male.
3. Dyspareunia.
4. Unexplained reproductive failure that may be due to:
   (a) Tubal spasm of psychogenic origin.
   (b) Immunoglobulins in cervical mucous of IgA, IgG, IgM type against semen or sperms of the husband.
   (c) Ineffective penetration of the ovum by the sperm based on psychodynamics of hostility.
   (d) Imperfect nidation of fertilized ovum in endometrium.
   (e) Improper transit of the fertilized ovum through fallopian tube causing ectopic pregnancy.
   (f) Abortion in 1st trimester.
   (g) Eclampsia in 2nd, 3rd trimester.
   (h) IUGR (intrauterine growth retardation) in 2nd, 3rd trimester.
   (i) Recurrence of all the above.

Reproduction is universal for human race; but it is tempered with cultural values and ego defenses. So, it is highlighted here as a classic illustration of bodymind unity.

Since sexuality is one behaviour that overrides the importance of most others, the readers are recommended the following masterpieces of the twentieth century.[23]

Notes

1. Candace Pert, *Molecules of Emotions*, New York, 1990.

2. Maier, S.F., Watkins, L.R., Fleshner, M., *Psychoneuroimmunology: The Interface between Behaviour, Brain and Immunity. American Psychologist*. 49; 1004, 1994.
3. Andrew, Baum, Robert, J. Gatchel, David S. Krantz, *Psychoneuroimmunology, Cancer, and AIDS: An Introduction to Health Psychology*, 1995.
4. Adler, R. (Ed.) *Psychoneuroimmunology*, New York, 1981.
5. Storb, cited by Adler, R. (Ed.) *Psychoneuroimmunology*, New York, 1981.
6. *Ibid*. (Ed.) *Psychoneuroimmunology*, New York, 1981.
7. Simonton and Simonton, *Getting Well Again*, New York, 1980.
8. Lusher C., Nicoli, B., Malenca C., and Muller B., Synaptic plasticity and dynamic modulation of the postsynaptic membrane. *Nature Neuroscience*, 3; 545-67, 2000.
9. Eric Kandel A new intellectual framework for psychiatry? *Amer.J. Psychiatry*, 155; 457-469, 1998.
10. Carew, Hawkins and Kandel, *Science*, 219; 397-400; 1983.
11. Hawkins, R., Abrams T., Carew, T. and Kandal, E. *Science*, 219, 300-405; 1983.
12. Walters, E. and Byrne, J. *Science*, 219; 405-408, 1983.
13. Kandel, E., From metapsychology to molecular biology: exploration into the nature of anxiety. *American Journal of Psychiatry*, 140; 1277-1293.
14. Rossi, E.L. and David, B. Cheek, *Mind-Body Therapy: Ideodynamic Healing in Hypnosis*, London, 1988, pp. 55-60.
15. Glaser, R., Kennedy, S., Lafuse, W., *et al*. Psychological stress induced modulation of interleukin 2 receptor gene expression and interleukin 2 production in peripheral blood leucocytes. *Arch. Gen. Psychiatry*, 4; 707-712.
16. Glaser, R. *et al*. Stress associated modulation of protooncogene expression in human peripheral blood leucocytes. *Behav. Neurosci*. 107; 525-529.
17. In this fertile ground for Nobel hunting, there are a few sad stories about the mean of the nobles. It is particularly sad from the feminist point of view since the victims were women. One such story is that of Crick and Rosalind Franklin. Crick utilized the crystallography methods of Rosalind even without acknowledgment; the more famous is one about Candace Pert and her professor and guide, Sol and other two, Hughes and Kosterlitz. Last three shared the Nobel prize to the exclusion of Pert (see pp. 101-02, ref.vi).
18. Brown, P., *Genomes*, New York, 1999.
19. Tolle, T.R. *et al*., *Immediate Early Genes in CNS*, New York, 1995.
20. Fernandes, J. and Hoefler, J., *Gene Expression Systems*, New York, 1999.
21. Lydic, R., *Molecular Regulation of Arousal States*, Boca Raton, 1998.
22. Ridley, M. *Genome, The Autobiography of a Species in 23 Chapters*, New York, 1999.
23. *Studies in the Psychology of Sex*, Volume 1-6 by Havelock Ellis available as Gutenburg Project; Free on line; William Masters and Virginia Johnson, Human Sexual Response (ii) Human Sexual Inadequacy.

6

Psychopathology I

Psychobiological Model

Psychology is a hybrid science. There are several areas here where there is no objective evidence of the proposed theories. And, yet they are of great relevance since they work in practice. Psyche itself has no objective reality: most people know conceptually that they have a mind. Such areas of great relevance to a hypnotherapist are: Freudian concept of levels of mind and, theories of structure of personality. Having understood them, we shall discuss psychobiological factors that affect them to produce a disorder or disease.

Levels of mind: topographical model. Freud

The *conscious* mind includes all the sensations and experiences of which we are aware at any given moment. Freud insisted that only a small part of mental life (thoughts, perceptions, feelings, memories) is contained in the realm of conscious mind. Whatever the content of conscious experience may be for a given person at a given time, it is the result of a selective screening process largely regulated by external cues. Moreover, it is conscious only for a brief time and can be quickly submerged into preconscious or unconscious levels as the person's attention shifts to different cues. In short the conscious mind represents a small and limited aspect of personality.

Subconscious mind is that content of the psyche that can be brought to awareness with some effort.

The deepest and major stratum of the human mind is the *unconscious*: thoughts, desires and impulses of which we remain largely unaware. Freud also believed that much of it was once conscious, but has been actively repressed–driven from consciousness because it was too anxiety provoking. Once these forces are pushed into unconscious mind, there is a great resistance within the individual to their ever becoming conscious. Hence, material in unconscious is completely inadmissible to awareness, yet it largely determines the actions of people. In fact, Freud believed that unconscious material may be expressed in disguised or symbolic form in our daily life through slips of tongue, misperception, accidents and seemingly 'out of character' irrational behaviour. Our underlying 'true' feelings and motives thus come up despite our efforts to hide them. It is no exaggeration to say that unconscious mind is the dynamic demiurgic force that drives people through out life. Psychoanalysis emphasizes the interpretation of fantasies and dreams as avenues for deeper understanding of the unconscious processes underlying behaviour.

The concept of unconscious mind is identical with that of *chitta* in Indian philosophy.

Personality

The discussion below is primarily based on Freud's construct. It is entirely hypothetical. However, without going into details of psychoanalysis, most psychotherapists would derive some intuitive understanding of a client's psychopathological perspective that may work around Freudian construct and, therapy based on them works. But as the work of a therapist progresses, he soon realizes that there is substance to various theories. Instead of subscribing to a particular school such as cognitive, behavioural or humanistic existential, most therapists will eventually learn to focus in finding out "as to where the shoe pinches" and how to get rid of it.

However a formal learning of theories beyond Freud to modern times is of great value in structuring the sessions and cannot be overemphasized. For examples, designing of a session will involve metaphors and, Carl Jung's concept of archetypes and collective consciousness will provide the therapist with appropriate models. Erik Erikson and Margaret Mahler's emphasis on childhood relationships will provide clues to maladies that arise during conflicts/maladjustment during that period. Knowing about the approaches of other neo-Freudians makes the therapist aware of socio-cultural impact on the personality.

For the egalitarian who wishes not to be trapped in speculative jargon of various schools, best recourse is to go with the basic understanding of Freud's construct and then, practice an eclectic approach revolving around Carl Roger and Abraham Maslow. People are what they are as a product of innumerable factors; they approach a therapist because they aspire to be better than what they are. They will try do their best up to self-actualization; creative insights generated in hypnosis are effective tools towards that goal.

Id, Ego and Superego

The concept of unconscious mental processes was central to Freud's early description of personality organization. However, during the early 1920s he revised his conceptual model of mental life and introduced three basic structures: Id, Ego and Superego. They correspond roughly to desire, reason and conscience.

- ***Id***

Id refers exclusively to the inherited, biological, and unconscious component of personality. It is without morals, or logic, and is driven by two instincts: Eros and Thanatos. They are individual's reservoir of psychic energy too, and remain basic to the individual throughout life. Operating on a primitive basis, it is free from all inhibitions. Id is ruled by the pleasure principle: the drive to immediately increase pleasure, reduce tension and avoid pain, which when pent up, creates tension. Immediate tension reduction is called the *pleasure principle*. In sum, the id is demanding, impulsive, blind, irrational, asocial, selfish, and finally, pleasure-loving.

Freud identified two mechanisms the Id employs to rid the personality of tension and obtain pleasure: *reflex action* and *primary process*. In the former, the Id responds automatically to the sources of irritation, thereby promptly removing the tension which irritant elicits. On the other hand, primary process is a psychological phenomenon whereby the individual reduces tension by forming the mental image of an object previously associated with satisfaction of a basic drive.

Obviously, the primary process by itself is not capable of reducing tension. Consequently, a new or secondary psychological process develops. When this occurs, the structure of the second system of the personality, ego, begins to take form.

- ***Ego***

Ego is a psychic entity that constantly strives in the service of the self to maintain balance between the irrational instinctive urges of the id and restrictive, forbidding forces of superego. In doing so, ego is constantly under tension to satisfy id and find ways to do so without over tripping the boundaries laid by superego.

Purpose of ego is to gratify the desires of the Id in accordance with the restriction of both outer reality and superego. It monitors and directs id's impulsive desires and in doing so, operates at conscious and unconscious levels of the mind. The ego stresses rationality, and balances the impulses of the id against the demands of the environment. It plans to satisfy the id in safe and realistic way, and helps the person to adapt to the real world. The id operates according to pleasure principle; whereas, the ego operates according to the reality principle i.e., gratification of the instincts can be delayed until the time when the most pleasure can be obtained with the least pain or negative consequences. According to reality principle, the energy of the id may be blocked, diverted, or delayed, all in accordance with the demand of reality and the conscience. The ego is able to separate wish from fantasy, can tolerate tension and compromise, and changes over time. Accordingly, it determines the expression of the development of perceptual and cognitive skills.

To sum up ego is logical, rational, and tolerant of tension, the "executive" of the personality: but is a poor rider on the swift horse of the id. Freud said:

> One might compare the relation of the ego to the id with that of between a rider and his horse. The horse provides the locomotive energy, and the rider has the prerogative of determining the goal and of guiding of the movements of his powerful mount toward it. But all too often in the relations between the ego and the id we find a picture of the less ideal situation in which the rider is obliged to guide his horse in the direction in which it itself wants to go.

It may be interesting to note that substitution of reality principle for pleasure principle is actually not a dethronement of the pleasure principle, but only a safeguarding of it. A momentary pleasure, uncertain in its results, is given up, but only in order to gain in the new way as assured pleasure coming later. This doctrine (ego defense) of substitution is powerfully mirrored in Indian religious traditions. People are asked for renunciation of earthly desires in this life in order to enjoy pleasures of heaven after death.

- *The Superego*

The superego represents moral branch of our functioning and is the internal representative of traditional values and ideals that we stand for and the punishments we expect when we violate the code. The main functions of superego are: to prevent the impulses of the id, to persuade the ego to replace moralistic goals, and to attempt perfection. A child is not born with superego. It develops through interactions with parents, teachers and other formative figures. Initially for child superego is simply what is prescribed as right or wrong by his parents. However, as the child grows, his superego enlarges to incorporate norms of his expanded social world including his peer group, neighbours, teachers, relations etc. The superego may be considered as an individualized reflection of society's collective consciousness. In a generalized way, we may term id as the biological component of personality, the ego as the psychological component, and the superego as the social component. Superego is as irrational as id but in the opposite direction. It is concerned completely with the good of society and perfection in an individual.

To emphasize again, the terms conscious, unconscious, id, ego, and superego are conceptualizations of psychic phenomena. We do not have id, ego, and superego as some physical entities inside us. They get meaning through the dynamics or process implied in them. Personality is determined by struggle among the instincts, logical thinking, and conscience. The three mental structures must work in some degree of harmonious balance for a person to be functioning in a healthy manner. This has to be socially acceptable.

The Dynamics of Personality

Freud believed that for psychological activity as with any kind of work, some form of energy is necessary and he termed it as psychic energy. He postulated that psychic energy might be transformed into physiological energy and *vice versa*. The point of contact or bridge between the energy of the body and that of the personality is the id and its instincts.

Instinct

Freud categorized instincts into two broad groups—the life instincts and death instincts.

Life instincts [Eros] cover forces necessary for life process and propagation of the species. Eros embraced not only sex drive, but also strivings toward union, creation, construction, integration and the cohesion involved in family formation. It also includes friendliness and cooperative undertakings, and the reproduction of new units, including human offspring. The form of energy by which the life instincts work is libido.

The death instinct [Thanatos] refers to person's unconscious wish to die or return to an inorganic state. It is a controversial and least- accepted part of the theory. Instead most analysts refer it as aggressive instinct, i.e. that humans have an innate drive or instinct to fight or to behave aggressively, just as they have physiologically based instincts of hunger, thirst, or sexual arousal. The death instinct embraced all the opposites of Eros- aggression, hostility and attack, striving towards destruction, disunion and disintegration, as well as decay of interpersonal relationships. All of them urge to lose individuality. Like sexuality, aggression poses many problems for the individual and for society. Learning its uses and control is one of the major tasks of childhood and adolescence.

An individual's behaviour is determined by the interplay of both these instincts. They work together and against each other and have a hand in everything a person does. The primary example of this is "sex" itself, where the libido is present, and varying degree of aggression too. The presence of intensely opposed strivings in human organism leads to all kinds of conflicting trends, including man's pervasive ambivalence. It includes such complex combinations as occurs in ordinary cooperative and competitive work and play, and in constructive and aggressive enterprise.

Development of Sexuality

Freud's major work on sexuality is the 'Three Essays in the Theory of Sexuality,' published in 1905, and then substantially expanded and amended as it went through six editions over the subsequent twenty years. The work has richness, complexity, and elegance which popularization has obscured. In his work,

Freud first brought out the narrowness of the conventional definition of sexuality; then he showed sexuality to have a complex and lengthy history and finally, in the light of this history, an emended definition was made. Before Freud, human sexuality was thought of as something that simply appeared at puberty. With his theory of psychosexual development, Freud attempted to show how sexuality begins in infancy as something related to, but also different from, adult sexuality, and how it developed through a sequence of stages. Final form of adult sexuality is influenced by a great number of pleasurable, sexual-sensual experiences that occur on the passage from infancy through childhood to adulthood. During this process, lasting personality traits and defenses develop.

Freud's theory considers personality development through five progressive psychosexual stages

Oral birth to 1 year
Anal 1-3 years
Phallic 3-5 years

Latency-6-puberty

Genital—starts on puberty and lasts till death.

First three stages are also called pre-genital stages. The name of the stage is on the basis of region of the body whose stimulation allows for discharge of libidinal energy. Age 5 years to puberty, though important, is not a developmental stage and is considered as latency period. As child grows he passes through different erogenous stages seeking objects or activities for stimulation and gratification. The shortfall or excess of such stimulation creates *frustration* and *overindulgence*, both leaving permanent impressions. Adulthood personality reflects childhood in terms of residual behaviour of that particular developmental stage.

Defense Mechanisms

We have understood ego as constantly striving to strike a balance between persistent, irrational demands of the id and the restrictive, deterrent denial by the superego. This causes tension. Freud thought that when tension could not be handled effectively by ego through the realistic methods, the individual would resort to defenses. These defenses are involuntary mental mechanisms that distort one's perception of internal and external reality to reduce subjective distress. But stretched beyond a limit, stress mounts, tensions built up, perception blurs further and, one is on the fertile ground of disorder and disease.

Ego defenses are brought into play when ego finds it difficult to do its task. Defense mechanisms help the ego to defend against anxiety and stress and, also to give some expression to unacceptable impulses in indirect, disguised form. On the other hand, they can be maladaptive in turning the person away from reality. Basically, whether a defense is adaptive or maladaptive depend on the extent of distortion, how pervasive it is, and the circumstances under which it occurs.

Vaillant [1971] has grouped defense mechanisms hierarchically, included within the "high adaptive level" of defenses of anticipation, altruism, humor, sublimation, and suppression. These adaptive mental mechanisms maximize gratification and allow conscious awareness of feelings, ideas and their consequences. Everyone, normal or abnormal, uses a characteristic repertoire of defense mechanisms.

The distinction between mental health and illness is not made in terms of whether or not there are defenses, for there are always defenses. The distinction is made in terms of whether the defenses promote the effective compromise of balance, or the ineffective denial of one of the two opposing forces.

Valliant's Classification

Vaillant (1971) has grouped defenses hierarchically according to the relative degree of maturity associated with them. Narcissistic defenses are the most primitive and appear in children and people who are psychotically disturbed. Immature defenses are seen in adolescents and some non-psychotic patients. Neurotic defenses are encountered in obsessive-compulsive and hysterical patients as well as in adults under stress.

Narcissistic Defenses

- *Projection*

Perceiving and reacting to unacceptable inner impulses and their derivatives as though they were outside the self. The person projects ones own unacceptable impulses on others so that others are assumed to harbour them. A hostile person perceives the world as a dangerous place; a sexually frustrated person interprets innocent gestures of others as sexual advances. On the psychotic level, this takes the form of frank delusion about external reality, usually persecutory.

- *Denial*

Refusal to accept the true nature of a threat. Belief that one will not contract cancer or heart disease although one smokes heavily. Psychotic denial of external reality, unlike repression, affects the perception of external reality more than the perception of internal reality. Seeing but refusing to acknowledge what one sees, or hearing, and negating what is actually heard, are examples of denial.

- *Distortion*

Grossly reshaping external reality to suit inner needs, including unrealistic megalomaniac beliefs, hallucinations, with fulfilling delusions, and employing sustained feeling of delusional superiority of entitlement.

Immature Defenses

Acting Out: There is direct expansion of an unconscious wish or impulse into action to avoid being conscious of the accompanying effect. The unconscious fantasy, involving objects, is lived out impulsively in behaviour, thus gratifying the impulse.

- *Blocking*

An inhibition usually temporary in nature, of affects especially, but possibly also of thinking and impulses. It is close to repression in its effects, but has a component of tension arising from the inhibition of the impulse, affect, or thought.

- *Hypochondriasis*

The transformation of reproach toward others arising from bereavement, loneliness, or unacceptable aggressive impulses into self-reproach and complains of pain, somatic illness, and neurasthenia. Existent illness may also be over-emphasized or exaggerated for its evasive and regressive possibilities.

- *Introjections*

The introjections of a loved object involve the internalization of characteristics of the goal of establishing closeness to and constant presence of the object. Anxiety consequent to separation or tension arising out of ambivalence toward the object is thus diminished.

Introjections of feared objects serve to avoid anxiety through internalizing the aggressive characteristics of the object, and thereby putting the aggression under one's control. The aggression is no longer felt as coming from outside, but is taken within and is utilized defensively.

- *Passive-aggressive Behaviour*

Aggression towards an object, expressed indirectly and ineffectively, through passivity, masochism, and turning against the self.

- *Projection*

Attributing one's own unacknowledged feeling to others; it includes severe prejudice, rejection of intimacy through suspiciousness, hyper-vigilance to external danger.

- *Regression*

A return to previous stage of development or functioning to avoid the anxieties or hostilities involved in later stages. This reflects a basic tendency to achieve instinctual gratification or to escape instinctual tension by returning to earlier modes and levels of gratification when later and more differentiated modes fail. Return occurs under stress to form of behaviour characteristic of an earlier period. An adolescent cries when forbidden to use parent's gadgets; an adult becomes dependent upon his parents following break up of his marriage.

- *Schizoid Fantasy*

The tendency to use fantasy and to indulge in autistic retreat for the purpose of conflict resolution and gratification.

- *Somatization*

The defensive conversion of psychic derivatives into bodily symptoms; tendency to react with somatic rather than psychic manifestations.

Neurotic Defenses

Controlling: The excessive attempt to manage or regulate events or objects in the environment in the interest of minimizing anxiety and solving internal conflicts.

- *Displacement*

Freud explained the dynamics of instincts through displacement. This concept represents shift from original object-choice to some other object due to difficulty in meeting first choice. Displacement of energy from one object to another is very important feature of personality dynamics. It accounts for the remarkable versatility of human nature. Freud suggested that the entire fabric of modern civilization is the product of displaced sources of libidinal and aggressive energy. Wars and prejudices represent displaced aggressive energy. There is transfer of ideas and impulses from threatening or unsuitable objects onto less threatening objects, e.g. A worker picks up a fight with a spouse after being criticized by his supervisor.

It is a purposeful, unconscious shifting from one object to another in the interest of solving a conflict. Although the object is changed, the instinctual nature of the impulse and its aim remains unchanged.

- *Externalization*

It refers to the tendency to perceive in the external world and in external objects the components of one's own personality, including instinctual impulses, conflicts, moods, attitudes, and styles of thinking. It is more general term than projection, which is defined by its derivation from and correlation with specific introjections.

- *Inhibition*

The unconsciously determined limitation or renunciation of specific ego function, singly or in combination, to avoid anxiety arising out of conflict with instinctual impulses, superego, or environmental forces or figures.

- *Intellectualization*

The control of affects and impulses by way of thinking about them instead of experiencing them. It is a systematic excess of thinking, deprived of its affect, to defend against anxiety caused by unacceptable impulses.

- *Isolation*

The intrapsychic splitting or separation of affect from content resulting in repression of either idea or affect or the displacement of affect to a different or substitute content.

- *Rationalization*

A justification of attitudes, beliefs, or behaviour that might otherwise is unacceptable by an incorrect application or justifying reasons or the invention of a convincing fallacy. There is self deceiving justification for unacceptable behaviour. A student blames her cheating on her teacher's leaving the room during a test; an employee, who is inefficient, says he quit the job to spare the boss.

- *Reaction Formation*

The management of unacceptable impulses by permitting expression of the impulse in antithetical form. This is equivalently an expression of impulse in the negative. Where instinctual conflict is persistent, reaction formation can become a character trait on a permanent basis, usually as an aspect of obsessional character.

- *Repression*

It consists of the expelling and withholding from conscious awareness of an idea or feeling. It may operate either by excluding from awareness what was experienced once at a conscious level (secondary repression), or it may curb ideas and feelings before they have reached consciousness (primary repression). Anxiety is ejected from awareness. A student forgets the date of a difficult examination; a patient in therapy forgets an appointment.

The Mature Defenses

- *Altruism*

The vicarious but constructive and instinctually gratifying service to others. This must be distinguished from altruist surrender, which involves surrender of direct gratification or of instinctual needs in favour of fulfilling the needs of others to the detriment of the self, with vicarious satisfaction only being gained through introjections.

- *Anticipation*

The realistic anticipation of or planning for future inner discomfort; implies overly concerned planning, worrying, and anticipation of dire and dreadful possible outcomes.

- *Asceticism*

The elimination of directly pleasurable affects attributable to an experience. The moral element is implicit in setting values on specific pleasures. Asceticism is directed against all "base" pleasures perceived consciously, and gratification is derived from the renunciation.

- *Humor*

The overt expression of feelings without personal discomfort or immobilization and without unpleasant effect on others. Humor allows one to bear, and yet focus on, what is too terrible to be borne, in contrast to that, which always involves distraction or displacement away from affective issue.

- *Sublimation*

The gratification of an impulse, whose goal is retained, but whose aim or object is changed from a socially unacceptable one to a socially valued one. Libidinal sublimation involves a de-sexualization of drive impulses and the placing of a value judgment that substitutes what is valued by the superego or society. Sublimation of aggressive impulses takes place through pleasurable games and sports. Unlike neurotic defenses, sublimation allows instincts to be channeled rather than to one damned up or diverted. Thus in sublimation feelings are acknowledged, modified, and directed toward a relatively significant person or goal, so that, modest instinctual satisfaction results. The channeling of primitive impulses into positive, constructive efforts occurs. For instance, a person paints nudes for the sake of beauty and art; a hostile person directs aggressive energies into competitive sports.

- *Suppression*

The conscious or semiconscious decision to postpone attention to a conscious impulse or conflict.

But there are times when defenses break down, and a glimpse of real truth ensues. These times occur when the person is in psychoanalysis/hypnosis through insight generation, or is severely debilitated, through psychological or physical stress. The accompaniment of breakdown in defense is acute guilt and anxiety—the feeling that life is about to end terribly and, indeed, should end for such a worthless person. The person cannot stay in such a state for very long and still maintain much integrity and organization. He is either restored to normalcy through what we may call psychological restoration of homeostasis or the defenses are reinstituted. Otherwise regardless of whether the source of breakdown was debilitation or psychotherapy—paradoxical though it may appear-catastrophe will result. Let us see as to how that happens.

Breakdown of Defenses: Process of Dyscreation

Creativity is generally ascribed to a positive meaning. Creating something means bringing out a product that is new and was not there before. When such a meaning is attributed to the process, aesthetic value is implied. Then, the new product is judged by the beauty of its form and expression that is likely to give joy to the observer. However, when applied to health, disease (psychic or physical) is to be seen as a product of a negative creative process. This implies that diseases do not occur, but are created by breakdown of ego defenses. It has validity as per our earlier discussion on psychology. It derives validation from two fundamental philosophical postulates in Indian ethos too.

The *Upanishads* conceptualized a life style devoid of any diseases. Such a life was nourished eternally from the universal source as.[1]

Let me be eternally connected to the Third Eye, so that, the life force gets enriched all the time.

And death was the culmination of cyclic process so that one was to depart as naturally as a ripened fruit separates from the plant. Connected to *the* universal source, there was no room for any disorder. However, if diseases do occur, there was a faulty connection to the universal source that maintained homeostasis. A clear consciousness was fundamental to the maintenance of homeostasis according to Charak, father of *Ayurveda.* In his masterpiece, *Charak Samhita,* he postulated an all-embracing hypothesis for pathogenesis of all diseases. He said, *pragyaparadha jayate sarva rogan*[2]: all diseases arise from faulty functioning of discriminating wisdom of intellect.

The diseases are generally classified into psychological disorders, congenital, traumatic, inflammatory, metabolic, endocrinological, immunological, new growths—benign and cancer—and degenerative. We understand the psycho-cybernetics of a large number of ailments and, even in what appears to be a mere accident, like the death of Princess Diana, one can surmise the faulty functioning of discriminative wisdom. Similarly, when we consider the infectious diseases or parasitic diseases like malaria, the understanding of waxing and waning of the immunological status of an individual during different levels of stress makes it evident that the ground is as important as the seed. However, it is still a far cry to the explanation of *all* diseases as arising from deranged psycho cybernetics. All the same, with the advances in the understanding of depth psychology, molecular biology and genetics, psychodynamics of many psychosomatic diseases are seen to be in congruence with Charak's hypothesis. The relevance of the proposition is now becoming clear in terms of cybernetic molecular biological pathways to a certain extent in many organic diseases too.

Let us see how.

Psychodynamics of Disease Creation

The Freudian concept of self as ego is all pervasive across the modern world now. The world is no more seen as a Mother Earth with all inhabitants as members of mutually interdependent family but as highly competitive combatants. Ego is crying out loudly, I for myself. Therefore, the ego truly functions as the guardian/servant of the self, constantly striving to balance the conflicting demands of id with the restrictive impositions of superego. What was seen by Freud in the study of his diseased subjects has come to be the normal pattern for most subjects of our times.

The balancing act by the ego turns out to be a tight rope walking exercise. Ego tries to function in the service of self. In the process, it tries to score a few tricks to satisfy id, under the impression that the superego is not watching. But in doing so, there is inbuilt threat to the self. This is the generic ground of anxiety that causes faulty perception. This vitiates action whose results are at variance with the self-centered calculations. Perceiving a further threat to self, ego mobilizes support of immature defense mechanisms. This further clouds perception, generating unsound concepts regarding the actuality. And a vicious cycle is brought about in one of the following ways:

1. Self → ego/superego/id → anxiety → stress → tension → increased acuity/clarity of perception → mature defense mechanisms → restoration to normalcy.
2. Self → ego/superego/id → anxiety → stress → tension → diseases of autonomic nervous system; IBS, myalgia, myofascial syndrome etc.
3. Self → ego/superego/id → anxiety → stress → tension → mobilization of immature ego defenses → faulty perception → wrong inference → wrong actions → temporary maladjustment → restoration to health.
4. Wrong actions → temporary maladjustment → further reinforcement → reaction formation → hostility to self and/society, stress → antisocial/criminal behaviour → breakdown.
5. Pathological breakdown, stress → psychiatric conditions/organic disease →
6. Derangement of cybernetic homeostatic molecular biological events → organic diseases, generalized (e.g. cardiovascular) or as per the targeted organ (e.g. thyrotoxicosis). →
7. For a prolonged period compounded with self rejection and hostility → autoimmune disorders →
8. Learnt helplessness → decreased immunity → cancer*.

To sum up, this is a brief narration of the negative creative play in the mind whereby disorder in imbalance of ego defenses is recreated as disease. Needless to emphasize, the figure is too simplistic. The above hypothesis is likely to give an impression that the author is a Freudian psychologist. (Far from it, the author, while celebrating the genius of Freud, believes that much harm that Freud has done to the civilization of the past century by creating a consumerist society was possible because only a genius of his size could wield such tremendous influence over the mankind). The model is given because that is one way to explain psychobiology of disease creation.

Alternatively, one may substitute stress as the causative agent of most disorders. That will satisfy the above paradigm and the materialist/dualist scientists too. Let us restate the position that though body-mind is one, the homeostasis and its breakdown in the body, do not function as a straight line algorithm. They are the bottom line of highly complex interactions.

It will be useful to remember that stress is the underlying cause: defense mechanisms are for coping with it. So, quantifying stress has been attempted by Thomas Holmes and Richard Rahe and is named as Social Readjustment Rating Scale (SRRS: See Appendix III) If one has more than 200 score in SRRS it becomes a powerful stressor situation. It may or may not damage organs depending upon the person's attitude (optimistic versus pessimistic), social support from family and neighbours, employment status, faith in religion, etc.

Social Readjustment Rating Scale[3]

Rank	*Life Event*	*Mean Value*
I.	Death of spouse	100
II.	Divorce	73
III.	Marital separation	65
IV.	Jail term	63
V.	Death of close family member	63
VI.	Personal injury or illness	53
VII.	Marriage	50[a]
VIII.	Fired from work	47
IX.	Marital reconciliation	45
X.	Retirement	45
XI.	Change in health of family membe	44
XII.	Pregnancy	40
XIII.	Sex difficulties	39
XIV.	New family member	39
XV.	Business readjustment	39
XVI.	Change in financial state	38
XVII.	Death of close friend	37
XVIII.	Change to different line of work	36
XIX.	Change in number of arguments with spouse	35
XX.	Mortgage over 10,000[b]	31
XXI.	Foreclosure of mortgage or loan	30
XXII.	Change in responsibilities at work	29
XXIII.	Child leaving home	29
XXIV.	Trouble with in-laws	29
XXV.	Outstanding personal achievement	28
XXVI.	Spouse begins or stops work	26
XXVII.	Begin or end school	26
XXVIII.	Change in living conditions	25
XXIX.	Revision of personal habits	24
XXX.	Trouble with boss	23
XXXI.	Change in work hours or conditions	20
XXXII.	Change in residence	20
XXXIII.	Change in schools	20
XXXIV.	Change in recreation	19
XXXV.	Change in church activities	19
XXXVI.	Change in social activities	18
XXXVII.	Mortgage loan less than 10,000[b]	17
XXXVIII.	Change in sleeping habits	16
XXXIX.	Change in number of family get-togethers	15
XL.	Change in eating habits	15
XLI.	Vacation	13
XLII.	Christmas	12
XLIII.	Minor violations of the law	11

a Marriage was arbitrarily assigned a stress value of 500; no event was found to be any more than twice as stressful. Here the values are reduced proportionally and range up to 100.

b In the mid-1960s, a mortgage like this was considered very large.

Homeostasis and Disease: A Bottom Line of Chaos

If we have to define them in physical properties, the correct choice is the physics of *Chaos*. When it comes to actual effects, let us see how even the classical physics has an element of indeterminacy about it. Suppose we have a finite accuracy and we do not know exactly where just one atom is, say to one part in a billion. Then it goes along and hits another atom and we find an even larger error in the position after the collision. Thus it gets amplified. Starting with a very tiny error, it can magnify rapidly as the collision of the billiard balls on the table.

No matter how precise, an arbitrary accuracy over a period of time makes accurate prediction impossible. And the time need not be very long (as seen in the calculations of the age of the universe); the time goes logarithmically with the error and it turns out that in what may be considered a tiny bit of time, we lose all the information and randomness may become obvious[4]. Thus, even in a system that should be governed by deterministic laws, only a slight change in a few of the parameters can alter the equation drastically. The end result can vary in unpredictable and seemingly random behaviour-chaotic fashion.[5,6,7] In such a system the equations that define the way the system would change with time are nonlinear. They are very sensitive too, so that a small initial difference may make an enormous change to the future state of the system. This has come to be known as butter fly[8] effect.

But it is commonsense that the cycle from disease to health is reversible. And the process of reversal is faster under hypnosis.

Caution! A Pathologist's Standpoint

Some two decades after the author has practiced hypnosis with good results, he happened to share them with an outstanding academician. Dr. Damodar Balar was onco-pathologist at Cancer Hospital, Ahmedabad. Short of ridicule, he asked: how have you forgotten the large lumps and bumps and massive cavities that we have studied in the course of natural histories of the various diseases? Should I remind you of the specimens of numerous organs that get studded with malignant metastasis? And so on it went.

A few years after, to my surprise, he sent an article from The New England Journal of Medicine[9] with a note that psychosomatic connections seem to be making some sense in view of linkages discussed over there.

Author has no hesitation to repeat again and again that at the material, emotional and spiritual levels, bodymind is one. But conceptual understanding can undergo quantum jumps; while therapeutic application has strategic limitations to manipulate complex molecular biological events. A therapist is aware of this all the time while accepting any case for therapy.

In nutshell, there is interaction of "nature" and "nurture" in the development of personality. Nature determines the basic drives/instincts in the human beings, where as nurture makes human beings human. A therapist has just a small, but pivotal role in nurturing.

Restatement: A Tribute to the Genus of Freud

Freud gave us a construct of psyche and personality more than a century ago. The advances in the field of psychology by sociobiologists, cognitive scientists, behaviourists, molecular biologists and geneticists have established the stature of psychology as a hybrid science; to the extent that it is called a pseudoscience at the back. Not one of Freudian theories can be proved to be scientific. Relevance of Freudian constructs is that they work in psychotherapeutic and hypnotherapeutic settings.

Freud's concepts regarding sexuality led to storms in his own life time and many of his followers parted company from him on this ground. Indians particularly frown on this aspect. The universality of his ideas can be glimpsed from the lives of some great Indians. Mahatma's grand son, Raj Mohan Gandhi, in his book, *The Boatman:Portrait of Gandhi* narrates the episode of Mahatma's affair with Sarla Devi. Pyarelal has so much more to say on Mahatma's sexuality in *Last Phase.* The veracity of pasychoanalytic truths is always open to question, yet, Eric Erikson won the Bookers Prize for his Freudian psychoanalytic work, *Gandhi's Truth.* And Sudhir Kakkar, Erikson's worthy pupil, is vastly admired in the West for his Freudian interpretations. The biographical work of Gopal Radhakrishnan, a historian and the son of Sarvapalli Radhakrishnan, about his father also draws a parallel in scooping and scavenging the affairs of his father. Indian instincts are no different from rest of humanity. But hypnotherapy should be culturally structured.

What Freud conceptualized long time back is now aptly mirrored in the present day modern civilization. The pleasure principle has overtaken most of the other values. Consumerism is the key word in the service of ego. So, it is now often seen that the tail (of id) wags the dog (the personality). The extent of the genius of Freud is evident from the fact that his construct of the personality, how so ever difficult to prove its scientific basis, is operational all across our present day civilization. Therefore, the reliance over the Freudian construct of personality as well as the understanding of the ego defenses in bringing about a therapeutic change in hypnotherapeutic strategy cannot be overemphasized.

However, a set of values may not have any intrinsic merit in the Kantian sense. Yet, the humanity and civilizations that built them were beautified to the extent that there were aesthetics of value system that extended beyond the gross pleasure principle. This we shall elucidate in Chapter on Psychology – Indian Tradition.

In the milieu of the culture and civilization, the personality of an individual functions to as to either flourish and flower or to fade. Here lies the importance of belief system of the subject. This is the focal point for planning the strategy for hypnotherapy.[10]

Post-Script to Chapter 6: Psychopathology I

Counseling and other psychotherapeutic models work on the basis of rationality and restoration to a rational state of personality. Towards this aim, discursive, persuasive, discursive, dialectical, reasoning, debating methods are utilized. Hypnotherapy, though generally considered as one of the psychotherapeutic method is distinctly different. Most people with psychodynamic disorders understand where the fault lies, but cannot avoid the behaviour! They know what the right action is but cannot follow it. A survey by American Psychological Association estimates a success rate in psychotherapy as low as 35 per cent. Hypnotherapy succeeds when others fail, since in this altered state of consciousness there is clear perception of immature defenses of ego. It also generates insight that may provide access to mature defenses of ego; though it cannot change the situation.

Say, a stock broker who has lost his wealth; may be he is on the verge of killing his family and committing suicide. This happens when the usual ego defenses such as projection of fault to others, denial of event, distortion and displacement of the situation as a dominating event or acting out, fail. The extreme step follows with failures of such other neurotic defenses as rationalization and externalization (that it occurs with everybody once in a while in stock market!).

The therapist cannot retrieve the losses; however he may utilize mature defenses in service of ego so as to alleviate depression, suppression of the impulse to commit suicide and recourse to activism, altruism and even humor.

Case Study 1

There are, as we have seen above, numerous biographies of Mahatma Gandhi. Several instances in Gandhi's life yield to psychoanalytical interpretation. Gandhi was a devout Hindu; the epic god Ram was his ideal; (When he was shot dead, "Hey Ram" were his last words). Gandhi utilized, and was helped by his peers to turn whatever immature or neurotic defenses of ego he came to experience, to a mature state of reconditioning. That led to the evolution and, unfolding of Mahatma within him.

To illustrate further: we mentioned earlier about Gandhi's attraction towards Sarla Devi. Let us see a bifurcation point here. Supposing he would have thought of following his inner urge towards the lady. He was known to follow this inner voice as is known, even in his political decisions. Suppose his choice was to go forward with this lady. The Indian cultural milieu as of now and more so then, revolves around the fidelity of the god Ram to a single woman. Whether his wife may have compromised or not with the situation (as is not uncommon) is inconsequential; there would have been no emergence of his personage as Mahatma.

In all human situations and more so in India, close intimate, frank, friendly advice from friends and relations works through indirect hypnosis as confrontational psychotherapy. Gandhi would have been surprised, astonished and, even shocked to receive a letter of admonition from his close friend C. Rajgopalachari, who cautioned him that this single occurrence, his public image of being a Mahatma would entireiy crash; the edifice that he was building, later to be known as the Father of the Nation, would vanish. Gandhi utilized the mature defenses of ego in service of his personality; such as altruism, self denial and asceticism. This preserved the ideals inwardly for his own moral defense and externally towards what he was shaping as his destination—his self actualization of the personality that he aimed to be. On the other hand, he had to struggle for sublimation of sex, up to the end of his life.

Case Study 2

The only son of a wealthy Non-Resident Indian, after a successful carrier in education and business arrived in India to get married to an Indian bride. This was in accordance to wishes of his parents. He as well subscribed to Indian cultural values and looked forward to a steady long lasting conjugal relationship.

He advertised in newspapers and, out of numerous responses, he got married to a girl who absolutely subscribed to all the values that the young man expounded; without a single question. After celebrating the marriage with ostentatious display of wealth, the couple moved to USA. The boy got his first jolt when it started showing that the girl had married a "Green Card" (Non-Resident Indians are given this card by American authorities, entitling them to be residents). Moreover, she was given to American life style.

The girl further tried to persuade her husband to draw money from his parents from India. She had a convincing argument that after all he was the only inheritor and it is now that they need money since they are in formative years. This resulted in ping pong visits to India by the boy.

Soon he was diagnosed with Irritable Bowel Syndrome. Sigmoidoscopy and Colonoscopy soon after revealed that he had Ulcerative Colitis. He was put on the drug Sulfasalazine and special diet for Ulcerative Colitis. The disease would abate while he was in India with his parents. It would relapse when he goes back to his wife in USA.

He was advised Total Colectomy in USA. When he was brought for therapy by his parents the psychodynamics were evident. The young man, a refined, sensible and highly intelligent man blamed only himself for dichotomy in his marriage situation. Though he was cheated, he took blame on himself. He not only accepted but defended his wife and family; that they have right to their own values.

The altruistic patient was asked to read The Art of loving by Erich Fromm. He understood that while forgiving others one has a duty towards oneself as well. In a few sessions his altruistic attitude was utilized to forgive himself as well and stop weeping, bleeding and cursing himself through his gut.

He divorced his wife. She was rewarded with ample alimony. He ejected the idea of living in alien culture milieu. He set up a software company in India, exporting products worldwide. He was persuaded to consent to marry again. Yet he remains unmarried after 6 years; no more ulcerative colitis.

Notes

1. *Tryambakam yajamahe, sugandhim pushti vardhanam;*
   Urvarukmiva badhanat, mrityo mukshi mamritat.
2. *Pragya* is comprised of three qualities: intellect, ability to bear and cope, and memory. It is comprehensively translated here as discriminating wisdom.
   * This is rather a simplistic narration of complex data accumulated over last 25 years in the field of psychoneuroendocrinology and psychoneuroimmunology.
3. Holmes and Rahe, 1967.
4. Feynman R.P. *Feynman Lectures on Physics,* New Delhi. 1996, pp. 1422-23.
5. Gleik James, Chaos, *Making of a New Science,* Harmondsworth, 1989.
6. Stewart Ian, Does God play dice? The mathematics of Chaos, Oxford, 1989.
7. Earnest Rossi, *Symptom Path to Enlightment.*
8. Initially, Chaos theory was introduced to forecast the unpredictable weather conditions. It suggests that dynamic equations governing the weather are so sensitive to initial conditions that fluttering of the wings of a butterfly would result in the occurrence of a hailstorm in other part of the world. That is why it is called *butterfly effect.*
9. Reichlin Seymour Mechanisms of Disease, Neuroendocrine–Immune Interactions, *The New Eng. Jour. Med.* 329; 1246-1253, 1993.

References

Breger, Louis (1974). *From Instinct to Identity.* The Prentice-Hall, Inc., Englewood Cliffs, New Jersey.

Durkheim, P. (1906). *Determination du Fait moral.* Revue de Metaphysique et de Morale. Quoted by Parsons, T. (1964). *Social Structure and Personality.* The Free Press of Glencoe, London.

Enns, C.Z. (1993). Twenty years of feminist counselling and therapy: From naming biases to implementing multifaceted practice. *The Counselling Psychologist,* 21 [1], 3-87.

Flugel, J.C. (1950). *The Psychoanalytic Study of the Family,* The Hogarth Press Ltd., London.

Fromm, E. (1982). *Greatness and Limitations of Freud's Thoughts,* Sphere Books Ltd., London.

Gurman, A.S. and Messer, S.B. (1995). *Essential Psychotherapies*. The Guilford Press, New York.

Hall, C.S., Lindzey, G. and Campbell, J.B. (1998). *Theories of Personality*, John Wiley & Sons, Inc., New York.

Hilgard, E. (1968). Psychoanalysis: Experimental studies. In d. Sills [Ed.], *International Encyclopedia of the Social Sciences*, Vol. 13, Macmillan and the Free Press.

Hjelle, L.A. and Ziegler, D.J. (1981), *Personality Theories*. McGraw-Hill Co., New Delhi.

Kelly, L. (1991). *An Exploratory Study of the Prevalence of Sexual Abuse in a Sample of 16-21 years old*. University of North London, London.

Parsons, T. (1964). *Social Structure and Personality*. The Free Press of Glencoe, London.

Pervin, L.A. and John, O.P. (1997). *Personality: Theory and Research*. John Wiley & Sons, Inc., New York.

Sandler, J. (1988). Psychoanalytic technique and "Analysis terminable and interminable". *International Journal of Psychoanalysis*, 69, 335-345.

Wollheim, R. (1985). *Freud*. Fontana Press, London.

— —. *Standard Edition of the Complete Psychological Work of Sigmund Freud*. Vol. XXI.

7
Psychopathology II
Medical Model

Axiomatically, disorders and diseases arise from malfunctioning of mind. *Bhagawad Gita* said: *manah sasti indriyani* (mind is the six sense organ); and, *Upanishad* described etiopathology in one *sutra: manahi eva manushyanam, karanam bandh-mokshabhyoho* (mind alone is the cause of bondage and liberation for human beings). Tibetan Buddhism postulated the mind as a mirror that constantly reflects, and yet, it tends to gather dust all the while.

Thus mind is an instrument through which we perceive the world; primary aim being survival. The world is an ever-changing environment demanding abilities of reacting and defending. This may need changing the inner or outer surroundings, for survival. The basic instinct of any living organism is to preserve itself. Hence, when an animal is confronted with a perceived dangerous situation – it reacts. The animal will use as many resources as needed, as much energy as possible, to deal with the threat. In the animal kingdom the rules of survival are simple—only the strongest survives. And what Charles Darwin postulated as the doctrine of survival of the fittest is seen covertly in human society too.

So far psychobiological model and medical model of pathogenesis work in parallel. However, medical model works on research in laboratories as well as clinical studies. Now, we shall follow the medical model that not only takes into account bodymind continuum, but also describes in detail as to how it is so. We shall have an overview of stressful situations, physical and psychological, that can derange the homeostasis to produce disorders and diseases. This is hard core science.

When faced with danger, main options are fighting (when the enemy is perceived as weaker, or when defending the cubs or herd) and running away or fleeing, (when encountering a fierce lion, for example). In the face of danger, the body changes its inner balance and priorities into a high physiological arousal, to enable these two functions – fight or flight. In human beings it is not so simple as in animals. Various psycho-social, cultural, religious, economic and several other factors can present themselves as a threat or stress. Yet we have much to learn about the coping strategies in this respect. But the basic response to such dangerous situations remains the same—fight or flight "F or F" response.

Interestingly, we all need stress in order to excel. Teams need stress in order to perform well, and in the right doses, stress can be very healthy, or even enjoyable. Such stress is known as good stress or eustress. However, when stress becomes excessive it can be very damaging. It can harm health, happiness, work performance, team spirit, co-operation, relationships and personal development. Such stress is termed as bad stress or distress.

Stress is how one reacts to pressures: it is subjective. We can learn to keep the pressures and get rid of the stress. We can learn to change anxiety to concern. We can learn to change distress to eustress.

Hans Selye[1], in 1936, as a medical student in Montreal, Canada saw that there were a host of signs and symptoms common to several ailments. Based on this observation, he conceptualized that these features were in the form of response by the body to the unusual demands made upon it so that it can maintain homeostasis. He introduced the phrase—Fight or Flight (F or F) response to stress. He also called it General Adaptation Syndrome. The agent that induced stress, he called as stressor. Selye was to eventually devote his entire life to the study of stress: till, (it is said) that he died in 1976 out of stress arising out of income tax matters!

Stress is a physiological response whose purpose is to mobilize reserves of the body. This recruitment is mediated through different mechanisms including stress hormones: thus it is the wear and tear our bodies experiences as we adjust to our continually changing environment: Stress is an individual's physical and mental reaction to environmental demands or pressures. Summarizing, stress is any disturbance that triggers stress response in human body!

The factors that contribute to the experience of stress—stressors—are many and varied. They can be broadly categorized into biological, social, cultural, psychodynamic (inner conflict), rational, experiential and spiritual.

Stress Response

Walter Canon first demonstrated elevated plasma catecholamines (CA) in cats exposed to barking dogs and identified the sources as sympathetic nervous system (SNS) and adrenal medulla—Sympathoadrenalmedullary (SA) System. He suggested that the role of CA (peripheral) was to redistribute blood flow and reorient metabolism towards production of glucose and free fatty acids etc. which provide energy for musculature to enable F or F response. Later Hans Selye demonstrated the importance of adrenal cortex and secretion of glucocorticoids (GC) in stress. The secretion of GC is the final stage in activation of hypothalamic—pituitary—adrenocortical (HPA) axis. This is stress axis.

The axis is initiated by secretion of corticotrophin releasing hormone (CRH) from hypothalamic neurons, mainly paraventricular neurones (PVN), with terminals in median eminence. This region of hypothalamus in turn receives afferent connections from limbic system and lower brain stem. CRH is transported by portal blood flow to anterior pituitary, which in turn secretes corticotrophin or adrenocorticotrophic hormone (ACTH). ACTH acts on adrenal cortex and causes secretion of GC (cortisol and/or corticosterone depending on species).

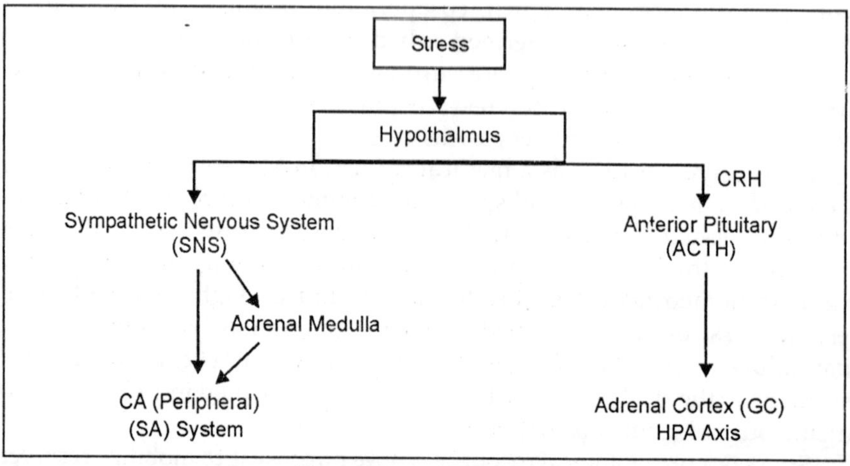

Fig. 7.1: Stress Response

As shown in Fig. 7.1, the manifestations of the F or F responses are mainly through two channels, nervous-sympathoadrenalmedullary (SA) system, a division of autonomic nervous system (ANS): and endocrine—HPA axis. The SA system affects many bodily functions instantly and directly, while hormones have slower yet wider effects on body. Both hormones and neurons communicate with cells and create the delicate balance between the body and its surrounding, through paired systems and feedback mechanisms.

Some of the effects of stimulation of SA system are:

- Increase in heart rate, cardiac output, blood pressure and respiration.
- Redistribution of blood flow—more to the muscles and heart, less to gut.
- Increase in blood glucose level as ready source of energy.
- Accelerating metabolic rate (increased BMR) for emergency actions.
- Thickening of blood—increased RBC to supply more oxygen, increase in WBC for better defense from infections and increase in platelets to stop bleeding quickly.
- Sharpening of senses and mental reactions.
- Secretion of endorphins—natural painkillers, providing an instant defense against pain.

All these actions prepare the organism to meet the emergency situation or challenge to fight or to flee. Virtually, the functions of all systems (e.g. the heart and blood vessels, the immune system, the lungs, the digestive system, the sensory organs, and brain) are modified to meet the perceived danger.

At times an individual can neither fight nor flee; he may just be full of fear. At such times, instead of 'F or F' response, there is withdrawal and conservation response. In such situations, there is increased susceptibility to illness/ infections. This can lead to organic disjunction or disease.

The stress response is part of larger physiological response known as the 'General Adaptation Syndrome' (GAS). GAS is comprised of three phases, which the body experiences in response to a stressor:

- Alarm
- Resistance
- Exhaustion

All phases are intended for short-term mechanisms of survival rather than long-term options. In the 'alarm' or 'fight/flight' phase, adrenaline and other related hormones are released in order to increase heart rate, blood and oxygen supply to the brain and muscles with reduced supply to digestive function. The 'resistance' phase releases hormones to sustain the body to fight the stressor and cope with emotional crisis, after the effects of the 'alarm' response have worn off. Prolonged exposure to these two stages can induce the third phase of 'exhaustion'. It is in this phase that the body is most run down, depleted and susceptible to disease. The body can cope a lot but under persistent stress will eventually fail, ironically due to those very physiological mechanisms that are designed to save it. And the continual release of stress related hormones could lead to enormous wear and tear on all the organs in the body.

So, short-term stress can be beneficial and lifesaving, however long term stress can have detrimental effects and lead to deterioration in health.

Role of Brain in Stress Response

Presently, other neurotransmitters as stress mediators are also identified. Besides the secretion of CRH by Paraventricular nucleus (PVN) of hypothalamic neurons, large numbers of other neurochemical changes are observed in brain during stress. The critical one is activation of cerebral catecholaminergic (CA) neurons. They include norepinephrinergic (NE), dopaminergic (DA) and adrenergic or epinephrinergic (Epi) properties. Other cerebral neurotransmitters like serotonin (5 HT), acetylcholine (Ach), gamma amino butyric acid (GABA) also appear to be released in stress (See Chapter 4). Release of these cerebral neurotransmitters can alter the activity of HPA axis. Many of these neurotransmitters act on structures in limbic system; which in turn is intimately connected with hypothalamus. *Limbic system could therefore be considered as a link through which stressors act on HPA axis.* Thus the stress axis can be better designated as limbic-hypothalamus-pituitary-adrenocortical (LHPA) axis.

It is possible that each type of stress stimulates specific region or neurons of brain, releases a specific neurotransmitter, which acts on different parts of limbic system, producing on one hand, a non-specific humoral response stimulating HPA axis and on the other hand a specific behavioural response for adaptation.

Cerebral CRH as a Central Coordinator of Stress Response

CRH secretion during the stress activates anterior pituitary coticotropin and increases the secretion of ACTH. Concomitant with ACTH, anterior pituitary also secretes b-lipotrophin (b LPH) and b-endorphins which provide negative feedback at multiple sites. CRH, ACTH and b-endorphin each have its own independent effects also. The figure shows schematic representation of role of brain in stress. It shows links between various stress mediators and responses.

CRH is found in neurons in many other brain regions, besides the PV hypothalamic neurons. *Intra cerebral administration of CRH* has widespread effects that resemble those observed during stress. These include endocrinal, electrophysiological, gastrointestinal, neurochemical and behavioural effects. Endocrinal effects are activation of HPA axis and SA system and inhibition of growth hormone (GH) and gonadotropin secretion. Electro physiological effects

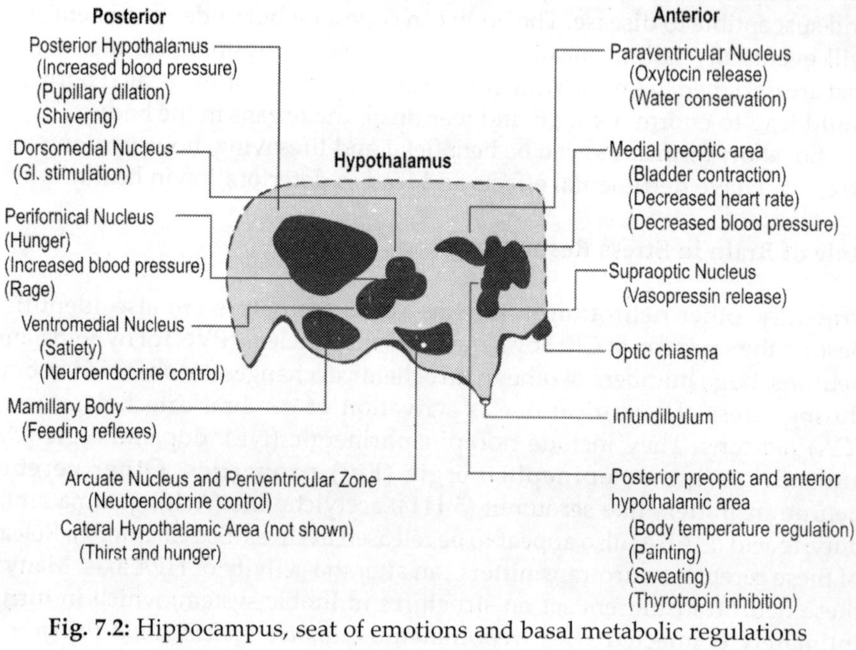

Fig. 7.2: Hippocampus, seat of emotions and basal metabolic regulations

include desynchronization of cortical EEG and activation of locus ceruleus NE neurons. In gastro intestinal tract complex changes in motility are seen. Thus, there is an important role of CRH in brain during stress. The role may be physiological, because blockers of CRH receptors prevent the normal responses to stress. Thus, cerebral CRH is suggested to be a central coordinator of response in stress.

Behavioural effects include anorexia, changes in locomotor activity, decreased sexual activity, anxiogenic effects on conflict behaviour and heightened response to treatments that normally induce anxiety or fear response.

Hippocampus and Stress

Repeated stress affects brain function, especially in the hippocampus, which has a high concentration of cortisol receptors. The hippocampus participates in verbal memory and is particularly important for the memory of 'context', the time and place of events that have a strong emotional bias. Moreover, glucocorticoids are involved in remembering the context in which an emotionally laden event took place.

Hippocampus regulates the stress response by inhibiting HPA axis. Many functional and structural changes are seen in the hippocampus during stress. These are reversible and short lived in acute stress but may be worse or permanent in chronic stress. Glucocorticoids (GC) may mediate these effects on the hippocampus. Persistent release of excitatory amino acid glutamate in hippocampus after stress may also be a contributing factor for neuronal damage – especially age related neuronal damage.

Stress in early life and neonatal handling influence the course of growth and age-related cognitive impairment. Early experiences are believed to set the level of responsiveness of the HPA axis and autonomic nervous system. These systems over react in animals subjected to early unpredictable stress and under react in animals exposed to good neonatal handling. In the former condition, aging of the brain is accelerated, whereas in the later, aging of the brain is reduced.

Amygdala and other related structures also play a role in stress.

The mediators of the stress have two modes of operation, fast and slow. Fast mode is driven by corticotrophin-releasing hormone (CRH) acting via CRHR-1 and produces the behavioural, sympathetic and hypothalamic-pituitary-adrenal (HPA) responses to a stressor. In the slow mode, urocortin (stresscopin) acts via CRHR-2 and facilitates behavioural adaptation. Current data suggest that MR controls the threshold or sensitivity of the fast CRHR-1 driven stress system mode and thus prevents disturbance of homeostasis, while GR facilitates its recovery by restraining, in these very same circuits stress responses and by mobilizing energy resources. It also prepares for future events by behavioural adaptation, storage of energy and metabolism.

Two modes of operation of Stress Mediators

> CRH-1 and 2 receptor (CRHR-1 and CRHR-2) systems drive the immediate (fast) response mode and late (slow) response mode respectively. MR determines the threshold or sensitivity of fast response. GR represents the slow adaptaive mode that terminates the fast response and that prepares for future through storage of energy and information.

Balance between the two is necessary for coping and adaptation.

Thus corticosteroid hormones secreted by the adrenal cortex are implicated in both modes—through their high affinity type 1 (mineralocorticoid receptors–MR) and lower affinity type 2 (Glucocorticoid receptors–GR) receptors that are co-localized in limbic neural circuitry. The balance in two stress system modes is thought to be essential for cell homeostasis, mental performance and health. Imbalance induced by the genetic modification or chronic stressors could change specific neural signaling pathways underlying psychic domains of cognition and emotion, anxiety and aggression. This *Yin-Yang* stress concept is fundamental for genomic strategies to understand mechanism of cortisol-induced stress-related disorders such as severe forms of depression and co-morbid diseases.

Protecting and Damaging Effects of Stress

At the onset of his discovery, 60 years ago, Selye recognized the paradox that the physiologic systems activated by stress do not only protect and restore, but also damage the body. Allostasis—the ability to achieve stability through change—is critical to survival. Through allostasis, the sympathetic nervous system (SNS), the hypothalamic-pituitary-adrenal (HPA) axis, and the cardiovascular, metabolic and immune systems protect the body by responding to internal and external stress. In contrast to homeostatic systems such as blood oxygen, blood pH, and body temperature which must be maintained within narrow ranges, allostatic (adaptive) systems have much broader boundaries. Allostatic systems enable us to respond to our physical states. (e.g. awake, asleep, supine, standing, exercising) and to cope with noise, crowding, isolation, hunger, extremes of temperature, dangers and microbial or parasitic infections. *Allostasis, therefore, is a protective mechanism by which body accommodates or adapts.* The price of this accommodation to stress can be allostatic load, which is the wear and tear that results from chronic over activity or under activity (maladaptation) of allostatic systems. *Allostatic load, therefore, constitutes the damaging effects of stress on the body.*

In both homeostasis as well as allostasis, hypothalamus plays a key role through the neuro-endocrine link.

Stress Response and Development of Allostatic Load

Stressful experiences include major life events, trauma, drug abuse and are salso related to the environment in the home, workplace, or neighbourhood. Acute stress (in the senses of 'fight or flight' or major life events) and chronic stress (the cumulative load of day to day stresses) can both have long-term consequences. The effects of chronic stress may be exacerbated by a rich diet and the use of tobacco and alcohol. They are reduced by moderate exercise.

Two factors largely determine individual responses to potentially stressful situations:

- The way a person perceives a situation
- Person's general state of physical health, which is determined not only by genetic factors but also by behavioural and lifestyle choices.

Whether one perceives a situation as a threat (either psychological or physical), vigilance or helplessness is crucial in determining the behavioural response—whether it is fleeing, fighting, or cowering in fear.

The core of the body's response to a challenge—whether it is a dangerous situation, an infection, living in a crowded and unpleasant neighbourhood or a public-speaking test—is two fold, turning on an allostatic response that initiates a complex adaptive pathway, and then shutting off this response when the threat is past. As discussed earlier, the most common allostatic responses involve the sympathetic nervous system (SNS) and the HPA axis. Activation of these systems cause release of catecholamine (CA) from sympathetic nerve endings and the adrenal medulla and secretion of corticotrophin (ACTH) from the anterior pituitary and cortisol from the adrenal cortex. Both catecholamine and glucocorticoids affect cellular events. Inactivation returns the systems to base-line levels of cortisol and catecholamine secretion, which normally happens when the danger is past, the infection is contained, the living environment is improved or the speech has been given. However, if the inactivation is insufficient there is overexposure to stress hormones. Over weeks, months, or years, exposure to increased levels of stress hormones can result in allostatic load and its patho-physiologic consequences.

They can be:

Individual differences influence perception of stress. Perceived stress leads to physiologic and behavioural responses, i.e. allostasis and adaptation.

Over a period of time, allostatic load accumulates. Such overexposure to stress mediators (neural, endocrine, immune) leads to adverse effect, i.e. disease.

Situations Associated with Allostatic Load

The first and most obvious is frequent stress (*repeated hits*). For example; surges in blood pressure can trigger myocardial infarction in susceptible persons. In primates repeated elevations of blood pressure over periods of weeks and months accelerate atherosclerosis, thereby increasing the risk of myocardial infarction.

In the second type of allostatic load, there is *lack of adaptation* to repeated stressors of the same type, resulting in prolonged exposure to stress hormones, as is the case of some of the people (10%) subjected to the repeated public speaking challenge, while majority of the people adapt to such repeated stresses in life.

In the third type of allostatic load there is inability to shut off allostatic responses after the stress is terminated (*prolonged response*). The blood pressure in some people fails to recover after the acute stress of an arithmetic test; and hypertension accelerates atherosclerosis. Women with a history of depressive illness have decreased bone mineral density, because the allostatic load of chronic, moderately elevated serum cortisol concentrations inhibits bone formation. Intense athletic training also induces allostatic load in the form of elevated sympathetic and HPA axis activity, which results in weight loss, amenorrhea and often related conditions like anorexia nervosa.

The failure to turn off the HPA axis and sympathetic activity efficiently after stress could be a feature of age related functional decline – the negative feedback effects of cortisol are reduced in elderly humans. A vulnerable link in the regulation of the HPA axis and cognition is the hippocampal region. According to the "glucocorticoid-cascade hypothesis" wear and tear on this region of the brain leads to dysregulation of the HPA axis and cognitive impairment.

In the fourth type of allostatic load, *inadequate responses* by some allostatic systems trigger compensatory increase in others. When one system does not respond adequately to a stressful stimulus, the activity of other systems increases, because the under active system is not providing the usual counter regulation. For example, if cortisol secretion does not increase in response to stress, secretion of inflammatory cytokines (which are counter regulated by cortisol) increases. The negative consequences of an enhanced inflammatory response are seen, for example, as high susceptibility to auto immune and inflammatory disturbances.

Factors affecting/contributing to allostatic load include, feeling of anticipation, worry, consumption of tobacco and alcohol, dietary choices and amount of exercise.

Anticipation participates in worry, anxiety and cognitive preparation for a threat. Anticipatory anxiety can drive the secretion of mediators like corticotrophin, cortisol and epinephrine and for this reason, prolonged anxiety and anticipation are likely to result in allostatic load. High Fat diet accelerates atherosclerosis and progression to non-insulin dependent diabetes by increasing cortisol secretion, leading to fat deposition and insulin resistance. Smoking elevates blood pressure and accelerates atherogenesis.

Stress and the Immune System

Links between psyche (behaviour), neuro-endocrine and immune systems are gradually unfolding. The result is a new branch of medicine—

psychoneuroimmunology—a relatively recent branch. The term was first introduced by Ader in 1980. Lot of work coming out since then clearly indicates scientific basis of interrelationship between psyche (behaviour), nervous, endocrine (neuro-endocrine) and immune systems—each affected by the other and in turn affects the other.

Glucocorticoids (GC) and Immune System

It is commonly said that stress impairs immune system—GC are known to suppress immune functions. The fact is significantly different and more complicated. Careful studies show that GC in normal physiological doses have noted stimulatory and permissive effects on immune system. Inhibitory effects occur at high (pharmacological) doses. Also, increase in GC level after acute stress does not last long. It rapidly returns to baseline (within 30 min) of cessation of stress. Further, there is an established immunologic "memory". If the immunologic memory is of a pathogen or tumor cell, the result of stress is presumably beneficial. If, on the contrary, the immunologic memory leads to an autoimmune response or allergic response, then stress is likely to exacerbate a pathologic state. Interpretation of experimental results also may be difficult because there may be direct as well as indirect effects of GC on immune system.

Catecholamines (CA) and Immune System

Experimental evidence suggests that catecholamines (CA) are intricately involved in immune system function. Some of these observations are:

CA in circulation may emanate from adrenal medulla (NE & Epi) and from sympathetic nerve terminals (NE). Sympathetic innervation has been clearly demonstrated in lymphoid organs like thymus, spleen and lymph nodes. Thus lymphocytes in thymus, spleen and lymph nodes may be directly exposed to these neuronal secretions.

Moreover, lymphocytes have both *alpha* and *beta* adrenergic receptors.

Interpretation of experimental data in vitro and in vivo has been difficult. Confounding factors contributing to complexity are manifold.

They are:

(i) compensatory increase in adrenal medullary CA after sympathectomy
(ii) redistribution of lymphocytes
(iii) compensatory changes in the number and kind of adrenergic receptors
(iv) coexistence in sympathetic terminals of various neuropeptides like vasoactive interstinal peptide (VIP), neuropeptide Y (NPY), substance P (SP), somatostatin etc.

Recent studies also suggest that CA released by SNS provide major mechanism by which the natural killer (NK) cell activity is regulated in vivo.

Other factors like CRH, ACTH, Endorphins, PRL etc. have also been shown to have effects on immune cells. Receptors for these are also found on immune cells. These neuropeptides and many others are also produced locally either by immune cell or by sympathetic nerve endings (coexistent with NE).

Immune System and Stress

Immune system in its turn also affects CNS—mainly through cytokines—interleukins 1 and 2 (IL-1, IL-2) and tumor necrosis factor a (TNFa). They activate HPA axis, thus, producing stress response. These cytokines can, therefore be labeled as immune messengers or immune transmitters. Activation of HPA axis by immune response indicates that immune system acts as sensory system. It signals brain to indicate the presence of a threat from external environment and triggers classical stress response.

HPA axis, in turn, provides the feed back mechanism *via* immune suppressive activity of GC. This inhibitory activity limits inflammatory responses and prevents immune system from over reacting, which may result in autoimmune problem.

Cytokines also have other varied effects on immune cells and on CNS. IL-1, 2 and 6, TNFα—all are pyrogenic. Fever is instrumental in fighting invading organisms. They are also behaviourally active. Some are sleep inducing (somnogenic), some decrease feeding, locomotor activity, exploratory activity and sexual activity. Sleep, hypomobility, anorexia, decreased libido may cause animal to hide and thus escape predators.

It may be that infections may cause breach in blood brain barrier, BBB, macrophages from periphery may invade and then proliferate in brain as microglia, which would synthesize IL-1. IL-1 acts as a potent growth factor for astroglia. It can cause astroglia proliferation, which then function to seal off the lesion and restore the damaged BBB. Thus IL-1 can have an important role of protection. But such episodes occurring repeatedly may be leading to Alzheimer's disease.

A variety of peptide hormones including CRH, vasoactive intestinal peptide (VIP), prolactin (PRL), somatostatin, ACTH, β-endorphin, β-lipotropin etc., also appear to be secreted by different immune cells and, immune cells also have receptors for these peptides. Thus, the terms neuropeptides, peptide hormones and immune peptides no more appear to be separate distinct entity. They appear to be released by, as well as act on, nervous, endocrine as well as immune system. Multiple sites of release, multiple effects of multiple peptides lead to multiple amplification loops that can act (stimulate or inhibit) on cascade of HPA and SA responses.

Mast Cells and Stress

Mast cells are present in all tissues of body, including brain. They are particularly active in atopic individuals (more prone to allergies). They are involved in allergic and anaphylactic reactions. Mast cells contain plethora of granules, with diverse actions. These include arachidonic acid products like prostaglandins, biogenic amines like histamine, chemo attractants, growth factors, neuropeptides, proteoglycans, proteolytic enzymes etc.

In brain, mainly in thalamus and hypothalamus, the mast cells are situated in close proximity with capillary endothelial cells and neuronal processes. Stimulation of brain mast cells leading to the release of their granules, could be by acute stress, nerve stimulation [by release of substance P (SP), nerve growth factors (NGF), opioids etc.], cytokines, hormones like ACTH and CRH, certain toxins, and viruses. Release of molecules like histamine and others can cause increased permeability and break down of blood-brain barrier (BBB). With this, other substances (could be cytokines also), are able to penetrate into brain and produce their effects. Other effects of molecules released from brain mast cells include direct effects on mood, anxiety etc. which are also some of the features associated with stress.

From discussion above, it is possible that acute stress activates mast cells not only in brain but elsewhere in the body also. This could be the basic of exacerbation of disease symptoms noted in some individuals associated with acute stress. Susceptibility of different tissue/organs of body may vary. Some of the examples of diseases that have connection are:

Mast cell degranulation in heart, leading to unstable angina & myocardial infarction:

- in intestine leading to irritable bowel syndrome;
- in bladder leading to interstitial cystitis; in skin leading to atopic dermatitis;
- in brain leading to migraine, multiple sclerosis and Alzheimer disease; and
- in lungs leading to asthma.

Pathways in Pathogenesis

The system of neuroendocrine regulation works this way. The peripheral components of the system are HPA axis, adrenomedullary sympathetic system and systemic sympathetic system. The central component is located in hypothalamus and brain stem which are connected with limbic system and cortex. Its main function is to maintain basal and stress related homeostasis. The system is responding to various signals or stimuli like neurosensory, circadian and blood borne signals through various information substances like TNF-α, IL-1, IL-6 etc. from various parts of body. It also responds to environmental stress including physical and emotional reactions.

Activation of this system heightens arousal, accelerates motor reflexes, improves attention and cognitive function, decreases appetite and sexual arousal and increases tolerance to pain. It also changes cardiovascular functions, metabolism and inhibits immune mediated inflammation.

CRH and noradrenergic neurons of central system innervates and stimulate each other. They are stimulated by serotonergic and cholinergic neurotransmitters and inhibited by GABA and POMC peptides which are responsible for analgesia that takes place in stress. CRH and AVP synergistically act on pituitary and secrete ACTH or corticotrophin. ACTH stimulates adrenal cortex to secrete glucocorticoids. Virtually all the components of immune response are inhibited by glucocorticoids like

1. Suppression of release of interferone, IL-1, 23 and 6, TNF-*alpha*, bradykinin, serotonin, histamin and enzymes such as collagenase and elastase.
2. Functions of subgroups of lymphocytes like Type 1 Helper T cells.
3. Damage to thymus and lymph tissues, reduced antibody production, poorer lymphocyte proliferation.

These responses help prevent over exuberant response of immune reactions which can become detrimental for person but on long term basis these can become the cause for development of immunological disorder like autoimmune diseases, cancer and AIDS.

Epinephrine and norepinephrine released by adrenal medulla and systemic sympathetic fibers affect immune reaction causing leukocytosis, lymphpenia and inhibition of natural-killer cell activity. The major immune organs like lymph nodes, thymus, spleen and intestinal Peyer's patches are supplied by autonomic nerve fibers. Lymphocytes also have adrenergic and cholinergic receptors on their surface.

Apart from these changes occur in response to stressful *stimuli* like decreased gonadotrophin and thyrotrophin secretion from pituitary in response to stress. This decreases secretion of releasing hormones from hypothalamus, causing decreased T3, T4 and sex hormones. Other hormones to be affected are prolactin and growth hormones. These changes in hormonal levels and subsequently altered milieu interior create different biochemical state for every stressor and *stimuli*.

This altered molecular biology is remembered by the system as state dependent memory and, by the brain as cortical engram. The immune system stores immunological memory too. These then become basis for development or progression of various diseases.

Immunoregulatory Effects of Hormones and Peptides

Many of the hormones secreted by HPA and respective target glands have immunoregulatory effects. The most convincing example is effects of glucocorticoids secreted by adrenal glands. Immune system is also affected by growth hormone and prolactin. Growth hormone deficient animals have thymic atrophy and are immune deficient and the effects can be reversed by supplementing growth hormone.

Prolactin through its receptors on lymphocytes stimulates the proliferation and secretion of cytokines. Estrogens increase the incidence of autoimmune disease in animals and humans. Substance P and substance K secreted by afferent sensory nerve terminals, stimulate immune cells to secrete inflammatory cytokines.

Hormones and Peptides found in Immune Competent Cells

Immune competent cells contain range of peptides, hormones and receptors associated with nervous or endocrine system. Lymphocytes contain POMC mRNA which codes for ACTH, endorphins and alpha-MSH. They also have receptors for various peptides, glucocorticoids and CRH. CRH is also secreted by monocytes. The secretion of neuropeptides and neurotransmitters by lymphocytes exert important paracrine and autocrine effects (Table 7.1).

Summarizing, two main recognition and defense systems of the body, neuroendorine and immune systems, speak the same language, that is, they can indeed talk back to brain and perhaps alter physiology and behaviour and *vice versa*.

Multiple effects of multiple molecules (stress mediators-hormones, neuropeptides, cytokines etc.—work as amplification loops at multiple sites and can enhance or inhibit the cascade of HPA and SA responses to stress. Both nervous and immune systems have memory—both can be conditioned—

Table 7.1: Immunoregulatory Effects of Hormones and Peptides

Hormone or Peptide	*Immune Function Affected*
Inhibitory	Lymphokine synthesis, inflammation
Glucocorticoids	Macrophage activation, synthesis of IgG and interferon-γ
Corticotropin	Activity of T-cells and natural killer cells
Chorionic gonadotropin	IgG synthesis, T-cell proliferation
α-Endorphin	T-cell proliferation, inflammatory cascade
somatostatin	T-cell proliferation and migration in Peyer's patches
vasoactive intestinal peptide	Fever, prostaglandin synthesis, secretion of interleukin-2
α-Melanccyte–stimulating hormone	
Stimulatory	
Estrogens	Lymphocyte proliferation and secretion
Growth hormone	Thymic growth, lymphocyte reactivity
Prolactin	Thymic activity, lymphocyte proliferation
Thyrotropin	IgG synthesis
β-Endorphin	Activity of T, B, and natural killer cells
Substance P	Proliferation T-cells and macrophages, inflammatory cascade
Corticotropin-releasing hormone	Lymphocyte and monocyte proliferation and activation

and can learn from previous adaptive experience or even unlearn the maladaptive behaviour.

This knowledge, far from complete yet, forms the basis of some of the methods commonly used for stress management. This also provides us further understanding of mind-body continuum and the scientific foundations of hypnotherapy.[2]

Post Script to Chapter 7: Psychopathology II

Derangement of psychobiological homeostasis from chronic stress, thus leads to a state of distress. This manifests in the form of a psychological disorder or psychosomatic disease. This is best illustrated by following case study.

We were teaching at a famous centre for treatment with Ayurveda. Most of the patients there had tried the ultimate with modern medicine and, having failed, they were at the centre, as a final destination. The chief asked us to visit a lady who was on ventilator support. She was a retired head of medical services in her State. Her diagnosis was Guillain-Barre syndrome. This is an autoimmune disease. The patients with low immunity are susceptible to the attacks of viral diseases. The patient with this syndrome suffer from a generalized paralysis of muscles all over the body and, when the respiratory muscles also get paralyzed, without ventilator support, the patient dies.

The psychodynamics were as follows:

> The lady was supported by her sister, a nonresident Indian, and a physician herself. The husband was away at work. His work was described as social work. The physician from USA plainly told us that three of them do not believe in hocus-pocus of hypnotherapy. They hardly believed in Ayurveda but, are there since the lady was not getting better with modern medicine.

Only through persistent subtle persuasion, the physician's sister from USA told more about the couple. The patient and her husband were idealist collegians in their youth. They paired up so us to serve the downtrodden. They became hardcore Marxists. The husband became a Party card- holder.

Their first shock came when they approached a general practitioner for getting fitness certificate for medical studies. The doctor charged them Rupees 5/each, issued a fitness certificate without even touching them!

During the medical studies they continued to be surprised and shocked by the callus and market oriented approach of most of the teachers. It was a sad realization that medical profession was not a noble profession, full of compassion and kindness but a market driven service industry.

After getting the medical degree, the husband took to the cause of farmers and landless labourers. He never practiced. Instead of a medical license, he got a license for gun. He would visit village after village, find out farmers who have been fleeced by money lenders. He would make the money lenders write

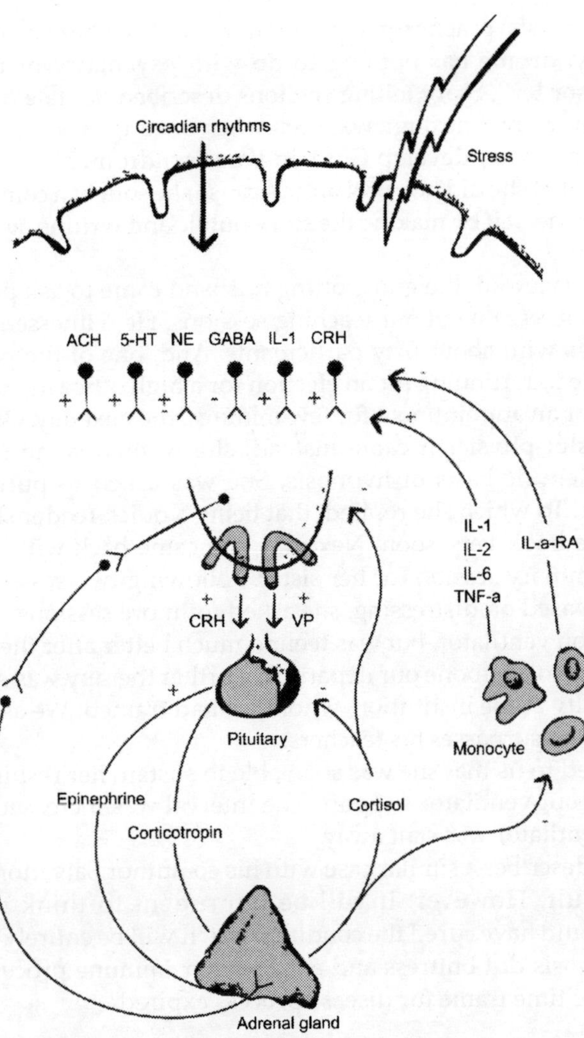

Fig. 7.3: Psychopathology II

of perpetual debt by putting, as an extreme threat, the barrel of his rifle on the temple of the lender.

The Guillain-Barre syndrome was the end result of struggle to bring about a revolutionary society since 30 years. Their commitment and devotion to their espoused cause was such that they had decided not to have any children. Whatever disjointedness that came about, in the process, was taken for granted.

The situation can be classically described as a couple of ants continuously donating the blood for the dear bleeding friend, the elephant.

The end result was that she landed with Guillain-Barre syndrome.

The therapy began with talking about science to the American sister; she had hardly known that there were over fifty thousand hypnotherapists (including psychiatrists) practicing hypnotherapy in USA. She exclaimed, "but Guillain-Barre syndrome has nothing to do with psychiatry or nor it is a psychological disorder". Story telling sessions described the tale of Candace Pert. A ray of hope, a breakthrough was seen when once again she asked, "Did Candace, you mean to say develop Guillain-Barre syndrome?"

We answered that she did not, probably because she sought a compensatory defense of the ego, herself by making the story public and writing, as a reward, a best-selling book.

After this interviewed, the gun-trotting husband came to ask permission whether he can witness one of our teaching sessions. He witnessed a session of group hypnosis with about fifty participants. And, one of the participant was, a high profile ladyrunning for an election for a high office in the country.

They asked for an appointment for few minutes, the next day. On that day the American sister-physician came instead; she wanted some references regarding the scientific basis of hypnosis. She was asked to purchase our inexpensive book. To which she replied, that being a quick reader she will be able to return the book very soon. Next day she came back with book and asked for a preliminary session for her sister. Following two sessions where the strategy was based on distressing, she asked for more sessions.

She was still on ventilator, but was feeling much better after the sessions. We were requested to postpone our departure. Further therapy was entrusted, to one of the faculty at the institution, whom we had trained. We assured the patient, that he even surpasses his teachers.

It was reported to us that she was soon able to sustain her respiration for few minutes without ventilator support. The interval was increased, so that, within a week, ventilator was sent away.

Ernest Rossi describes a similar case with his co-author Salvattore Ianotti with similar result. However, it will be imprudent to think that only hypnotherapy would have cured the condition but, it will be entirely scientific to state that hypnosis did buttress and enhance her immune process within such time that, the time frame for disease process expired.

List of abbreviations used

ACTH	Adreno-cortico trophic Hormone
ANS	Autonomic nervous system
BBB	Blood brain barrier
CA	Catecholamines
CRH	Corticotropin Releasing Hormone
CRHR	CRH receptor
DA	Dopamine
Epi.	Epinephrine
"For F"	Fight or Flight
GAS	General adaptation syndrome
GC	Glucocorticoids

GH	Growth hormone
GR	Glucocorticoid receptor
HPA	Hypothalamic-pituitary-adrenalcortical
LHPA	Limbic-hypothlamic-pitutary- adrenalcortical
IL	Interleukin
MR	Mineralocorticoid receptor
NE	Norepinephrine
NGF	Nerve growth factor
NK	Natural killer
NP Y	Neuropeptide Y
PRL	Prolactin
PVN	Para ventricular nucleus
SA	Sympathetic adrenal medullary
SNS	Sympathetic nervous system
SP	Substance P
TNF	Tumor necrosis factor
VIP	Vasoactive intestinal peptide

Note

1. In his heydays Selye has been compared to Einstein.

Bibliography

Akil, H and Morano, M., *Stress. American College of Neuropsychopharmocology: The Fourth Generation of Progress* (on line): http://www.acnp.org/G4/GN401000073/Nav.htm

Bruce, McEwen, Protective and damaging effects of stress mediators, *The New Eng J. Med.*, Vol. 338 (3) 171-179, 1998.

Ciirousos, G.P.: The Hypothalamus-Pituitary-Adrenal Axis and Immune Mediated Inflammation, *The New Eng. J. Med.* 332; 1331-1361, 1995.

David, De Wied and Pieter, A. *Van Keep: Hormones and Behaviour, in Hormones and the Brain*, 1980, pp. 103-205.

De Kloet, R.E., Hormones, Brain and Stress, *Endocr. Regul.*, Vol. 37 (2) 51-68, 2002.

Friedman, H., Psychoneuroimmunology, Stress and Infection, CRC Press, 1995.

Hans, Selye, *The Stress of Life*, New York, 1956.

——, *The Stress without Distress*, New York, 1974.

Lewis, C.E. *et al.*, Psychoneuroimmunology of cancer – Mind and body in fight for survival, 1994.

Morimoto, R, *Stress Induced Gene Expression*, available on line:

Reichlin, S., Neuroendocrine Immune Interactions, *The New Eng. J. Med.* 329; 1246-1252, 1993.

Rossi, E., *The Psychobiology of Mind body Healing*, New York, 1993.

Theoharides, T.C., Mast Cells and Stress A Psychoneuroimmunological Perspective, *J. Clin. Psychopharm.* Vol. 22 (2), pp. 103-108, 2002.

www.grc.uri.edu/progams/2001/stress.htm

8
Psychosomatic Diseases

Association of psychological factors and organic medical diseases has been firmly accepted during last three decades. It has been realized now that almost every medical illness on earth is influenced by psychological factors. PFAMC accounts for 30 per cent of outdoor illnesses and 50 per cent of indoor patients. This is so even when nonspecific psychophysiological symptoms like diaphoresis, palpitation, dyspepsia, diarrhoea, urinary frequency, vasovagal attack and other autonomically mediated symptoms are also not included amongst PFAMC as detailed below.

Psychological and behavioural factors affecting medical conditions[1]:

I. Psychophysiology
   (a) Physiological reactions to psychological and behavioural variables.
   (b) Biological regulatory mechanisms associated with behavioural and psychological variables:
      (i) Psychoneurophysiology
      (ii) Psychoneuroendocrinology
      (iii) Psychoneuroimmunology
      (iv) Psychocardiology.

II. Effects of concurrent psychiatric illness on the course and outcome of medical disorders.

III. Behavioural risk factors for disease and injury:
   (a) Personality variables
   (b) Cigarette smoking
   (c) Dietary habits
   (d) Alcohol and substance abuse
   (e) Hazardous sexual behaviour
   (f) Risk-taking behaviour (accidents, injury)
   (g) Noncompliance with medical treatment
   (h) Violence, suicide, homicide
   (i) Stressful or disruptive life change

Since, the relevance of psychological factors listed above is now well accepted, full diagnosis for labeling the composite illness has to be made as per guidance laid down below.

DSM-IV diagnostic criteria for psychological factors affecting general medical condition:[2]

I. A general medical condition (coded on Axis III) is present.
II. Psychological factors adversely affect the general medical condition in one of the following ways:
   A. The factors have influenced the course of the general medical condition as shown by a close temporal association between the psychological factors and the development or exacerbation of, or delayed recovery from, the general medical condition.
   B. The factors that interfere with the treatment of the general medical condition.
   C. The factors that constitute additional health risks for the individual.
   D. Stress-related physiological responses precipitate or exacerbate symptoms of the general medical condition.

Choose the name of diagnosis based on the nature of the physiological factors (if more than one factor is present, indicate the most prominent):

Mental disorder affecting general medical condition (e.g., Axis I disorder such as major depressive disorder delaying recovery from a myocardial infarction).

Psychological symptoms affecting general medical condition (e.g., depressive symptoms delaying recovery from surgery; anxiety exacerbating asthma).

Personality traits or coping style affecting general medical condition (e.g., pathological denial of need for surgery in a patient with cancer; hostile, pressured behaviour contributing to cardiovascular disease).

Maladaptive health behaviours affecting general medical condition (e.g., stress-related exacerbations of ulcer, hypertension, arrhythmia, or tension headache).

Other or unspecified psychological factors affecting general medical condition (e.g., interpersonal, cultural, or religious factors).

Illnesses included as PFAMC

Somatization disorders, conversion disorders, hypochondriasis, dysmorphic psychiatric illness and substance abuse diseases, are solely based in psyche. So they are not considered as PFAMC.

List covers only common illnesses:

(1) Gastrointestinal diseases:
- Esophageal motility disorders
- Peptic Ulcer
- Irritable Bowel Diseases
- Crohn's Disease
- Ulcerative Colitis

(2) Cardiovascular diseases:
- Hypertension
- Coronary Heart Disease
- Arrhythmia

(3) Pulmonary Diseases:
- Asthma
- Hyperventilation Syndrome

(4) Endocrine Diseases:
- Diabetes Mellitus
- Hyperthyroidism

(5) Rheumatological Diseases:
- Rheumatoid Arthritis
- Fibromyalgia

(6) Skin Diseases:
- Atopic Dermatitis
- Chronic Urticaria
- Soriasis
- Pruritis ani and vulva

(7) Neurological Diseases:
- Migraine
- Headache

(8) Malignancy

(9) Patient on Hemodialysis

For each one of these, association of various types of psychological abnormalities as a predisposing cause is identified. (Examples: suppression of anger with hypertension; type—A personality with ischemic heart disease) However, data derived in these studies are based on retrospective analysis and have no full-proof scientific evidences. However, this does not contradict the basic fact that psychological factors do play a major role in initiation, length of illness, prognosis of diseases, length of hospital stay and cost of illness in case of PFAMC.

PFAMC arises because of several factors:

(A) ***Psychological factors:*** *Stress*: Acute or Chronic or sustained. There is enough evidence to prove that both acute and chronic stress cause tremendous pathological changes in the body and play important roles in organ damage: either in initiation or perpetuation.

Depression: Superficial or deep

— Anger
— Guilt
— Denial
— Dependency
— Repression or for that matter, failure of ego defenses of all varieties.

(B) Psychiatric diseases
(C) Personality traits
(D) Behavioural causes
(E) Environmental and social causes
(F) Genetic susceptibility and organ sensitivity

Behavioural causes

(1) smoking, alcohol and drug abuse
(2) obesity and overeating
(3) unsafe sex
(4) noncompliance with medical advice

Genetic susceptibility: it is found that PFAMC is common in other family members. Even organ specificity has been suggested like stomach illness and cardiovascular-proneness, etc.

Management of PFAMC

It may be unwise for a hypnotherapist, not having medical training to deal alone with these conditions. A primary physician or a psychiatrist may be associated with. Hypnotherapy is then offered in tandem.

(1) *Role of Primary Physician*: If patient-physician relations are good, either because of long-standing association or a fortunate happening of compatibility, the primary physician can treat not only the medical condition but also use his common-sense and general medical skills to deal with psychological factors and also steer his patient toward altering his behavioural problems. For 30 per cent of PFAMC, this has been found to be successful. If a physician assesses that psychological factors are daunting and deep, he should have no hesitation in not only referring the patient to psychiatrist (if not at the first visit then at a subsequent visit) and also convince the patient to go to a psychiatrist. The primary physician should also be aware of the fact that some drugs given for medical illnesses can also cause psychiatric symptoms. He should also be aware of drug interactions between drugs prescribed by him and drugs prescribed by psychiatrists.

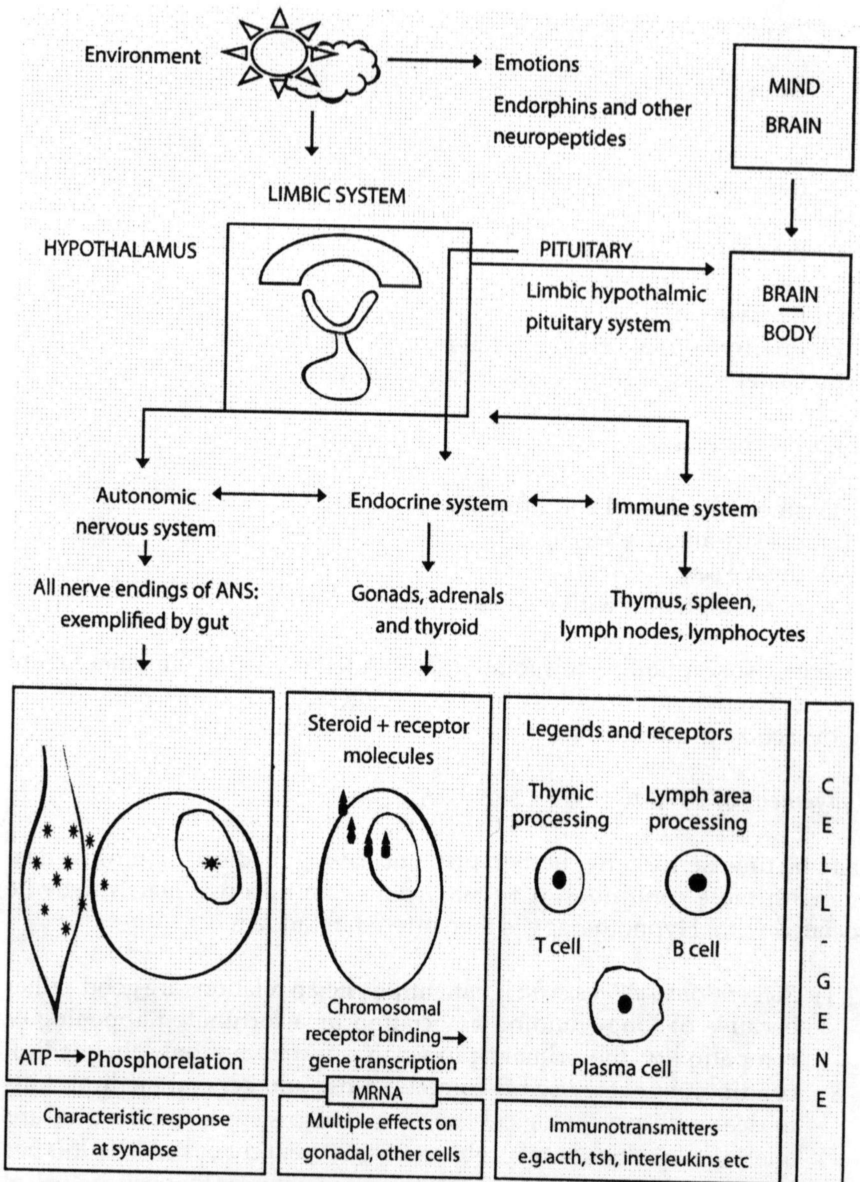

Fig. 8.1: Cybernatics Feedback to Limbic – Hypothalamic - Pituitary Axis

(2) *Role of Psychiatrist*: Many methods have been suggested for psychiatrists to treat PFAMC and none of them seems to be fully effective. Psychiatrists are likely to find them time-consuming. This is a situation where hypnotherapist may well fit in.

The various methods for treating these patients are:

(a) Psychopharmacology
(b) Psychotherapy
(c) Cognitive therapy
(d) Biofeedback methods
(e) Relaxation techniques, meditation and yoga
(f) Hypnosis

However, one must be aware that these methods will not always have long-lasting effects on a patient's lifestyle and so recurrence of PFAMC is highly likely.

Notes

1. Stoudemire, A., Hales, R.E., "Psychological and Behavioural Factors Affecting Medical Conditions and DSM-IV: An Overview." *Psychosomatics,* 32: 5-13, 1991.
2. *American Psychiatric Press Textbook of Psychiatry.*

9
Genetic Basis of Psychobiology, Psychotherapy, Hypnotherapy

In 1953, one morning James Watson went early to his laboratory and as he was clearing the mess on his table, it suddenly struck him. Yes, it was to be a double helix! (Chapters on Creative Process). He quickly went about arranging his data in a state of elation and in the same evening, along with his collaborator, Francis Crick, mounted on a table in a pub-to announce the discovery to the world. The same was published in Nature immediately thereafter.[1] Prof. Hargobind Khurana did not find a suitable job in India on his return from USA. That was good fortune so that he went back to USA. There he was to win the Nobel Prize[2] for discovering the genetic code in 1966. A little less than 50 years after Watson and Crick's revolutionary finding, two separate teams of geneticists across the Atlantic decoded the entire genome of the human species. We seem to know the function of almost all the genes as well as their precise location now. It may be the colour of our iris, or the finely tuned manufacture of complex enzymes, or the gross behaviour, the genes dictate what we are.

At this point of time, the fact has raised existential questions regarding ontology. Are we predetermined to be and act in the way that we do? If genes are the determinants, is there any place for free will? There is a definite yes for the free will, as long as we decide what to think and feel. What we think and feel influences our genes. And there seems to be a better way to influence our genes through the altered state of consciousness—hypnosis. Let us see how.

Basic Facts about Chromosomes and Genes

Body, cells and genes follow all laws of physics and chemistry without exception.[3,4] So our thoughts and emotions must have actual physical (electromagnetic) and chemical basis in the brain. They are created as physical events—as molecular biological chain events and though they seem to be abstract, they have tale tell fingerprints in brain.

Genes that a child has inherited have already created platform to land this knowledge. Genes rapidly recreate intellect that is accumulated over generations. And the information that genes carry has been preserved and passed on, not only through the generations, but, across the entire path of evolution.[5]

Our experience and emotional involvement in an event can activate neurogenesis-new set of neuronal interaction throughout our lifetime. This happens with turning on genes to modulate response, growth developments and healing. This can be recalled and reframed by modifying and reconstructing at genomic molecular level through our brain with the inputs of emotions and thoughts that are specifically directed. Rossi[6] saw new approaches to stress, psychotherapy and healing arts with the use of hypnosis. If the nature creates us to be what we are, it is thus that we co-create ourselves.

Proteins are structural, functional and regulatory units of the cells of the body, tissues and organs and usually they perform a unique function. Enzyme, hormones and antibodies are all proteins. It was thought that each gene encodes for one protein only (RNA–ribonucleic acid). With post transcription editing, now it is known that one gene can code for several proteins. Genes thus form a template for the production of proteins. That protein then, through its product, by feedback loop signals gene again.

Gene is deoxyribonucleic acid (DNA). It is a part of chromosome that is involved in expression of a single protein. DNA is the borderline between living and nonliving. This is so because DNA can replicate itself. With advancement in understanding of the functioning of DNA molecule, variations in the definition of gene have come about. But said in simple terms, a gene is a DNA sequence that codes for functional RNA chains. Some of the functional characteristics of genes are:

- Genes are mutable units. Somatic genes after damage or error in replication can change and produce altered protein.
- Genetic diversity of Homo sapiens is determined by polymorphism, mutations, and recombination of genetic material during cell division and epigenetic events.
- Genotype is inherent gene structure. Phenotype is physical expression of gene often modified by epigenetic events caused by environment.
- The genes accomplish task by sequential expression and turn off. But some genes like the housekeeping genes are always on.[7]

Gene Classification as per Function

Genes are classified according to the function. Their time of expression is also variable as a group. From table 9.1, we see immediate relevance to hypnotherapy. In order to do so, we shall first understand gene expression.

Gene Expression

Not all genes are active all the times. Housekeeping genes are working most of the time but other genes spring into activity as per the specific demand of the environment that is perceived through the brain. And accordingly, they cease their activity too. This particular aspect is of paramount importance since that has relevance to creativity in hypnotherapy. This we shall see a little later. First let us understand gene expression.

Table 9.1: Gene Expression

Gene family	*Time of expression*	*Major function*
1. Housekeeping genes	Daily, almost all times	Metabolism
2. Clock genes	Circadian	Synchronization with day and night cycle
3. Immediate Early genes	Seconds, minutes	Psychobiology and extended realms of Body-mind
4. Activity-Dependent	Minutes to hours	Memory and learning
5. Behavioural state related	Hours	Wake, sleep, dream and mood
6. Intermediate and early active	1-2 hours	Immune
7. Late activated	4-8 hours	Response to environment

A particular molecular biological event targets a particular gene. In response to it, double strand DNA unwinds. Now, the actual process of new protein synthesis starts. A multifunctional enzyme, DNA polymerase, then creates a template called messenger RNA–mRNA.

Gene Transcription and Gene Translation

Since mRNA is a template, it carries all the information that the original DNA sequence in the gene has; except that it is not able to replicate itself. What has now come about is that a master copy of the genetic DNA is made out. This process is called gene transcription. After some modification, m-RNA enters cytoplasm from nucleus and binds to ribosome in endoplasmic reticulum. Ribosome can be compared to a printer head and several copies are made by printing from it. That way, the ribosome, now bound to mRNA, using transfer RNA-tRNA-translates the message given by DNA and assembles amino acids in m-RNA specified sequence to produce peptide. This process is called gene translation.

Central Paradigm of Gene Activation

- Proteins are building blocks of body. They are parts of enzymes also. Proteins consist of chain of amino acids. Body plays with 20 amino acids. By phosphorylation proteins can be activated. Proteins are extremely versatile. Methylation, acetylation and glycosylation can change the activity of proteins.

- Amino acids are obtained from digested food. Body can manufacture some amino acids but some essential amino acid must come from food and such amino acids are called essential amino acids. Every protein has specific sequence of amino acids.
- Chromosome is a coiled chain of polymer of deoxynucleic acid –DNA-packed in double helix form for compactness within nucleus of cell.
- Four nucleotides, namely adenine, thiamine, guanine and cytosine in varying sequence make different genes and in so doing will encode information. It may be said that ATGC make alphabets of genomic information.
- DNA is polymer of four nucleotides paired as AT and GC arranged on sugar phosphate backbone. DNA has double strands except in sex chromosomes. So each gene has two copies. Like a rope, two strands are coiled as double helix. Only one strand is used for transcription.
- Codon is trinucleotide sequence e.g., ATG, CTG GGA etc. that code for each amino acid, to start translation and stop translation. Possibly 64 combinations write up entire instruction.
- Messenger RNA acts as template. It is transcribed from one strand of chromosome and nucleotide sequence is complementary. A-T and G-C are complementary pairs. Messenger RNA is further processed with removal of unnecessary genetic material and tail is added.
- Francis Crick, soon after the discovery of double helix, in 1956, defined this pathway for the flow of genetic information and labeled it as central dogma. He stated it simply as: Duplication DNA > transcription > RNA > protein.
- Thus, a gene produces a specific protein. The protein after attending its function, directly or indirectly through cell receptor and signal transduction, influences expression of that gene in a cybernetic loop. This is a feed back mechanism. Sequential expression and deexpression of gene accomplish a particular task in controlled fashion.
- House keeping genes are under negative control and, are expressed all the time unless switched off by repressor protein. Genes under positive control are expressed only if activated.

Immediate Early Genes (IEGs)

About 100 immediate early genes (IEGs) are known by now. They do not require a full cycle of new protein formation to bring about the effects of their expression. Therefore, they have particular relevance to psychodynamic interplay. The functions of IEGs are almost of a nature of fantasy. Their role needs to be further explored in relation to altered states of consciousness. Coming into play in a very short time, varying from few seconds to a couple of minutes, they further cause the expression of immediate activated genes. Even an empathetic touch can promote healing through the activation of IEGs. This becomes obvious when we see the functions of IEGs like *c-fos, jun-4, c-myc* and *max*.[8] They are most likely to yield fertile results when explored during the altered states of consciousness.[9, 10] The test is simple as it is done on a sample of DNA from leucocytes in the blood. However, it is not easily available and is expensive.[11] The gene expression is not ubiquitous; that is a valid objection. So, it may not express in all the cells of the body at a given time and, could be tissue specific. That makes the research sophisticated.

Relevance to Hypnotherapy

All that happens in the body has to be in accordance with the natural laws. DNA, the interface between the living and non-living, in all its "plays" must also confirm with these laws and, we have the evidence that it does.

Altered states of consciousness are different expression of behaviour. A different pattern of brain functioning is evident on fMRI of the subjects under hypnosis.[12] Genes dictate our behaviour. So, there must be a differential expression of genes for the different states of consciousness. We know that IEGs are concerned with the state of arousal. Similarly, it is established that there is gene regulation of sleep and dream states.[13] So, there must be differential gene expression of a different state of consciousness that hypnosis is. That it is indeed so is being proved by empirical research on meditative states.[14]

A single cycle of gene expression takes about 90-120 minutes. The therapeutic sessions by Milton Erickson lasted for a similar duration.[15] Apart from several distinguishing features of his therapeutic strategy, this time duration may as well be the important factors.

Most psychotherapists programme their session for a duration of 20 minutes. This is the time needed for the expression of intermediate activated genes. That would mean that in a session of this duration, the behaviour modification is further carried out by the effects of activity dependent, behaviour state related, intermediate activated genes. They may be causing expression of late activated genes that may last indefinitely.

Rossi[16] considers each session of hypnotherapy a creative process. The process is initiated by IEGs and is taken over by intermediate acting genes that relay it to the late activated genes and, so on. The process may carry on from several hours to indefinite time, Rossi charts the process as per the circadian cycle that may last from 90-120 minutes. The chart is reproduced elsewhere.

There is as of yet no direct study as to how hypnosis may influence proteome; however, if it were to influence gene expression, it surely will influence proteomes. Of course, genes dictate the synthesis of proteins and so, it stands to reason that there would be the way that the genes regulate proteome too. In fact, this may provide an easier and less expensive way.

Say, instead of studying the expression of melatonin regulating genes (2 in numbers), it is easy to estimate the levels of melatonin in blood.

Emergence of the (w)Holisitc Paradigm, Psyche, Brain, Systems in the Body, Cells and Genes.

Des Cartis is blamed for introducing a separate, dualistic mind and body paradigm. It is now time to give him credit for his axiomatic assertion, "I think, therefore, I am (this body)." The circle is turning full, not with philosophical speculation but by the advances in the scientific understanding so, that, the mind and matter are seen to be the same stuff.

We saw the convergence of psyche and soma with the enunciation of general adaptation syndrome by Hans Selye.[17] Discovery of various hormones that have obvious psychological effects buttressed the mind-body linkage. Forty years after Selye, when Candace Pert[18, 19] discovered endorphins and, subsequent discovery of several information substances (See earlier Chapters) being secreted by the brain, hardly any further proof was needed for her to proclaim that there is but one entity; i.e. *bodymind*.

However, still a major question remains to be answered. The behaviour is genetically determined. The genetic inheritance cannot be changed. So, how can psychotherapy modulate behaviour?

Consciousness, Brain Plasticity and Neurogenesis

It is platitude to say that neurons do not regenerate nor do they multiply. However, their synaptic connections do grow and multiply[20] in response to genetic expression of behaviour state related genes, as well as late activated genes. It also provides a clue that how we can create ourselves a new as per the programme that we desire. This explains how fresh learning can generate psycho-cybernetic replays that delays the ageing. That also explains how hypnotherapy works. To quote, Eric Kandel,[21] (Nobel Laureate 2000):

It presumably does so by producing changes in gene expression, that alters the strength of synaptic connections and structural changes that alters the anatomical pattern of interconnections between nerve cells of the brain.

With the advances in molecular biology, Rossi and Cheek[22] hypothesized a psyche-gene connection in 1983. It was documented in their classic book, Mind-Body Therapy. Further research was needed over the next 15 years to convert their philosophical vision into a probability. How does an order by the brain in terms of an idea to requite a particular behaviour? It undergoes transduction into molecular biological events of intricate subtlety and, return is granted in the form of explicit behaviour (ideodynamic transformation). We can hypothecate how is the genetic play for the same brought about. Let us see this most fascinating evolution of the (w)holistic scientific paradigm step by step.

The milestones of the research in this area have been as follows:

- Carew *et al.* (1983),[23] Hawkins *et al.* (1983)[24] and Walters and Byrne[25] described the information transduction within cells as activity dependent neuromodulation. This was brought about by secondary messenger systems such as camp, Ca^{++} and diacylglycerol.

- Kandel[26] in 1983 in a seminal work, described the passage from metapsychology to molecular biology.
- Rossi, independently of his own, in 1983, 1985 and 1986,[27] hypothesized mind gene connection and postulated that as molecular basis of therapeutic hypnosis. This was indeed a giant leap forward based on logical positivism. It still needed to be buttressed by empirical evidence.
- Glaser *et al.*,[28, 29] deriving from the experimental results, documented the path of information transduction in 1990 as: primary messengers from neuroendocrine system → trigger cell receptors → initiate a cascade of secondary messengers → mediation of gene transcription → mRNA production → protein synthesis and other information substances that act on their specific receptors.
- During the concluding decade of the last millennium, there have been a torrential cascade of path breaking research. There have been Nobel[30] prize winning contributions. Rather than cataloging them here, reference is made to the monograms.[31, 32, 33, 34, 35]
- Nobel prize for physiology and medicine 2004 narrows the gap between the genetic arousal and sense perception as well as memory of an experience. Richard Axel and Linda Buck have explained how people can smell a lilac flower on one fine spring morning and recall the smell years later.
- They discovered that about 1000 genes were responsible for this. The genes give rise to a huge variety of proteins in the cells of the nasal mucosa that are responsible for a particular smell to be sensed by the brain.

And with this latest pointer, it is difficult not to narrate a spectacular case out of the few cases of anosmia that we have successfully treated. In brief, the story is:

A professional lady, aged about 40, with two children was brought for therapy as she had lost the sense of small since past seven years. She was teaching biochemistry at a college. The loss occurred around the time that she was working towards her Ph.D. and was a severe professional handicap.

In history taking it was soon evident that the period around her Ph.D. work was highly stressful with the demands of the teaching job, care of the young children as well as running the house. In giving up her sense of smell, she has "genetically engineered" a coping mechanism to off load some thing special.

After putting her in deep trance, she was age regressed to the period prior to the stress times. By eliciting the ideomotor signaling, it was confirmed that now she was at a period when her sense of smell was intact, by making her "sense the smell" of some of the common aromatic compounds she worked with as well as the smell of flowers of her choice. She was then age progressed to the present time, but with selective ablation of the stressful time.

Following the session, when she reached her sister's home, she suddenly told her, Oh I never knew you had *parijat*[36] in your garden!

This lady was followed after a lapse of three years. She has now retained the sense of pungent odors: fine smell is lost.

Notes

1. Watson and Creek, Molecular Structure of Nucleic Acids, A Structure for Deoxyribose Nucleic Acid, *Nature*, 737-38, 1953.
2. Weeber, E.J., Levenson, J.M., Sweatt, J.D., Molecular Genetics of Human Cognition, *Mol. Interv.* 339; 36-91, 2002.
3. Watson, J.D., Hopkins, Roberts, Steitz and Weiner, *Molecular Biology of Gene*, Fifth Edition, Menlo Park, 1996.
4. Guyton, A.C. and Hall, J.E. *Textbook of Medical Physiology*, 1996, pp. 27-39.
5. Ernest Lawrence Rossi, Bhaskar Vyas, and Kathryn Lane Rossi *et al.* What Makes Us Human? A Neuroscience Prolegomenon for the Philosophy of Evolution and Consciousness http://network.nature.com/groups/transcience/forum/topics/5202; creating consciousness-chapter three
6. Rossi, E.L. *The Psychobiology of Gene Expression*, London, 2000.
7. *The Science Behind the Human Genome Project*-Web pages that define some basic genetics concepts and explain how the Human Genome Project was implemented. Defines chromosomes; genome and proteome.
8. Rossi, 2002, *Psychobiology of Gene Expression*, New York, pp. 11-22, 2002.
9. Now DNA microarrays are available. Several thousand molecules of different sequences are put on a simple slide and they are matched against those present in the leucocytes in the blood/cells in the tissues. A reaction like the one between the information substance like a hormone and receptor accrues. This identifies the gene that is being expressed.
10. Ever since Ernest Rossi personally told this to the editors, we plan our therapeutic sessions for 90 minutes; at least the first one. The reinforcement is through listening to a recorded cassette, daily. This is further enhanced by weekly follow up sessions till the lasting therapeutic change is brought about.
11. David Atkinson, Salvatore Iannotti, Mauro Cozzolino, Stefano Castiglione, Angela Cicatelli, Bhaskar Vyas *et al.* A New Bioinformatics Paradigm for the Theory, Research, and Practice of Therapeutic Hypnosis; *American Journal of Clinical Hypnosis* 50:2, October 2007.
12. Amir Raz, Melissa Lamar, Jason T. Buhle, Michael J. Kane, Bradley S. Peterson, Selective biasing of a specific bistable-figure percept involves fMRI signal changes in frontostriatal circuits: A step toward unlocking the neural correlates of top-down control and self-regulation; *American Journal of Clinical Hypnosis*, Volume 50, Issue 2, 2007.
13. Rebeiro, S., Goyal V., Mello C., and Pavlidas, C., Brain gene expression during REM sleep...Learning and Memory, 6; 500-08, 1999.
14. Jeffery A. Dusek, Hasan H. Otu, Ann L. Wohlhueter, Manoj Bhasin, Luiz F. Zerbini, Marie G. Joseph, Herbert Benson, Towia A. Libermann: Genomic Counter-Stress Changes Induced by the Relaxation Response, On line Plus One.

15. Ever since Ernest Rossi personally told this to the editors, we plan our therapeutic sessions for 90 minutes; at least the first one. The reinforcement is through listening to a recorded cassette, daily. This is further enhanced by weekly follow up sessions till the lasting therapeutic change is brought about.
16. In this fertile ground for Nobel hunting, there are a few sad stories about the mean of the nobles. It is particularly sad from the feminist point of view since the victims were women. One such story is that of Crick and Rosalind Franklin. Crick utilized the crystallography methods of Rosalind even without acknowledgment; the more famous is one about Candace Pert and her professor and guide, Sol and other two, Hughes and Kosterlitz. Last three shared the Nobel prize to the exclusion of Pert (*see* pp. 101-02, ref.vi).
17. Hans Selye, *The Stress of Life*, London and New York, 1956.
18. Pert Candace, The Wisdom of the Receptors: Neuropeptides, the Emotions and Bodymind, Advances Vol. III, No. 3: Summer 1986.
19. Candace Pert, Molecules of Emotions, Why You Feel the Way You Feel, London, 1997.
20. Lusher, C., Nicoli, B., Malenca C., and Muller B., Synaptic plasticity and dynamic modulation of the postsynaptic membrane. *Nature Neuroscience*, 3; 545-67, 2000.
21. Eric Kandel A new intellectual framework for psychiatry? *Amer.J. Psychiatry*, 155; 457-469, 1998.
22. Rossi, E.L. and David B.Cheek, *Mind-Body Therapy, Ideodynamic Healing in Hypnosis*, 1988.
23. Carew, Hawkins and Kandel (1983) *Science*, 219; 397-400.
24. Hawkins, R. Abrams T. Carew T. and Kandal E. *Science*, 219,300-405; 1983.
25. Walters, E. and Byrne *J. Science*, 219; 405-408, 1983.
26. Kandel, E. From metapsychology to molecular biology: exploration into the nature of anxiety. *American Journal of Psychiatry*, 140; 1277-1293.
27. Rossi, E.L. and David B. Cheek, *Mind-Body Therapy, Idcodynamic Healing in Hypnosis*, London, 1988, pp. 55-60.
28. Glaser, R., Kennedy S., Lafuse W., *et al*. Psychological stress induced modulation of interleukin 2 receptor gene expression and interleukin 2 production in peripheral blood leucocytes. *Arch. Gen. Psychiatry*, 4; 707-712.
29. Glaser, R. *et al*. Stress associated modulation of proto onco gene expression in human peripheral blood leucocytes. *Behav. Neurosci*. 107; 525-529.
30. In this fertile ground for Nobel hunting, there are a few sad stories about the mean of the nobles. It is particularly sad from the feminist point of view since the victims were women. One such story is that of Crick and Rosalind Franklin. Crick utilized the crystallography methods of Rosalind even without acknowledgment; the more famous is one about Candace Pert and her professor and guide, Sol and other two, Hughes and Kosterlitz. Last three shared the Nobel prize to the exclusion of Pert.
31. Brown, P. *Genomes*, New York, 1999.
32. Tolle, T.R. *et al. Immediate Early Genes in CNS*, New York, 1995.
33. Fernandes, J. and Hoefler J. *Gene Expression Systems*, New York, 1999.
34. Lydic, R. Molecular Regulation of Arousal States, Boca Raton, 1998.
35. Ridley, M. Genome, The Autobiography of a Species in 23 Chapters, New York, 1999.
36. A flower occurring in India with delicate fragrance.

10

Psychology: Indian Perspective

The Master Piece of *Raj Yoga, Patanjali's Yoga Sutra* is a classical treatise of psychological practice. Moreover, many other texts dealing with Indian philosophy and metaphysics also elucidate psychology in a significant way. Most of the principal *Upanishads, Bhagawad Gita* and *Yoga Vashishtha* can be viewed as dealing with psychotherapy. The last two mentioned texts are Master Minded programmes for psychotherapy of depression. *Upanishads* are taught around the parables, which are metaphors in indirect hypnosis. Besides, there is a psychological construct that has survived for 5000 years and is still valid in its revelation and interpretation of human mind.

Of course, there is no scientific validation of this psychology: primarily because Indians have not included them in the curricula at the Universities. Psychology as a discipline has suffered when it was not included in planning by the first planning commission soon after independence. There is no national council and instead of one, there are a few, each claiming to be national. The scientific research can follow after primary study. What is of relevance is that here is a model that works in hypnotherapy. But the constructs have been subjected to a rigorous critic through elaborate logical systems like, *sankhya, yoga, Nyaya, Vaisesika* and *purva-mimansa.*

Though the texts were bracketed with Indian Classical Philosophy, various psychological constructs that were postulated or evolved were not mere philosophical speculations. The structure may have been hypothetical but the designs were as valid as, or probably more than, say, Freudian constructs of personality. While the psychologists at the national level are toiling to separate philosophy from psychology, a brief summary is merited here. This is helpful to understand Indian psyche and can be integrated with therapy.

There is a different kind of motivation towards a distinctly different goal than what is perceived in Western texts. The highest motivation is–quite antithetical to the concept of ego in the service of self–is *praptti*–total surrender to the Divine. The concepts that lead to this kind of motivation are built step by step as follows:

Personality Constructs

There are four components: mind (*manah*); unconscious mind (*chitta*); *buddhi* (intellect) and *ahankara* (ego, I the doer).

- ***Body-mind as Single Entity***

Mind is considered as a dialectic faculty that tries to understand by comparison and contrast. So, it is the cause of bondage as well as liberation.[1] It is described as the sixth sense organ.[2]

- ***Chitta***

Chitta is the store house of all memories.

- ***Buddhi***

It corresponds with intellect. It is a discerning tool with faculty of rational discrimination. Intellect when taken together with the intuitive wisdom, is called *Pragya.* In a normal person functioning of *pragya* is clear. Such a person is healthy. All diseases arise from the faulty functioning of *pragyna.* Clouding of the faulty functioning of *pragya* is poignantly and poetically depicted in *Bhagawad Gita* as

> "Pondering on the objects of senses, a man develops attachment, from attachment springs up desire, desire gives rise to anger. From anger arises delusion. From delusion unsteadiness of memory comes about, this results in destruction of intellect. From destruction of intellect, a person perishes".[3]

- ***Ahankara***

Though it literally translates as ego, the meaning is different from the Freudian construct. This is best illustrated from the concept of two birds on a tree.[4] One is just watching; doing nothing else. The other one is engaged in activity and is eating the fruits too. One is, I, the seer. The other is I, the doer. While this reflects the unresolved understanding of self-reference in the brain even as of to-day, the *Upanishad* has taken the cognizance of the faculties to observe and act to drive at a point further. The birds are perched on a tree that represents the universe. In the process, there is only an artificial doer: it is nothing without and apart from the universe around it.

Ego strengthening is taught as a necessary step in hypnotherapy. Indian model may not decry it in therapeutic process: it is utilized in *Bhagawad Gita* as well as *Yoga Vashishtha* to bring Arjuna and Rama out of depressed state.

However, ego and ego boosting can assume a form of vanity. The *Bhagawad Gita* says,

> "Egoistic persons perform action with self glorification, obstinacy, filled with the pride and intoxication of wealth, in ostentatious manner. When a person is filled with egoism, because of his sense of power, insolence, lust and wrath, through malicious hating such a person hates the Divine in himself and others".[5]

They arė then, considered to be at the root of misconception about the reality according to Classical Indian philosophy. "I, my self, am a part of the universe and so I am the Universe",[6] would be the appropriate ego boosting suggestion in Indian context.

Ego defenses cloud perception and distort reality. Rather than taking recourse to any kind of neurotic or mature ego defenses, even the average Indian feels more comfortable to think that the interconnected universe has nth number of intangible forces; so he is really not the doer of any action but is just an instrument. "Ego diminution" carried further may be seen by Freudian psychoanalyst as an escape mechanism in the service of ego itself! Whether this is a kind of neurosis or altruism is of not of much consequence to the therapist. For him, it is a handy tool to absolve his client of a crushing sense of guilt that arises from the accountability of each individual's action.

- ***Alternate Paradigm of Self***

The apparent I as my self is an illusion. The real self is a part of Self that is Brahman. *Mandukya Upanishad* says, *Atma* and *Brahman* are one. *Aham brahmasmi.*

Bhagawad Gita[7] says,

> "The senses are subtle, more subtle is mind; yet finer is intellect. That which is beyond intellect is the Self."

Every individual self (*jiva*) is a particle of the universe (*brahman*). This particle has all the characteristics of the root, i.e. *brahman*. It manifests in the form of *tanmatras* that are 24 in number (Five sense organs, five organs of action, five *koshas,* as discussed below, five kinds of breaths, *antahkarana, atma* and *paramatma* etc.). The relevance to hypnotherapy lies in the fact that the ailment may be seen as arising out of any of these faculties and may be aimed at restoring the proper functioning of the same.

- ***Yet Another Paradigm of Self***

The physical self as is evident in the physical form is composed of five sheaths. They are:

1. *Annamaya kosha*—physical body–The eating disorders truly belong to this physical form. And the corollary can be extended to include such forms of ailments where primarily the gross physical form is affected.
2. *Pranamaya kosha*—vital or energy body–This is subtle. The concept goes that the body is permeated by different kind of energy forms that get conducted through the body *via* energy channels. The qualities of the various kinds of *Pranas* are vividly described in *Ayurveda.* In the philosophical/psychological literature of Sri Aurobindo, this is referred to as the functioning of the vital.
3. *Manomaya kosha*—mental body–Of course, this is the most dominant in terms of producing psychosomatic ailments. The faulty perception is ascribed as the important cause of ill-health.
4. *Vigyanamaya kosha*—A state of over mind consciousness–This is the faculty of discriminative wisdom or intuitive insight that only human beings are gifted with. In the therapeutic set up insight generation belongs to this realm. Though all individuals are gifted with the faculty of insight, it is impaired during stress and such other conditions where emotional connotations impair it.
5. *Anandamaya kosha*–A state of bliss–This is what is observed in the state of profound meditation. Some semblance to this happy state is seen during profound hypnotic trans too.

Gunas

Each individual is a distinct personality and the law of averages does apply. Primarily there are three qualities, *sattva, rajas,* and *tamas.* They do not function in isolation. Each individual is supposed to have a dominant trait at different times. To be specific, *sattva,* connotes an attitude of righteousness and truthfulness; *rajas* stands for agility an motion while *tamas* is for inertia. Different combination in the quantitative composition make for a particular personality.

The therapeutic relevance is to identify the dominant trait and utilize it in the therapeutic structuring of the specific programme in the context of neurolinguistic programming. It has to be emphasized that there are no qualities in the sense of virtue or demerit of the *gunas.* The quality that is valued is to go beyond all these traits so as to have a clear perceptual vision.

Motivation

There are four kind of motivating drives: *Dharma, Artha, Kama* and *Moksha.* This is in sharp variance with the various motivational constructs in Western psychology. They defy hierarchy and are operational at all phases of life. So, it is enjoined upon all the individuals to pursue the attainment of wealth, fulfillment of desires in the righteous way (according to *Dharma*) so as to finally aim at liberation from bondages of all kinds so as to avoid rebirth. Desire for *Moksha* in covert or overt forms is a powerful motivation for Indians. As mentioned above, the ultimate tool to attain *moksha* is surrender to divine.

Ashramas

Considering the life span of 100 years, it is divided into four equal segments: *brahmacharyashrama, grihasthashrama, vanaprasthasrama* and *sannyasa.* Now, the duration of the segment obviously varies. Of clinical relevance is the differing motivational drive in different phases. This is almost akin to Erik Erickson's phases of life. During third phase, the individual still carries on the life of a house holder, but there is supposed to be a radical shift in the motivation. That is *lokasangraha,* working for the larger social good.

Lokasangraha

Having fulfilled the desires and discharged the duties, the needs have shrunken to a bare minimum. Beyond this age, the individual has gathered and mastered several skills and, has learnt about the intricacies of life. He has gathered wisdom. All this are social assets now. Work at this stage gathers fruits for the benefit of larger social interests. The concept is distinct from philanthropy or charity.

This may or may not be evident in clinical set up and there is quite some overlap from the Western cultural milieu. I for myself as the main motivation has already emerged with most Indians. However, it is of tremendous archetypal relevance and works as such in therapy.

- ***Rebirth***

Again the belief is strong and has archetypal significance.

- ***Theory of Karma***

It is supposed to be as much fundamental to the functioning of the affairs of the world as Newtonian Physics. Each *Karma* has a *consequence,* so that, all events and relationship are *karmic* connections. More often than not this works out in the service of the client as a suitable explanation to the hidden ways that the life unfolds and treats the individual.

- ***The Concept of Energy Centers***

This is discussed in the Chapter on Archetypal Symbols.

- *Different forms of Pranayama*

There are numerous kinds of breathing exercises. Each of them leads to difference benefits. The commonest form that is very conducive to the induction of trance is simple deep breathing in the ratio of one to one inhalation and exhalation. For those who have practiced before coming to the therapy, incorporation of an interval, as in the practice of *anuloma—viloma pranayama* is helpful in deepening the trance.

Belief is fundamental to psychotherapy. All that is mentioned above is to be taken without a value judgement and the belief of the patient is the sole arbiter in the matter of choice. The therapeutic subtlety lies in strategic utilization.

Consciousness in Indian and Buddhist Traditions

These traditions treat mind as a function of the brain. Consciousness in the Indian tradition as well as "subtle mind" of the Buddhist tradition are different from the mind.

Classical Indian Tradition

Beginning with *a priori* assumption that, at the beginning there was one single immutable consciousness that has manifested in various forms in the entire universe (cf. Big Bang origin of the Universe, a mathematical point from where everything has originated in the Universe), the Indian Classical thought arrives at the derivation that all the conscious manifestations in the world are one at the source and so are interconnected that way. This is best explained by a quotation from the *mahimnastava,* a hymn to *Siva,* when translated reads as:

As sea is the goal of all rivers, so thou art the ultimate goal of different paths, straight and devious, which men follow, according to their different tastes and inclinations.

A prayer, based on the Unitary nature of human consciousness, which is the fundamental postulate of *Vedanta* is recited as,

- O Hidden Life, vibrant in every atom,
- O Hidden Light, shining in every creature,
- O hidden Love, embracing all in Oneness,
- May each, who feels himself as one with Thee,
- Know he is also one with every other.[8]

A human being is thus a part of the Cosmic Whole, not only as one with every other, but also with the entire Universe. This provides the fundamental basis of the action based on compassion. The unity of the individual consciousness *(atman)* with the cosmic universal consciousness *(Brahman)* is best summarised by axiomatic sayings from *upanishads* as:

Aham Brahmasmi[9]—I am the Ultimate—Absolute (Consciousness)
Tat tatvamasi[10]—You are the Ultimate—Absolute (Consciousness)
Ayam atmabrahma[11]—This *atman* is Ultimate—Absolute (Consciousness)
Pragyanam Brahma[12] —The intelligence (Consciousness) is the Universe.
Sarvam khalu idam brahma[13]—All this is verily consciousness only.
Ekamevadvitiyam[14]—Consciousness is the only one, without a second.

Buddhist Tradition

The Buddhist philosophy postulates two levels of mind: coarse mind and subtle mind. The coarse mind is the product of the processes of the brain and that way there is a basis to its materialistic proposition that can be processed through the storehouse of memories (of this life).

Coarse mind is the mirror that, at the best, reflects the *sanskara,* i.e. cultivated and acquired values. And a mirror that gathers dust, does not reflect any light.[15] Subtle mind of the Buddhist tradition,[16] or consciousness, as we may call it, is fundamentally pristine and pure. It is indestructible. It leaves the body at death and reincarnates again and again. That is the cycle of rebirth. In the process, it may evolve to higher spiritual states to reach the state of *Bodhisattva.* Such an enlightened consciousness reincarnates at will for the betterment of sentient beings.

Some enlightened beings attain highest state of consciousness when they become Buddhas. All of us are capable of being a Buddha. The Buddha does not reincarnate, He goes into a state of *nirvana* from where there is no return.

The Dalai Lama classifies the natural phenomena in threefold: (i) that can be directly apprehended, (ii) that can be known by logical inference and, (iii) that are based on someone else's testimony or authority.[17]

While one would want to have recourse to the first category almost all the while, it is commonsense that it is impossible. For the sake of clarity, it has also to be kept in mind that the direct apprehension is subject to be clouded by the projections of mind.

But the Freudian precept that mind sees what it wants to be seen in the way it would like it to be is a common affliction of scientists and philosophers both.

At the onset we postulated that all diseases/disorders arise in the mind. This was a broad generalization based on ancient Hindu wisdom. Needless to say, both seed and soil are necessary variables. Swine flu will not occur without infection with the virus: malarial parasites are the causative organisms for malaria. They occur in a few in an endemic population since those who get sick had a predisposition in terms of stress that is fertile soil.

The same is true for autonomic nervous system disorders, hormonal disorders, and even malignancy. The data regarding association of

Table 10.1: Tabulation of the concepts

	Materialist Proposition	*Eastern Traditions*
Consciousness	It is the function of the specific areas of the brain. But no idea as to how does it arise. Vanishes as the specific part of the brain dies.	Consciousness is subtle mind. It never vanishes. It reincarnates. Or it merges into *sunyata* at *nirvana*
Philosophical Postulate	Epistemological and empirical; Causality and change accepted as the basis of phenomena except at the level of quantum physics where randomness and chance are the rules	Epistemological and empirical; no inherent existence of any phenomena; but the law of causality and change is immutable. Only by the cessation of all *karmas* can one go to *nirvana*
Specific Feature	Falsifiability is the specific feature by which most advances in knowledge of phenomenology has advanced	Envisages a fourth state of consciousness whereby one can generate the subtle mind which can transcend the ordinary dimensions of space and time.

psychological stress with unexplained reproductive failure[18] and breast malignancy[19] is well documented.

This will justify application of hypnotherapy holistically to almost all illnesses. A subtle understanding of the psychodynamics and deft strategic manipulation can be learnt with practice as most surgical residence make to be surgeons.

Notes

1. *Shvetashvatara Upanishad.*
2. *Manah shashti indriani. Bhagavad Gita.*
3. *Bhagavad Gita* II, 63-4.
4. *Kena Upanishad.*
5. *Bhagavad Gita* XXVI, 17-18.
6. *Soham, Soham!* Or, as sung by Shankaracharya, *aham Brahmasmi* as mentioned in the text below—*Sidananda roopa, Shivoham, Shivoham!*
7. *Bhagavad Gita* III, 42.
8. This short poem, by Annie Besant, that come to be Universal prayer of The Theosophical Society.
9. *Brihadaranyaka Upanishad.*
10. *Chhandogya Upanishad.*
11. *Brihadaranyaka Upanishad, Mandukya Upanishad.*
12. *Taittiriya Upanishad.*
13. *Chhandogya Upanishad.*
14. *Chhandogya Upanishad.*
15. Madame Blavatsky, the Founder of Theosophical Society, who derived her inspiration from Tibetan Buddhism, coined this metaphor to distinguish between mind and consciousness.
16. The Buddhist tradition uses the words coarse mind and subtle mind.

17. The Dalai Lama, Consciousness at Crossroads, ed. By Zara Houshmand, New York 1999, p. 169.

Bibliography

Dalal A.S. *An Introduction to the Psychological Thoughts of Sri Aurobindo: A Greater Psychology*, Pondicherry, 2004.

S. Radhakrishnan, *The Hindu View of Life*, Oxford, 1950.

K. Ramakrishna Rao, Anand C. Paranjpe and Ajit K. Dalal, *Handbook of Indian Psychology*, Delhi, 2008.

18 (a) Vyas Rajni, Adwanikar Geeta, Hathi Leena, Vyas Bhaskar, Parikh, R.D., Psychodynamics of Unexplained Reproductive Failure, *J. Obstet. Gynecol. Ind*, 2002; 52: 35-38.

(b) Rajni Vyas, Gita Advanikar, Leena Hathi, Strategic Psychotherapeutic Intervention in 554 Couples With Reproductive Failure, *J.Ind. Med Assoc.* To be published in 2013.

Abstract:

This is a report of clinical study of 554 couples with reproductive failure during the period 1978-2005 where psychodynamic situations were seen to be causative factor/s and, in addition to the standard therapeutic measures, psychotherapy was added in treating them.

This clinical study is probably of longest duration reported so far reported in literature. Over a period of 28 years, in a peer group comprising of three gynaecologists, it reports consistently sustained success rates that are unsurpassed. This is achieved by a simple insight that psychodynamic tensions can so imbalance the physiology that it may not reveal in laboratory tests and yet block the fertilization and, it is reversible psychotherapeutically.

The success was in terms of pregnancy. This occurred in 397 couples. Within six months, success occurred in 213 couples, within 7-12 months in 65, within 1-2 years in 92, and, a further 27 succeeded by persisting with us for more than 2 years. This gave an overall success rate of 397 out of 554 (71%).

A drop out is considered a failure for the purpose of the study. Within 6 months 58 couples dropped out. Subsequently, 50 dropped out within 7-12 months, 35 within 1-2 years and 14 dropped out after more than 2 years giving an overall figure of failures as 157 (29%).

A persistent, unprecedented high success rate in the study establishes that "unexplained" reproductive failure is psychodynamically triggered and is reversible with appropriate psychotherapy.

These couples have no anatomical defects, but their reproductive physiological functions got deranged as a result of stress in their environment.

These seminal studies are positive proofs of Mind-Body continuum as well as to and fro conduit of the psychodynamic information and its translation into *soma.*

(c) Vyas Rajni, Adwanikar Geeta and Hathi Leena, Vyas' Modification of Huhner's Test : An Innovation for Immunological Infertility, *J. Obst. Gyn. of India,* Vol. 53; No. 4, July/August 2003).

(d) Maitri, C. Shah, Sejal H. Thakkara & Rajni B. Vyas, *American Journal of Clinical Hypnosis*, 54; 116-123, 2011.

Abstract:
The clinical application of hypnosis has been effective in obstetrics. Intrauterine growth restriction and oligohydramnios are dreaded complications of pregnancy that may result in preterm deliveries causing increased perinatal morbidity and mortality. In this longitudinal prospective study, clinical hypnosis was used in addition to the conventional medical management in such pregnancies. The perinatal outcome was compared with the control group wherein hypnosis was not used. The hypnosis group had a significantly shorter preterm delivery rate (p =.004) and fewer incidence of low birth weight babies (p =.009). Significantly reduced operative intervention in terms of lower rate of caesarean section (p =.008) was also observed in the experimental group. Hence, the use of clinical hypnosis as a viable adjunct to medical management is suggested to help to prevent neonatal morbidity and foetal loss. A multicenter randomized, controlled clinical trial is encouraged in this area.

19(a)Fashoyin-Aje, L.A., Martinez, K.A., Dy, S.M. New patient-centered care standards from the Commission on Cancer: opportunities and challenges. *Journal of Supportive Oncology* 2012; e-pub ahead of print March 20, 2012.

(b) Lutgendorf, S.K.. Sood, A.K., Antoni, M.H. Host factors and cancer progression: biobehavioural signaling pathways and interventions. *Journal of Clinical Oncology*, 2010; 28(26): 4094-4099.

11
The Indian Psyche

The mind is conditioned by its environment. So, its facets are moulded by inputs from a particular culture. To that extent, one is tempted to assume that there may be an Indian psyche. But even a cursory glimpse on the social, economic, political and cultural cauldron that India is, and has been, makes one wonder whether there can be any consistency in Indian psyche over a period of time or regional frame. Yet, there are a few salient features that do have a relevance to therapy. The hypnotherapist will do well to keep this in mind.

Economics of Illness/Ill Health

A large section of Indian society lives below the poverty line. And a still large section lives on the verge of the poverty line. An illness may tilt the balance. For the middle class with ill-defined measures of social security, any kind of treatment is a further hardship that adds stress to already stressful state of illness. This is a constraint that the therapist can do very little about. But some how the juggernaut of Indian health care non-system carries on! John Galbraith was astonished at the remarkable smooth functioning of an anarchy! Indian therapeutic situation has counter points of strength: if these are reinforced with high level of competence and finely tuned strategy, the economics are not deterrents to success.

Social Systems in Tradition and Transition[1]

- *Family*–One of the most favourite pipe-dream of idealist Indian is the world as a single family. The classic joint family with a ruling patriarch has disappeared; but some variation of form still survives with its supportive and compromising propositions. Family feuds are more of norm than the exception. The brothers are supposed to be sharing, stand united; and doting and protective to the sisters: yes, that it what is said in the scriptures. The archetypal structure of the elder son being the crown prince prevails. Animosity of the cousins is natural propensity as derived from the epics. It is archetypal inheritance, so denial is to be viewed as a reinforcement unless proved otherwise.

- *Gender issues*–Female sex is the second sex. The girl child is more often than not an inferior child: she being the preferred child is a rare instance. Woman has been sung in the *vedas* as *yatra naryastu pujyante, ramante tatra devatah*![2] But did not *Manusmriti* say something more practical about the way women should be treated?

Following independence, Hindu law is reformed that gives equal property rights to women. The violation of law is more frequent than its practice. Female foeticide is illegal: it is in practice. The craving for a male child verges on the madness. This cuts across the social and economic strata. The psychodynamics of neurosis reverberates across the emotional brain as well as on the hormonal axis. (See the Chapter on Infertility)

Gender equality is not an Indian issue: inequality is global. It is yet to happen that a woman becomes president of America. To illustrate, let us recall a story from the office of a multinational company somewhere in New York.

The real life story goes as:

> A man went to see the CEO of the company by appointment and he was a few minutes early. In the ante-room, he found two ladies working on the office computer side by side.

He said: I am so and so. I have come to see the CEO.

A lady: What can I do for you?

The man: Oh Honey, you already are sweet as you are. I would rather talk to the gentleman.

The lady: So would I have liked to talk to one. Never mind. I am the CEO. State your business, Sir!

In one survey by International Labour Organization, it was found that 80 per cent of the work was done by women globally. The figures for the Indian woman will exceed even that.

To illustrate:

A middle aged daughter of a former vice-chancellor, having a doctorate herself, asked her father: Dad, why did you have to give me such high education if my morning was to begin by fetching the milk and warming it up and so on? Dad replied, Wait till your children grow up. The things will be different then. We met the lady some 20 years later: she is still doing the same except that now she has found a niche for herself to go around lecturing about gender equality!

This is about a couple of Indian origin settled in the U.K. The wife, a kidney transplant surgeon, told us: After long hours at surgery, she would come home to find her dentist husband waiting for her to come and prepare a cup of tea. One day she arrived rather washed out.

The husband showed concern and asked, Darling, you looked worn out today. Do you want something?

She answered: Yes, I want a wife!

Role of daughter in law – She is the last one to eat in the house: though most families believe that the family that prays together, stays together. She has to sub-ordinate. Assertion of individuality is offence that can be punishable with even with a death sentence! Though it cannot be a rule, instances abound. If not homicide, the commonest cause of suicide in a married young woman is torture by the in laws.

An NRI lady friend of ours of high academic merit told us that her father-in-law told his son that in their aristocratic tradition, daughter in laws with such outrageous behaviour are burnt alive.

The archetype cuts across the social levels. We illustrate therapeutic relevance as:

- A former prime minister of India had an errant daughter in law thrown out of her house with her baggage strewn on the public road!
- For her infertility clinic, Dr. Rajni Vyas will run down to be sharply in time. She will give priority to young women, so that, they may be able to return early. At the end of the clinic, she saw many of them still merry making, whiling away their time in the corridors. Their explanation was that the hospital is a good excuse to be away from the mother-in-law!
- A wife of a high professional, advised to take complete bed rest for premature labour at about 32 weeks of pregnancy. She failed to carry on much further. Following delivery of a premature baby, she confided to Dr. Rajni Vyas that bed rest was out of question since there was a ritual to be conducted for the coming occasion in the in laws family and she prepared some 30 kg of sweets squatting on the floor. Following the delivery of third female baby, husband did not appear for two days at the hospital.

Dowry, in covert or overt form, is a treasured tradition.

Modern Indian Youth

Still the majority of the youth are the products of large family: a few have been a single child or with one sibling. The later class aims at excellence: the previous class toils hard and do achieve excellence that often surpasses the privileged peers. Hard work still remains a value and virtue. The feelings of inferiority of pre-independence time is gone: there is India shining for every Independent citizen of independent India. The master skills of imitating are still there and powerful, so that, often the imitation surpasses the original. The classic example is Bollywood vs. Hollywood. But the real change is in bursting out of a spirit of innovation that is fast changing the scenario of the entire fabric of Indian society. The classic illustration is soft ware revolution and biotechnology.

Lure of affluence is now counterbalanced with the happiness index in the young minds. Many young graduates shirk from the jobs with multinationals abroad to settle with even pastures at home. Saving habits of older generation are considered primitive.

Love marriages are few and far between. Crashes here are more common than in traditional arranged marriages. Most youths would not wish to defy their parents and would marry as per their wishes.

Modern Young Indian Woman

She is aware about the bias against her sex and has her own defense mechanisms to cope with it. So neurosis is a way of life. Most of them may not know Kalpana Chawala or Kiran Majmudar—or, was it that you are misquoting Kiran Bedi – but they want to assert for sure. And alas! So many of them do so by putting themselves on fire!

She is a classic example of *the survival of the weakest!* Or, is a symbol of fire and strength of *Durga.* She looks towards older mammas as those who faced and survived the hard toils of the bygone times; but in the process have accumulated wisdom.

Modern Young Indian Man

He knows life is difficult and would still want to dream of being able to idle away his time. He is nurtured and doted upon by the mother: it is his right to be in bed till late in the morning. He is latently aware that he is the torchbearer of his family name: there in lies his strength. What ever the laws of the land may be, he is sure that he is the legal heir to the family wealth: often enough he asserts this right before the demise of parents!

When married he expects the wife to deal with him in the same way as the doting mother reared him with; but her currency may be different; and then, she is just not okay! His dream girls are from Bollywood. Yet he is aware that the girls whom he interviews (or rarely, proposes in a love relationship) for marriage ask embarrassing questions like what he can provide per month. His masculinity is threatened at college and at work by hard working females who usually score over him. They certainly do not tolerate his natural urge for male domination and whisper "male chauvinist pig" loud enough between their giggles for him to listen. One of his other pet dreams is to make it big on the stock market. He invests without understanding even the fundamentals and when loses, suffers from impotence and infertility.

Worship of the Mother Deity is common in most families. Oedipus complex haunts the young man in the close family set up. It has taken a large toll before he grows in his marriage.

- *Hobbies*: Indian contingent was over 500 sportspersons to the last Olympic Games. There was only a single bronze medal won. A group of 18 students represented India at the last Science Olympiad. All 18 won medals. When interviewed as to whether they would pursue a career in science, all of them said no!
- *Social Fabric*: Caste system is unique to India where a child inherits a social status by merely being born to a class of the society. This is since ancient times and the emphasis is highlighted in the recent times because of preferential treatment of certain backward castes.

Numerous studies by social scientists have highlighted the caste specific personality traits, skills and rituals that can be very useful for the hypnotherapist. Study of behaviour of various sub castes has the traits of sophisticated social science: an understanding is useful in therapy.

- *Rituals*—For an average Indian, the day begins with a ritual and ends with the same. If probed deeply, they are portent with meaning, but are ordinarily conducted mechanistically. In most households, there is worship, and though there may be plenty of gods on the shrine, a particular deity is a favourite. (see the chapter on Archetypal Symbols). Celebrations account to large number: there is celebration of death too! Celebrations do mean expenses; they have to be incurred even by soliciting debts. Since the rituals and celebrations are metaphoric and have stories built around them, they too yield hypnotherapeutic rewards.
- *Character*—An average Indian has no qualms of conscience with double dealing. The religion is to be followed ritualistically, the gods have to be worshipped so that they remain expiated and ethics are what philosophers spin fine yarn with. There is no quarrel with that: the matters of the world are different. You have to be "practical". Corruption is a global phenomenon and if we practice it as a way of doing quick business and fast work, that saves cost for every one. Even within the inner precincts of high temples, jumping queue by bribing tout priests is official. What benefits most people, most of the time—*bahujana sukhaya, bahujana hitah* (It translates as: One that benefits many and makes most of them happy is okay)—is good to follow!

And lying is also necessary to make matters smooth. Did not even *Yudhishthira* lie at least once! Yes, lying and bluffing are no vices for an average Indian.

The relevance to therapy is that despite of such a practice, Indians do have a moral streak and a conscience that peeps out often. And it does bite to cause neurosis and neurotic breakdown.

- *Superstition*: This is as common as pollution. So, it is better labeled by the therapist as a belief system. Belief in the destiny verges to the extent of fatalism. But the dichotomy is evident here too. *Ishwarpranidhana* (meaning surrender to God) is okay: but does not the *Gita* preach that we have to act, act and act? Astrology is widely believed and astrologers are consulted on good and bad occasions. The science of *vastushastra* has always been there, we were not aware that non-practice of this can bring about misfortune. Now, that misfortune does not abate, the walls and the doors should be broken down and reset.
- *Sankalpa:* It is usual to barter with God. The belief generated by this practice can be so strong as to generate results. *Sankalpa* in the form of daily, regular fortnightly or other form of cyclic practice for a local or distant pilgrimage has therapeutic relevance.
- *Sex*: The older generation was brought up in the shadows of towering influence of Mahatma Gandhi, (who honestly tried to be puritan all his life and imposed it strictly on his followers), with Victorian age ideas regarding sex. Following the arrival of television, Bollywood values prevail. Love at the first site does occur; it does not always lead to a catastrophe! Sex outside marriage is a taboo. But violations abound. Since marriage is a value in itself, marry in haste and suffer at leisure is a common practice. Exposure to sex in the school children is increasing but teenage pregnancies in unmarried girls are not. The reason is that the termination of pregnancy is legal. By the time of graduation, at least 30 per cent of the young adults have had sexual exposure. Incest is a common source of childhood trauma, usually not reported.
- *Marriages*: Most marriages are arranged marriages; they survive better. The scenario is different in villages, mid size cities and metropolis. The metropolis is governed by pragmatism and eclectics. There is wide spread pseudo-secularism. The cultural conflict is highly stressful in inter-religious marriages and yes, in marriages outside of the caste too, the cultural conflict compounded by parental involvement as a duty, can also be a potent and widely prevalent source of conflict. The choice of a suitable partner is getting difficult and recourse to the advertisement in *The Times of India* and other news papers is frequent. The choice is most of the times advertised along the caste base.

Rama, with the ideal of one wife, is an archetypal hero. The escape route is easy: give up this God in favour of Mohammad, adopt Islam. And who really cares to practice religion any way! Philandering is frequent, more often than not, wife knows about it and, as long as he looks after the family affairs, expenses and is kind to the children, puts up with the grievance. The lies and manipulations that accrue are what the life is meant to be; neurosis can be lived with: in case of de-compensation with neurotic breakdown, the doctors will take care!

The wife should be a model *Sita.*

- Divorce is abhorred—Tolerance is a national virtue and young people could go up to tremendous length of stress to preserve marriage.
- *Lure of the foreign lands*—No one has seen heaven above earth, developed nations seem to be heavens on the earth. All kinds of trickeries and manipulations are a game. For professionally qualified, it is an escape route from surfeit, deceit and intrigue. Broken families and lost values are nostalgia for the diasporas. A syndrome that is being termed as the syndrome of the parents of NRIs has come to be.
- *Guru*—Most families have at least one. Their contribution to the mental health is immense. They have undergone a professional orientation. So there is a latent psychotherapeutic skill. Sexual exploitation of women is common.
- *Muslim Community*—The wounds of partition still silently bleed. The communal divide has widened. There are a few intercommunity marriages: the successful examples are illustrative. Usually, they are riddled with problems. The minority psyche manifests in the form of irrational fears, phobias and belligerence. Triple *tallaq* is a nightmare for most women. *Maher* can be pittance. Muslim personal law board is a powerful body: *shariat* is the law. *Fatvas* by the maulavis have to be followed. Communal riots have caused many post traumatic stress syndrome.

Notes

1. Sudhir Kakar: The Indian Psyche comprising The Inner World, Shamans, Mystics and Doctors and Tales of Love, Sex and Danger, Delhi, 1996.
2. It literally translates as: The Gods like to play where women are worshipped.
—*Manusmriti*, III. 56.

12

Philosophical Perspectives on Design of Strategy for Hypnotherapy

Before enunciating and exploring further panoramas of hypnotherapeutic transformation, it is necessary to pause here. Psychology is aptly defined as the science of mind. Science is concerned with the objective facts about the various material aspects of the phenomenal world. This leads to a paradox. Science is concerned with quantification and analysis. Mind has no matter. The material that is there in mind is in the form of software. How would the qualities of the mind yield to quantitative classification and analysis? Therefore, some would classify psychology as soft science, hybrid science etc. The best criterion is the one that is applicable in real life. We believe most of the divisions in various schools glorify only the individuals: even NLP and hypnosis are same. Even today, therefore, psychology is much akin to philosophy. Science is that which can be proved wrong: philosophy can be discussed endlessly.

What is relevant is how a particular discipline can be useful in the service of mankind. Since mankind is vast and variable, there would be no uniform mind set. Mind is conditioned by the environment; the environment can have innumerable variables that condition the mind.

A social environment is generated as per archetype and norms accepted by a group through the interactions. A larger community comes to adopt what we call as culture. Each and every culture has its own thought. This in turn generates very values. Values become a way of life for those who are fortunate enough to live according to them: the same value system can become a royal road to strife for those who are courageous enough to rebel against the conditioning of the mind. At a personal level, it can bifurcate into a neurotic breakdown or lead to enlightenment. While enlightenment is the fundamental attribute of all human beings, most of us need to find a reconciliation through introspection: when this fails, of course hypnotherapeutic help is one of the finest tool of our times.

But hypnotherapeutic strategies cannot be a standard structured format for one and all. This is why there is a division in the discipline of psychology such as Indian psychology, Western psychology, psychology of tribal people etc. Divided thus, it is possible to identify mindsets given to a particular culture and in a larger context, to a given civilization. Scientific facts of hardcore science like mathematics or physics are universal. The softwares in the mind of people will vary. There is enough evidence to deduce generation of value systems from various motivations. The understanding of the entire gamut of neurotic compensations comes into operation in psychodynamics at the time when a client seeks help. There is no litmus test for deciphering psychodynamics: even psychoanalysis cannot yield absolute facts. This is based on assumptions and can be dangerous, It can collapse any time and, the patient may quit therapy. That is alright: but not so if the disappointed depressed subject jumps of a multi-storeyed building.

Therefore, for evaluating value systems and the values generated there from for each and every client, we have to establish certain *a priori* norms. They are the fundamental values given in the personality and the environment of the individual. Therapist need to know and understand the value generating systems in a given case.

Satyam vada (speak the truth), *dharmam chara* (follow the right path) and such axioms serve this purpose admirably. But there are a few, very few universal norms. The difficulties arise when the subjective interpretations of such axioms twist them beyond the context. The evolution of the motives can not be traced as a straight line while interpreting data either through the statements of formal logic or statements of science. Moreover, the poetical, emotive, pictorial or aesthetic has a tremendous relevance to life processes and happenings at the societal-personal-cultural scene and must be accounted for.

Philosophy is indeed a tool to evolve the value generating system. But there has to be wholistic view and acceptance of the interdependence and interconnectedness of the individuals and societies. Not to account for the fundamental unity of human aspirations would lead us to believe that the ultimate constituents of the world are just "facts". There would then be no place for abstraction like value or beauty. It will also eliminate the intuitive and the mystic altogether. And, there are no isolated facts in the world; even a subatomic anti-particle automatically changes its axis of rotation no sooner the axis of rotation of the corresponding one is changed.[1]

As a counter-point, hermeneutic approach of interpreting through various facets of the personality of the client is likely to provide a better perspective for the design of the therapeutic strategy. It can be more conducive to find a solution; based on the premise that there are facts only in relation to other facts.

This involves brainstorming for the therapist and, brain storming does, indeed produce novel solutions. An experience of certain amount of muddle-headedness well known to creative people undergoing creative process does result in crystallisation of ideas following a rigorous mental shake-up. Muddle-headedness is common to both; therapist and the subject: both of them will need to come out clean following therapeutic session. At the end of therapy, there may be a reconciliation from the conflict and strife with return to normative function life; there may be a personal attitude (psychologically speaking, a personality trait) to strive, to struggle, not to find and not to yield[2]; there may be a shift to a different–higher order of values that one may call spiritual. Ernest Rossi calls this a Symptom Path to Enlightenment.[3]

Search for values and their meaning is thus perennially on, as man does not live by bread alone. No sooner the urge of man is satisfied for the elementary needs; he turns towards abstract questions.[4] In so exploring he has to find the yardsticks-parameters with which to measure the worth and the good. While the trade and commerce is the cause of physical movements the search for the meaning and values is the principal motivating factor in the movements in the minds.

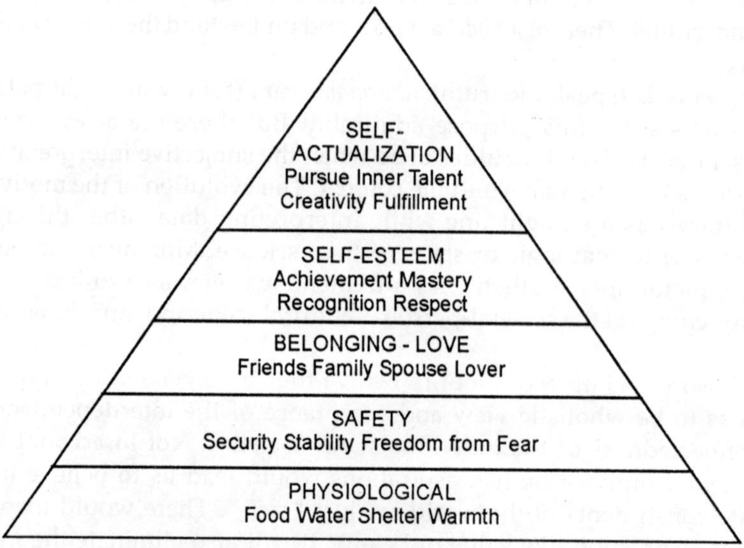

Fig. 12.1

Abraham Maslow postulated five levels of needs. The ascending triangle has also expanded now to include transcendental needs as follows:

1. *Biological and Physiological needs*—air, food, drink, shelter, warmth, sex, sleep, etc.
2. *Safety needs*—protection from elements, security, order, law, limits, stability, etc.
3. *Belongingness and Love needs*—work group, family, affection, relationships, etc.

4. *Esteem needs*—self-esteem, achievement, mastery, independence, status, dominance, prestige, managerial responsibility, etc.
5. *Cognitive needs*—knowledge, meaning, etc.
6. *Aesthetic needs*—appreciation and search for beauty, balance, form, etc.
7. *Self-Actualization needs*—realizing personal potential, self-fulfillment, seeking personal growth and peak experiences.
8. *Transcendence needs*—helping others to achieve self-actualization.

What Maslow said is common acceptance with the Western model of life style. Paradox will focus the message from this chapter when we reflect on Indian models, like Mahatma Gandhi!

Resolution of such strife occurs through the shifting of the parameters to that of realisation of beauty and harmony. Aesthetic appeal either in the external form or, in the intuitive appreciation of an idea. This can make man free from the turmoil of the search. This can end what poets have called their depression, as the Dark Night of the Soul.[5] Insight from the therapy is like the break of the dawn. An alternate tool is thus found because, "A thing of beauty is joy for ever".[6]

Faith as a Tool

The reconciliation thus arrived through the aesthetic appeal does not yield to the logical analysis or metaphysical reasoning. It turns out to be a matter of conviction, which may translate into belief. This may transcend to being a faith. The dynamics of aesthetics cannot be defined; beauty is beautiful.

Such an experience is a gratifying grace and while strife and turmoil in every day life carry on the basis of dialectics and reason, man may seek a meaning beyond transience, which he finds in aesthetics. An aesthetic endeavour is not only pleasing but is an end in itself.

Aesthetics as the Basis of any Therapeutic Strategy[7]

Beautification of life is culture. While the task of understanding the meaning of life is an onerous and, never ending, it is indeed a great pleasure to beautify the existence. Once the existence is sustained through the fulfilment of primary needs, the process of beautification brings various structural forms into existence. This at the individual level will bring about a charismatic personality. Their collective ensemble in a group, society or nationality will come to signify the excellence. No matter what may be the belief of a spectator, the sculptures depicting the pantheon of gods and goddesses in the ancient Hindu temples, the Buddhist paintings in the Ajanta caves, the sculptures, paintings and architecture of the Greco-Roman period; and to come to the contemporary period, the British Museum and the Louvre, (and the cover page of this book) signify the appreciation of boundless creative excellence of the entire human race: and thus become a heritage of values for the generations to come.

Symbols and their Message

The appreciation of aesthetics is invariably an intuitive experience and its expression in the form of externalisation is symbolic. The symbols thus connote essentially an abstract experience, which may take the form of institutions as expressed by the architectural designs or conceptual forms like the universities and societal systems. However, let it not be missed that the Idea is the first reality. Subsequent complexity of the conceptual forms compounds in the formulation of the language and literature, in the enunciation of and the practice of a religion and, if a society claims to have arrived at the understanding of meaning of life, as most religious societies do, in propagating and authenticating that notion. The notions propagated over a period of time will become deeply rooted so as to be recognised as the "philosophy"—way of life, of that particular society.

Symbols thus evolved through the search for values. They tend to be substituted for the meaning. This is particularly so when the imagery has intuitive and experiential elements to it as in a religious experience. Symbolic imagery establishes its identity with energy sources in the entire being of the individual. It does generate dynamic, unconscious forces.[8] The consciousness is then surcharged with vibrant and turbulent energy. That is indeed very powerful. This is the basis of *tantra, vajrayana, kundalini yoga* and *Kashmir Shaivism.* It is the basis of transformation through trance in hypnotherapy. The exposition of the process of functioning of *ichchhashakti* and *kriyashakti* in the form of *Shakti*—feminine energy, provide pathways to any creative pursuit. But then, this is culturally determined, as there are several varieties of religious experiences.[9] However, all of them, including hypnotherapy have this cataclysmic spiritual quality.[10]

Culture as the Fountainhead

The edifice of the present day society rests on the cultural foundation; on the values that evolved in search of valid parameters to judge good and no good and bad and ugly. This process itself is pleasant to pursue since the pursuit of the meaning of the existence or the deciphering of the enigma of the Nature is far too complicated a task for the most to be preoccupied with, in day to day life.

Conclusion

It remains for the philosophers to speculate and construct articulate concepts, to intelligently formulate hypothesis, logically to find proofs and scientifically to falsify them. Philosophy, thus, is the mother of all sciences. When pursued with the aspiring intention of understanding the world, it opens up pathways to empirical research in finding the normative systems for generation of values; when explored with the motivation of flaming activism to change the world for better, as Karl Marx would want to have it, it ignites revolutions. When pursued with the aspiring intention of understanding the hypnotherapeutic world, it yields strategies that transform the individual personality.

Sri Aurobindo said, A moment sees what ages toiled to express!

Notes

1. Einstein Podosky and Rosenthal phenomenon for the entangled particles.
2. A quote from *Romain Rolland.*
3. Ernest Rossi, *Symptom Path to Enlightenment.*
4. Saul McLeod Maslow's *Hierarchy of Needs,* published 2007, updated 2012.
5. Saint John of the Cross, "Dark Night of the Soul" A poem and a treatise he wrote commenting on the poem Sixteenth Century.
6. John Keats.
7. See the Cover page by Jyoti Bhatt in the Context of the discussion here.
8. This is indeed the physiological foundation of meditation through *mantra, sutra* and symbols. Sound and images have neurolinguistic correspondence with body systems. Through a technique in Mahayana Buddhism, *Kalachakra* meditation, one visualizes 928 images of gods and goddesses in a rapid succession so as to extract essence of symbolic virtue of each one of them into one's being.
9. William James, *Varieties of Religious Experiences.*
10. Rupa Dave, Hypnosis is One of the Varieties of Religious Experiences, Presentation at the 7th National Conference of Society for Clinical and Experimental Hypnosis: Psycho-philosophical perspectives, 2009, Baroda.

13
Healing and Rejuvenation

Transformation through Trance, a Creative Process

What is understood about the process of transformation form a disorder/disease to normalcy by utilization of hypnotherapy is a matter of mystique and mystery. Several hypotheses are advocated; most of them are speculative enough to be accounted as philosophic. We do not delve upon them. Hard core laboratory research is scanty. The account below is our own: it is scientific to the extent logical positivism can be. Inference is drawn from a long unchartered course in practice for over 30 years. We have noticed the following possible ways that trance brings about transformation: from disease to health and from mundane to spiritual as well. Bottom line of all theoretical probabilities is the heightened state of suggestibility. This is unique to hypnosis in contrast to carious forms of psychotherapy available. This is fundamental to the success of command therapy.

Order Out of Chaos: Reversal in Hypnosis

A quick reversal of the pathology that may have lasted for a long time is possible during a reasonably short period of time with hypnotherapy. The mechanism of reversal may lie in any one or several traits of the altered state of consciousness that we call hypnosis. They are: 1. It is the prime state of consciousness where positive creative processes find expression and flowering. 2. It is the fertile ground for generation of insight. 3. In this state the boundary between real and surreal gets blurred so that there is automatic preference for the positive against negative traits. At the organic level, 4. There is reversal of stress. 5. A possibility of genetic transmission to neuronal network and brain plasticity occurs. Let us elucidate this in more details.

1. *Hypnosis as a Ground State of Creativity; Preference for the Positive*

It is no exaggeration to state that all creative work, be it a work of the aesthetic kind like painting or literary work like writing poetry or work of scientific invention occurs in a state which is akin to hypnosis. The verbal, grammatical language of the left brain is replaced by the symbolic contents which have meaning of their own: all the same the symbols do carry a message that some how, some where in the nervous system finds transcription and translation into ordinary every day usage. Poets have described their creative process as descending from somewhere; the painters are known to work under some kind of frenzy. Given to the discussion in the scientific framework, we may refer to some of the data concerning the scientists. Let us refer to the creative process as described by Einstein himself.

Einstein describes the experience of intense creativity through insight and intuition in response to a query from Hadamard, a fellow mathematician of his times.[1] Einstein has admitted to getting into a different state of mind in his creative moments. He has described it as thinking with the symbols. This is reproduced verbatim as:

My Dear Colleague,

In the following, I am trying to answer in brief your questions as well as I am able. I am not satisfied myself with those answers and I am willing to answer more questions if you believe this could be of any advantage for the very interesting and difficult work you have undertaken.

(A) The words or the language, as they are written or spoken, do not seem to play any role in my mechanism of thought. The psychical entities, which seem to serve as elements in thought are certain signs and more or less clear images that can be "voluntarily" reproduced and combined.
There is, of course, a certain connection between those elements and relevant logical concepts. It is also clear that the desire to arrive finally at logically connected concepts is the emotional basis of this rather vague play with the above-mentioned elements. But taken from a psychological viewpoint, this combinatory play seems to be the essential feature in productive thought—before there is any connection with logical construction in words or other kind of signs that can be communicated to others.

(B) The above-mentioned elements are, in my case, of visual and some muscular type. Conventional words or other signs have to be sought for laboriously only in a secondary stage, when the mentioned associative play is sufficiently established and can be reproduced at will.

(C) According to what has been said, the play with the mentioned elements is aimed to be analogous to certain logical connections one is searching for.

(D) Visual and motor. In a stage when words intervene at all, they are, in my case, purely auditive, but they interfere only in a secondary stage as already mentioned.
(E) It seems to me that what you call full consciousness is a limit case that can never be fully accomplished. This seems to me connected with the fact called the narrowness of consciousness.

The investigations so far suggest that during hypnosis, the right hemisphere becomes dominant. It has been observed from the split-brain patients of Roger Sperry that the right brain is involved with those kinds of brain functions as we term as creative. However, what is the method of transcription that Einstein and such other creative geniuses would have evolved to put their symbolic creations into ordinary language or mathematical formulae remains an enigma.

Regardless, this seems to be happening in the hypnotherapeutic process much in the same way!

2. *Hypnosis as the Fertile Ground for Insight Generation*

We do not know, as of to day, as to how insight occurs. But most people know when they have insight. When one arrives at such a moment, there is an eerie feeling of elation and joy of discovery. Various scientists and philosophers give interesting accounts with a common factor that a different state of consciousness is involved.

- *Revelation from a Background State*

Penrose[2] conjures a background state of silent activity at such moments of insight. This is based on his own experience. After detailed discussion about the possibilities of various physical designs of the creative process of consciousness, he explores the field of intuition that leads to fascinating discussion of consciousness at the moment of mathematical discoveries. He describes a moment of flash while his conversation stopped with his colleague at the time of crossing a street. He solved a mathematical problem concerning the center of black hole in his mind in that short time. This has been perplexing him for quite a while. But on resumption of conversation after the street was crossed, he forgot all about it. However, he continued to feel a strange feeling of elation around him. He had to chase that feeling for quite a while as to what was its cause till he realized that the cause was the sudden resolution of a long-standing riddle.

It is a common knowledge that generation of insight is not accomplished by any amount of toil that goes in the process of didactic, dialectic, and discursive logic. This is restricted to the left hemisphere functioning of the brain. Insight strikes like a flesh of lightening. Poetical truth and justice are experienced by the mankind since ages but may not qualify as empirical evidence. There are several notable examples in the field of science. Discovery of benzene ring by Kekule through a dream is interesting. He dreamt of serpents forming a ring by holding each other at the tail end. So did Singer dream of spears with a hole at the proximal end to invent the sawing needle. Archimedes' "Eureka, Eureka" is still reverberating in history. We now call it *A-ha* experience. The latest is the discovery of DNA code by Watson and Crick. To quote Watson[3]:

When I got to our still empty office the next day morning, I quickly cleared away the papers from my desk top so I would have a large, flat surface on which to form pairs of bases held together by hydrogen bonds.... I saw all too well that my prejudices led nowhere.... Then I saw that both pairs could be flipped flopped over...

And there are many such other instances from ordinary life too. The fact that the insights came without didactic, dissective, dialectic reasoning does say something about an extraordinary occurrence. It is not possible to tap such an event at will. Even if it is an altered state of consciousness, we can only deduce that such an alternate/differential/quantum jump processing does occur in the brain.

Insight can be in the nature of self-reflection: it may be a look within oneself. Generation of insight into ones personality is a standard modality of all forms of psychotherapy. Jung and Jose Silva (the author of *Mind Control Method*)—they are separated in time and space and academics—created a model of insight generation by having a dialogue with an imaginary person. Jung described this as transcendental function that served as a tool in all forms of creativity and healing.

- *Numinous Images and Guiding Angels: Insight Generation*

Jung's subjects experienced a kind of luminosity during transcendent imagination. The numinous images came up in these subjects spontaneously and their spiritual quality made Jung to think that this was a way to connect to divinity or God. Some of the most interesting examples of the creative process through imagery show the generation of ecstatic states and heightened insight that are familiar in the literature of mysticism[4,5]. Jose Silva[6] has popularized his "mind control" method where he employs a councilor. But in contrast to numinous images that Jung's subjects experienced, Silva may employ the image of Sophia Loren! What is of relevance is a dialogue that one establishes with such images that leads to insight generation to resolve ones conflicts. We have been using this technique for hypnotherapy and employ such images that suit the subject's sensibilities. The process does require reinforcement and the insight may not occur as instantaneous flash; but eventually it does arise either as a flash or a gentle trickle of a ray of light.

Such flashes come about from the activities of unconscious mind. But it is much more than a mere uncovering of the unconscious. Is it an exploration of unconscious mind? Unconscious mind stores what mind has already known, was found repugnant and has repressed it. It cannot provide generic ground for something fresh and new that is the essential feature of creativity and invention. It is evidently clear that this is not the function of ordinary state of consciousness. More often than not, unconscious mind deals with ugly things that need to be repressed and need be relegated to the dark recesses of mind. So, it may not connote well with the creative experience that may win a Nobel Prize. But it suits well with the tortured or contorted psyche of a sick person who needs to intuitively understand the pressures from his/her unconscious mind. It is probable that the healing under hypnosis is through the "unconscious" understanding of the unconscious mind through a subtle, not directly discernible process. However, there is a cue. That is about the feeling of elation.

- *Truth is Beauty and Beauty is Joy*

Elation is a feeling of being "high". Like Penrose, Heisenberg has also described this feeling on the discovery of uncertainty principle.[7] Perhaps every one has experienced such elation once in a while. Who does not feel "high", when face to face with a reality that is transcendental? A discovery or invention is creativity incarnated and it takes one face to face with a new dimension of reality. Reality so experienced is beauty personalized and a thing of beauty is joy forever. From an entity that is not quantifiable, consciousness, we are led to further abstract realms of aesthetics. The most ardent and unabashed advocacy for the equivalence of a good theory to a thing of beauty comes from Dirac[8] who is the youngest Nobel Laureate so far and (therefore) having the largest number of his students who received Nobel Prize. He claims that it was his keen sense of beauty that enabled him to *divine* (the word is as used by Dirac) his equation for the electron. That is because Truth is beauty and beauty is joy.[9]

So intuition is not just a delayed recall. Nor it is plumbing or ploughing of the unconscious. It seems to arise from a background state of silent rumination over a problem for a length of time. Let us consider each moment of reflection. At every moment of ideation, numerous brain cells will engage in electrical activity with varying potentials that shall generate electromagnetic/quantum electrodynamic field. Since thoughts/emotions reverberate all over the body in the form of molecular biological events, all thoughts and emotions act as agents for the generation of a quantum electrodynamic field – QED—in the brain/nervous system. Several such fields then superimpose to arrive at the flash. Intuition thus be said to be the product of the super-impositions of several QEDs. This is put in the form of a chart by Rossi.[10] That corresponds with the four phases of creative process described by Ramachandran in his contribution about the creative process. It confirms to Ericksonian model of ideal time duration of a hypnosis session. We believe it will not be long before the chart will be validated by the studies of arousal and other genes under hypnosis. Since the play of genes may continue in a modified form for an indefinite time, post hypnotic suggestions have long lasting effects. Therefore, we have modified Rossi's chart as shown below it.

We have arrived at a step where we can now conceive intuition being a creative endeavour. What is of further relevance is that such a processing is facilitated by altered state of consciousness/hypnosis. While one cannot cultivate intuition so as to reveal itself at will, it can at least be approached through the help of a hypnotherapist.

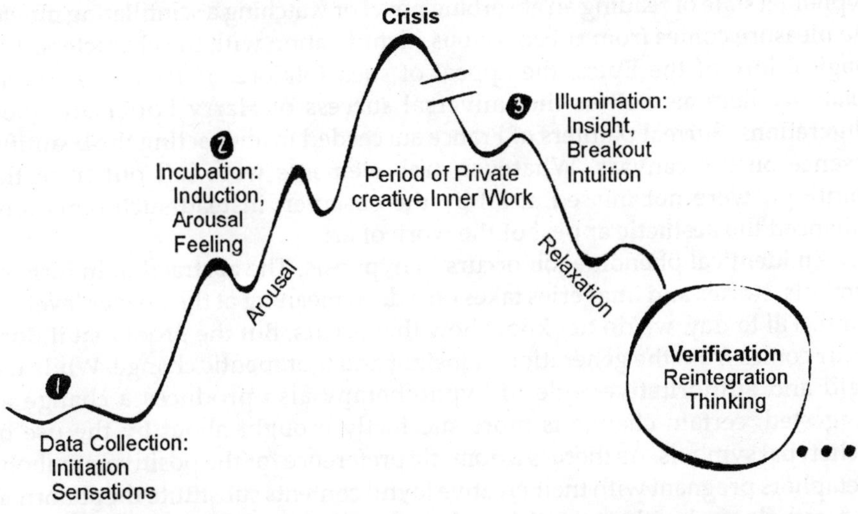

Fig. 13.1: A Classical Hypnosis Session of ninety minutes Duration
Source: Original diagram from Rossi.

The four stages of the creative process in psychobiologically oriented psychotherapy in the upper part of the diagram is a utilization of one of the natural 90-120 minute ultradian rhythms that take place throughout the 24 hour Circadian rhythm. This also corresponds with many hormonal messenger molecules of the endocrine system such as growth hormone, stress hormone cortisol and the sexual hormone testosterone. They have typical circadian peaks at different times of the 24 hour cycle.

Author's modification of the above based on psychobiology of gene expression following a hypnotherapeutic session

3. *Blurring of the Boundaries between Real*[11] *and Surreal*

Apart from the effacing of the conventional structure of time and space, hypnosis is characterized by an extraordinary feature. That is the blurring of boundaries between what we commonly understand as every day reality and what one may think as pure imagination. The nature of reality has been a matter of much philosophical speculation. Plato conceptualized the mankind as chained men in a cave who gathered the view of the outside world from the images that the shadows of the world reflected on the walls of the cave. Shankaracharya, the father of Vedantic philosophy, propounded the world as an illusion and attributed the Reality to somewhere beyond. They are joined by none other than true material philosophers of our day, quantum physicists, who are unanimous in one hypothesis that we do not as yet know what is Reality.

We all have enjoyed the fairy tales and liked to read fiction. And in the hypnoidal state of reading an absorbing novel or watching a scintillating movie, the pleasure comes from subconscious identification with the characters. The magical lure of the Epics, the appeal of such folklore, as *Panchatantra* and *Anderson Tales* as well as the universal success of Harry Potter are good illustrations. Surreal painters of France succeeded in abstracting the beautiful essence on the canvass. Whatever drab elements were left out from the paintings, were not missed at all by the observer: instead such omissions enhanced the aesthetic appeal of the work of art.

An identical phenomenon occurs in hypnosis. The abstraction in form of symbols, stories and imageries takes on a deep meaning at the deeper levels of mind. Till to day, we do not know how that occurs. But the proof that it does occur comes from the generation of insight and therapeutic change. While the rigid and authoritative style of hypnotherapy also produces a change as suggested, certain change is more succinctly brought about by the use of archetypal symbols. As there is axiomatic preference for the positive, symbolic metaphors pregnant with their creative joyful contents substitute the abnormal and pathological with normative and rejuvenative process.

- *Archetypal Symbols as Metaphors*

For the human beings collective unconscious mind is time and again manifested in group actions[12]. Where from the information is derived? Jung ascribes it to dynamic demiurgic forces in the collective unconscious mind. But where is the collective unconscious mind? Where does it reside and how does it operate? We do not know. But the influence of archetypal symbols is seen to be deeply pervasive not only in a cultural group but in entire human race as can be seen from the dream contents.

The psychodynamic forces operate through the retrieval, revival, renewal and regeneration of the archetypal symbols. These processes are brought about by the forces that lurk alive in the various layers of the consciousness. They are truly the driving forces of personality, society, civilizations and history.

Whatever may be the psychodynamics of their operation, utilization of archetypal symbols is profoundly effective in hypnotherapy. And what is crooked, warped, contorted, fragmented or twisted undergoes metamorphosis when superimposed with near isomorphic archetypal symbol so that a (w) holistic paradigm that is in consonance with wholesomeness and beauty

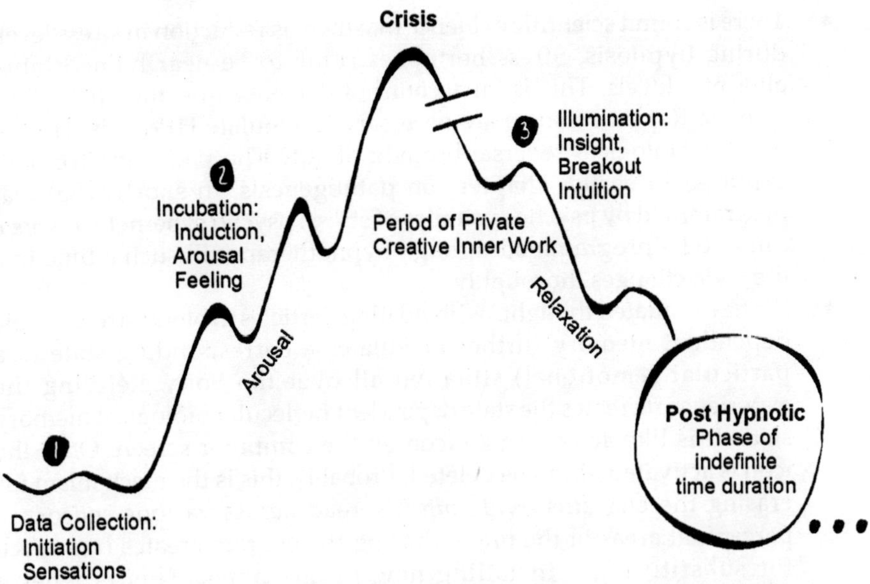

Fig. 13.2: Authors Modification based on Psychobiology of Gene Expression

emerges. The symbols may be in the form of universal images like sun for the father as the protector and the earth as the mother as the source of nourishment and energy. They may be culture specific as Vishnu as a protector, Shiva as the destroyer and Brahma as the creator: or Christ and Buddha as the embodiment of compassion. In the state of hypnosis for a child brought up in the Western Tradition, Santa Claus will gift him/her with a comfort chamber where it is so easy to breathe or for a child brought up under the influence of Indian tradition, Ganesh comes alive under hypnosis so that his sweets have qualities that can stop his/her enuresis.

- *Automatic Preference for the Positive*

Though difficult to explain, it is well established that negative suggestions do not work under hypnosis. So much so that, it is emphasized that the usage of language should be in positive sense. This correlates with the positive contents of the symbols too. When the positive contents of the symbols overlap the aberrant discreative perceptive images, there is a preferred unconscious choice that undergoes transmutation to the positive messages incorporated in the symbol/s.

4. Reduction of Stress: Conversion to Eustress

Taking recourse to medical model discussed earlier, we emphasize the following:

- There is sound scientific evidence that there is reduction in stress levels during hypnosis. Stress hormones come to be near homeostatic–allostatic levels. This is on account of decrease in sympathetic over activity. Repeat sessions are necessary to regulate HPA axis. How is this physiological reversal brought about? The pathways we have explored in earlier chapters on pathogenesis. In short, what was programmed by psychodynamics of stress, psycho cybernetic reversal can also be programmed through hypnotherapy till such a time that life style changes thoroughly.
- We have equated thoughts with floating particles in blood stream. State dependent memory further postulates a corresponding state to a particular (emotional) situation all over the body. Reliving the experience recreates the state dependent molecular biological memory state. It is like activating an icon on the computer screen. Once the icon is activated, it can be deleted. Probably, this is the mechanism for erasing the engrams (wide *infra*) spread across various sensory–perceptual areas of the brain. Erasing the engram creates free space for substituting – installing new programmes. This is what a hypnotherapist does when he makes the subject relives a traumatic experience, erases it with selective ablation of past and reconstructs a pleasant experience as a replacement.

Brain works like a computer in several aspects. The analogy may not just be a simile. This may be just as it is. And, in the matter of speed, it is indeed as fast as a computer.

5. Genetic Transmission to a Neuronal Network: Brain Plasticity

The genes dictate all forms of behaviour. Behaviour is executed through the operations of the brain and the nervous system. The brain continues to record all the events as they occur in their various sensory inputs. Penfield, a neurosurgeon, demonstrated that specific memory might be evoked by stimulation of a particular area of the brain by a microelectrode. He postulated the existence of engrams in the brain—'cortical patterns' that preserve the details of a particular experience, as in a file. This is one of the first steps towards a physiology of the mind. The nature of the pattern, the mechanism of its formation, the mechanism of its subsequent utilization, and the integrative processes by which it is brought into the substratum of consciousness—these will some day be translated into a physiological formula. Such a formula is bound to have a cybernetic role for the genes incorporated into it. We shall have to wait for a decade or two for laboratory validation.

Arousal by a symbolic content that has been incorporated within the self, encompassing the entire physiological structure, can cause a cascading of molecular messenger molecules. These molecules seem to be the key notes for the behaviour patterns that replicate what the symbol signifies. This process does seem to have a genetic connection in the form of activation of early arousal genes and further play of genes.

Neurolinguistic programming explains the mechanism of transformation through brain plasticity.

Every kind of new conceptualization involves novelty of brain connections. While the existing neuronal network constantly recreates its circuitry, and thereby innovates new pathways for executing a command, stereotype behaviour classically illustrates how some conditioned reflexes get further engraved. This applies to unwanted and unavoidable habits such as smoking.

With hypnosis, there is development of new synaptic connections. The command may remain the same, its execution changes its transmission via the synaptic routes. For instance; a command by the brain? synapses at neuronal cells A, E, H → synapses at P, T, Z cells → Execution is modified through neurolinguistic programming as, a command by the brain → synapses at neuronal cells A, E, H → synapses at cells M, O, R, S → Modified execution quite different from previously expressed behaviour. This is how the subjects with paranoid traits and obsessive compulsive traits undergo change. So will be effected the changes in other behavioural patterns.

6. Creative Visualization as Conscious Meaningful Thought Process

Creative visualization is one of the hypnotherapeutic modes of 'visual experience'. A person experiences imageries in his/her imagination. Imagination itself is a process of transforming thoughts. Imagination as it has been usually understood is a power to call up images. More importantly it is one of the inner senses of realization. When this realization grows into something new, may be a novel idea, a new concept, a better way of doing things, or into an aesthetically pleasing product, the visualization may be termed creative.

Creativity is initially formed in imagination. As Tagore illustrates it, "For a man by nature is an artist; he never receives passively or accurately in his mind a physical representation of things around him. There undergoes a continual adaptation, a transformation of facts into imagery, through constant touches of sentiment and imagination."[13] A creative genius–or an ordinary individual experiencing hypnosis—is very much conscious about sensing creative ideas that form in his imagination. In his imagination he tries to conceive imageries for a better representation. At the beginning, he *feels* about it but his intention is to have a *perspicuous* representation that is more significant. Representation involves emotion, feelings, sentiments through which the artist in any subject nurtures the gestate images.

A creative state undergoes *transformation* in the process of formulating new ideas. That is to say, the content of a creative state gets modified till the artist realizes that the piece of art is complete. The modification is a 'sustained interplay'[14] among the emerging imageries and their applications. The sustained interplay is process between the convergence and divergence of various mental states. The self-regulative function among the imageries precisely brings out the *cognitive flexibility* of realizing the content of mental states. For instance, we can think of a musician trying to put notes in the instrument. The person repeats the notes again and again till he gets fine-tuned playing the notes. The painter works on the canvas repeatedly with colour and line many times till he is satisfied. The process of modification therefore is a shift from an *imperfect* creative state to a *perfect* creative state. The modification of mental states *persists in time* which could be linguistically translated in terms of the verb 'to happen' or 'may happen'.[15]

When a person is involved in creating something new, he is aware of the experience that he undergoes. The feeling of that sensibility is a mode of realizing something and then expressing it. The form of sensing and form of describing is nothing, but a process of transformation of experience, which results in joy, pride, something new which we call transforming too. This transformation of thoughts is a part of thinking whether it is verbal to visual or visual to verbal. The content of visual experience of thought and the expression of the experience of thoughts are meaningfully connected. As Searle interprets, "There are perceptual experiences, they have intentionality, their intentional content is propositional in form; they have mind to the world direction. The properties which are specified by their intentional content are not in general literally properties of perceptual experiences."[16]

Searle emphasizes that there is an intentional feature embedded in structuring the content of experience. He maintains that the semantic characterization of the content of experience flows from the *intentionality* of consciousness. The "eyes" see what the mind knows and is looking for. Secondly, intentionality bridges the gap between the mental representation and linguistic representation. There could be an isomorphic relationship that persists between the two levels of representation and intentionality remains as a connecting principle between them.

The flow of intentionality constitutes a field of experience. In the field of experience a person comprehends the meaning that s(he) tries to disclose. An artiste's willingness to have a perspicuous representation of thought signifies not only the pictorial features of thoughts but also the process of experiencing. The content of the experience is to give a *meaning* to the piece of art. Thus, looking for a meaning in the representation of thought is a self-referential feature of intentionality. For instance, while playing few notes, a musician keeps on modifying the notes for a better tune. Here, being conscious of tuning and opting for possible modifications are due to the self-referential feature of consciousness. That is, intentionality is involved in showing the directedness from *mind to the world,* i.e., playing of the notes shows flow of intentionality from thought to action; whereas, listening to the tuning shows the *world to the mind* direction. The intention flows from the *subject pole* to the *object pole* and *vice versa* which constitutes the field of experience.[17] The shift of visual fields would show the manifoldness of intentionality transforming the visual fields and entering into different realms of experience. That is, precisely how one talks about the experience of *solitude* in the presence of others. Although the shifting of visual field is the process of the change in sequence of thoughts, still it is due to the intentionality that acts in the *background* of consciousness.

7. Cerebration of Hypnotic Suggestions

One of the axiomatic principles of philosophy is that a thesis gives rise to its antithesis. The creative discourse between the two gives rise to synthesis. Two schools of philosophers argue whether the creative process is with a meaning attached to it or it is just a grammatical progression of an algorithm like what the computer does. Hypnosis is the generic ground of creativity. For the hypnotherapist, both kinds of brain processing are evident. A beautiful expression from a human mind may be so full of meaning that the generations explore it. The distorted and contorted manipulations of an obsessive compulsive personality, or a paranoid subject and at the extreme, a schizophrenic are neither with any beauty nor there is any meaning.

This is illustrated by the following example. What happens to the mind/ in the brain of the person who creatively attempts to visualize the image of Goddess Sarasvati? Visualization of the creative symbol of Sarasvati in all its magnificent splendor and associated paraphernalia expounds a meaning of learning and erudition, serenity, peaceful joy and creative wisdom in the minds of all belonging to the Indian ethos. In the process, it may facilitate learning and scholarship. Such interpretation contributes to the semantic thesis of Searle. However, as the process is transcribed in the brain cells, it will have to undergo several stages of molecular biological events in progression. This will be particularly so when the holographic integration of inputs of all the senses happens. The memory in the brain is in the form of engram over a wide area of the brain. So, as the meaning to the creative visualization of a symbol becomes obvious, interaction between nth number of engrams is most likely to have occurred by the time that the creative process has yielded a result.

And let us see a step further about intentionality and motivation in creative process. Motherhood is a creative process across the animal kingdom. Regardless of various stages of brain development, nurture of the new born is universal. A mother in some of the lower categories of animal kingdom stays near her eggs, overtly hidden by her under a heap of leaves created by her, even though she has no hands. In the process of creative protection that lasts for about two months, she goes without food for days together. She leaves no sooner the eggs are hatched. Even when such a mother has no cerebrum and would hardly have anything comparable to the human thalamus, the instinctual behaviour has to be guided from somewhere, be it genes or brain centers. Is there no intentionality/motivation in what she is doing? Can this be only a grammatical reading of the physical laws?

Therefore, intentionality and motivation are prime movers in the therapeutic process. No subject can be hypnotized against his/her will. And hypnotherapy shall yield better results when the subject is experiencing creative images that have been heavily loaded with archetypal meaning. To make this more explicit, let us revert back to the Chinese Room thought experiment.[18] Even if the translation from English to Chinese and from there to Japanese were to follow mathematical rules, there appears to be "a ghost in the Chinese Room"—borrowing the concept from Arthur Kowstler[19] who understands the meaning at the same time as it translates. Hypnotherapy transmutes the meaning to a higher creative order too. If we were to extend the analogy, transferring the data from one programme of the software to another programme like WordStar files to Word would be purely mathematical without involving any deciphering of the meaning by the computer. This is analogous to directive, command hypnotherapy and so it will extend results in the syntactical sense only.

Rejuvenation: An Illustration

In all societies and cultures, there are recurring instances as to how some people happen to rejuvenate themselves. We narrate an example:

Mr. M.B., a middle aged structure engineer in his late fifties, rushed into my rooms along with his wife. Both were agitated, flushed and almost panting. Some time back, he had pain in the left side of chest while he was in USA and was diagnosed as unstable angina. He rushed back home and following examination by his physician, was advised to undergo by-pass surgery. He was a diabetic poorly controlled with insulin. Both were frightened of heart surgery and wanted to find out a way out.

I explained to them that heart surgery is safe now a day. And the physician who has recommended the surgery is an astute one. When I failed to assuage their fears, I told them that there is an alternative: to undergo a few hypnosis sessions, consult another physician who is a believer in conservative therapy and follows Dean Ornish's programme, start gradual exercises as per his advice, learn meditation and. Change the life style. Being a scientist, he demanded me to explain how it helps. Using the currency of his own profession, I told him that the difference between clogged drains and blocked arteries is the simple fact that the living tissue has a capacity and software for rejuvenation. These not only can by-pass the block by opening up the collaterals, but can recanalize the blocked vessels.

It is six years past this evening. He gets up at 4.00 a.m. in the morning and drives his car to a near by temple. After the prayers, he leaves the car and walks about 3 km. to *Yoga Niketana* and does his prescribed quota of *asanas* at an even pace. The he meditates at least for 20 minutes before walking back to the temple to pick up his car. Apart from the change in the physical format of his day, he has changed his mind-set from highly ambitious to that of thanks giving for the gratuitous graces, the greatest of them all being spared coronary by-pass surgery. The bonus is that his diabetes is no more: he is off insulin and on regular diet.

Notes

1. Hadamard J. *The Psychology of Invention in the Mathematical Field*, Princeton, 1945.
2. Roger Penrose, *The Emperor's New Mind*, London, 1990, pp. 541-47.
3. Pelletier K.R. *Toward a Science of Consciousness*, New York, 1978, p. 106.
4. Rossi E. and Nimmons D. *The Twenty Minute Break: The Ultradian Healing Response*, New York, 1991.
5. William James, *The Varieties of Religious Experiences*, Edinburgh, 1901-02.
6. Jose Silva, *Mind Control*, New York, 1980.
7. Chandrasekhar S. *Truth and Beauty, Aesthetics and Motivations in Science*, Chicago, 1987, p. 64.
8. Dirac P.A.M. Pretty Mathematics, *Int. J. Theor. Physics*, 21. 603-5, 1982.
9. (cf. with the concept of *sat-chit-ananda*, meaning Truth-Consciousness-Bliss as a primordial expression of Reality in Indian Classical tradition).
10. Rossi Ernest, Sleep, Dream, Hypnosis and Healing: Behavioural State Related Gene Expression and Psychotherapy, *Sleep and Hypnosis*, 1, 141-55, 1999.
11. This book is not the right place to discuss the nature of Reality. The word real connotes the ordinary sense of actuality that we observe in our every day life.
12. Bhaskar Vyas and Rajni Vyas, *The Collision of Culture*, Delhi, 2000, pp. 19-23.
13. Tagore says creativity shows an intentional communication with our own self. It is a 'modification of our relationship' till we have perfect imageries. The imageries are the product of our feelings, sentiment and imagination. Rabindranath Tagore, "The Artist", *The Religion of Man*, (Hibbert Lectures 1930), Calcutta, 2000, p. 76.
14. Shear explains that the 'sustained interplay' is a process of reaching at a new idea. Johnathan Shear, *The Inner Dimension: Philosophy and the Experience of Consciousness*, New York, 1990, p. 120.
15. Stout makes this distinction while stating that processes are metaphysical categories *persisting in time* 'though they do not have temporal parts' that do not happen in time. Rowland Stout, "Processes", *Philosophy*, Vol. 72, no. 279, January 1997, p. 19.
16. John Searle, *Intentionality: An Essay in Philosophy of Mind*, Cambridge, 1983, p. 41.
17. J.N. Mohanty, *Self and its Other: Philosophical Essays*, New Delhi, 2000, p. 73.
18. Hypothetically, a person is made to sit isolated in a room. The person knows English but he does not know either Chinese or Japanese. Instructions are given in English to the person. He is asked to match Chinese scripts with Japanese scripts that are given separately in two different baskets. By reading the *rules* (algorithm) the person successfully correlates the scripts. Though the person succeeds in matching the scripts he still does not literally understand. He does not derive any meaning from the exercise except that he has done some work. This proves the point that the syntax is not sufficient for semantics, and minds have semantics."
19. Arthur Koestler, *The Ghost in the Machine*, London, 1967.

14
Indications, Applications and Contraindications

Before stating what all conditions can be alleviated or cured by hypnosis, it is necessary to elucidate what are the modern criteria of evaluating a drug or a modality for its efficacy.

Let us first take the example of a drug trial. After identifying the drug in its chemical form, it goes several stages of experimentation with the animals. The effects on all the organs are looked up. Its toxicity is precisely calibrated. After all such results are statistically significant so as to produce desired results in animals; the drug is put to clinical trials with double blind samples. There are rigid ethical protocols. And, after multicentric validation, the drug is put in the market. The cost of a trail of single molecule is about 1.5 billion dollars. The time frame is from 10-15 years. And, most drugs get outdated in about 20 years.

Now, let us see about a modality. Psychoanalysis came into vogue and was fashionable in West for earlier part of twentieth century. No doubt, several people benefited as far as their psychological symptoms were concerned. It never came up to the level of being called scientific. No body can prove a psychoanalyst wrong, but any body can come up with a different psychoanalytic interpretation. Enormous time extending over several sessions was needed and even costs proved prohibitive. Now, it is on the wane.

Hypnotherapy has a history of over 200 years. Its principal use was in the area of psychology. However, when its widespread physiological parameters were further validated experimentally, its scope has widened. This is accepted now by the medical profession in West. Yet, it will take time for testing its efficacy for each and every condition. Double blind studies will have to be conducted so as to qualify it as scientific rational therapy.

The conduct and assessment of hypnotherapeutic trials is difficult. Hypnosis is an altered state of consciousness. So, it is subjective. Even when there are objective criteria available for deciding the level of trance, subjective perception of the process varies to a great extent. Moreover, a qualitatively and quantitatively different amount of work is done by different subjects apart from the levels of trance they are in. And, it also varies from session to session.

Meanwhile, the current level of research has shown that during the process, different areas of the brain get activated as seen in fMRI studies. Now, that gene expression studies have become cheaper to conduct, precise information about the gene activation along with better understanding of the changes in brain plasticity will provide further understanding of reversal of diseases and process of rejuvenation.

Since there is no formal regulation of training in India and, Indian Medical Association has yet to recognize its utility; a lot of teaching and therapy is done by people who call themselves trainers and masters. They would probably be doing some good since hypnosis is easy to induce and non-directed hypnotherapy also works. The feel good factor is ubiquitous. And, a random cure may also be seen. Placebo effect is well proven.

So what is applied by hypnotherapist today is based on the results of its clinical applications by his teachers, peers and by himself. What is achieved by one may not be duplicated by all the others; the same results may not be achieved in a similar patient; yet, in group therapy a large number of subjects are seen to benefit; to that extent it remains an art.

It may be stated as a generalization that hypnosis can help focus attention, rethink problems, relax, and respond to helpful suggestions. Hypnosis relies mainly on your ability to concentrate and on the faith and trust you have on hypnosis and the therapist....Hypnosis can alter perception of pain and other sensations and gain some control over emotional and physical responses...Hypnosis can help control chronic cancer pain, menstrual pain and headaches; make labour and child-birth more comfortable; decrease the amount of medication needed during surgery; and shorten surgery recovery time...Hypnosis has been shown to alleviate the symptoms of irritable bowel syndrome and those of asthma. Subjects can gain control of unwanted behaviours such as tobacco smoking, bed-wetting, nail-biting, teeth-grinding, phobias, overeating, and difficulty in sleeping.[1] These types of random observations are frequent in literature. On the other hand, results of clinical trials verge on the bizarre.

What is derived from the phenomena in hypnosis, it can be derived that hypnosis can have its application in enhancing memory and creativity, in restoring normalcy to psychological disorders and to control of those conditions that are primarily due to autonomic nervous system disorder. There is clear evidence of stress alleviation and therefore, all conditions associated or due to stress itself may be definitely helped. Hormonal dysfunction may not be restored to normalcy: but hypnosis will help in treating it. The beneficiary effect of hypnosis in autoimmune diseases may occur after prolonged therapy but where there would be no definite treatment there is a chance and hope. We examine these possibilities in detail.

- *Memory and Creativity Enhancement*

This matter has been discussed in detail in Chapters on Phenomena in hypnosis as well as in Transformation in trance.

- *Pain*

The commonest symptom that the patients seek relief from is pain. Before we discuss the use of hypnosis for its relief, let us revise a few physiological facts. Factors affecting response to pain are:

- Attitude to pain that is developed in early childhood by parents or guardian
- Personality type
- Individual tolerance
- Age
- Gender
- Social learning
- Socio-cultural background
- Environment
- Level of anxiety, fear, stress
- Neurotic compensation and neurotic defenses

Pain is a body language. The semantics of this language are modified by any or all of above. This is proven from the fact that in at least 50 per cent of the subjects under study, more than 50 per cent of pain relief is experienced with a placebo. The placebo effect is well known and better understanding is still emerging with the help of advanced scanning methods about the exact location of the areas involved. The frontal and prefrontal lobes seem to be the sites of action for placebo effect.

The description of pain by the subject by using various adjectives is noted. It may be described like aching, biting, binding, burning, corroding. Crushing, cutting, dull, grinding, gripping, heavy, hot, numb, nauseating, penetrating, piercing, pinching, sharp, shooting, smarting, spasmodic, splitting, squeezing, stabbing, throbbing, tingling, twisting. This helps in not only in establishing a diagnosis but also in rapport building, planning a strategy for therapy and insight generation.

The following agents are causative for pain sensation:

1. Damaged tissue releases certain chemicals (bradykinin, serotonin, histamine, K ions, ATP, ADP etc.) of which bradykinin is the most powerful in causing tissue damage pain. These chemicals stimulate chemical pain receptors and cause pain. But they also reduce the

threshold for excitation for mechanosentitive and thermosentitive receptors.

2. *Ischemia*: Blockage of the blood flow to the tissues causes severe pain. Pain is caused due to accumulation of lactic acid in tissues due to anaerobic mechanisms during ischemia. Other agents such as bradykinin, proteolytic enzymes may also be released.
3. *Muscle Spasm*: It causes pain due to direct stimulation of mechanosentitive receptors as well as indirect effect due to spasm of blood vessels.

There is an emotional component to pain. It is accompanied by unpleasantness. Long standing pain causes irritation, frustration, depression etc.

Pain Sensation Transmission to the Brain

The mechanism of pain perception is both local and central. Pain sensation has a dual pathway, one for the fast pain and other for the slow pain. This is transmitted by two different types of fibers; one type, fast relaying sensations to the sensory cortex and the slow type, to the thalamus and other centers located lower.

A few fibers from spinothalarnic tract terminate in reticular areas of the brain stem, but most of them pass upwards and terminate in ventrobasal complex of thalamus along with dorsal column pathway. A few fibers terminate in posterior nuclear group of the thalamus. From thalamus, fibers pass to the basal areas of brain and to the somatic sensory cortex.

When tactile receptors are also stimulated along with fast pain fibers, localization of fast pain is exact. If only pain receptors are stimulated, localization is poor.

Pathways for Slow Pain

Fibers transmitting slow pain terminate very widely in the brain stem in one of the three areas: (a) reticular nuclei of medulla, pons, mesencephalon, (b) tectal area, (c) periaqueductal grey region. From reticular areas impulses are transmitted to intralaminar nuclei of thalamus, into certain portions of hypothalamus and adjacent areas of basal brain. Localization of pain transmitted in this pathway is poor.

There is an analgesic or pain control system of brain. In this analgesic system several transmitter substances are involved especially, encephalin and serotonin.

Many fibers from periventricular area and periaqueductal grey area release, encephalin. Fibers terminating in the spinal cord and originating in raphe magnus nucleus cause release of serotonin. This serotonin acts on local cord neurons that secrete encephalin. Encephalin causes presynaptic inhibition of both types of incoming fibers, where they synapse in dorsal horn. This is done by blocking calcium channels in the membranes of the nerve terminals. This analgesic system blocks the pain signals at the initial entry point to the spinal cord. It can block many local cord reflexes that result from pain signal. e.g. withdrawal reflex.

Role of Opiate Receptors and Endorphin in Modulating Pain

Endorphins are the neuropeptides, which resemble morphine and they show activity on various opiate receptor known as Delta, Kappa (k), and min (m). These receptors when stimulated by endorphins inhibit pain pathways (create analgesia), cause sedation, euphoria and wide range of other activities as caused by morphine.

The area called periaqueductal gray, located around the aqueduct between the 3rd and 4th ventricles of midbrain, is filled with opiate receptors, making it a control area for pain. By breath watching (*pranayama*), it is hypothesized, that a subject is able to plug into the periaqueductal gray, gaining access to it, he is able to reset pain threshold. Thus by conscious breath watching (technique employed by yogis) one cause the peptides (endorphins) to diffuse rapidly throughout the CSF, in an attempt to restore homeostasis. Endorphins, the body's natural opiates, as well as other kinds of pain relieving substances achieve diminution of pain. The release of endorphins can also be brought about through modulation of the state of consciousness as in hypnosis, meditation etc.

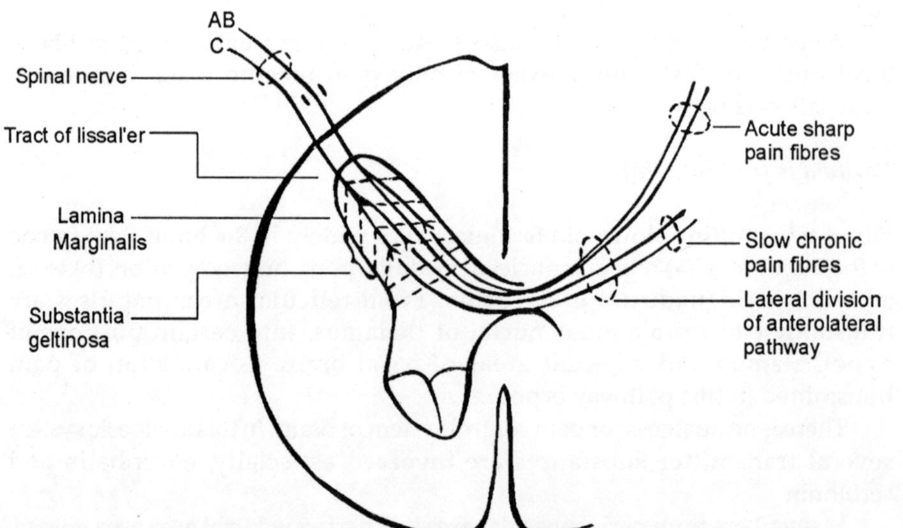

Fig. 14.1: Need for Different Strategies for Pain Relief Transmission of "Acute-Sharp" and Slow-Chronic" Pain Signals through the Spinal Cord

Pain is a protective mechanism. Therefore, before alleviating it, diagnosis, evaluation and assessment are done. Any kind of pain can be tackled with hypnosis. But the treating person has to know what exactly he/she is dealing with.

Patient with chronic pain will require multidimensional approaches. If the cause is established it should be known and is useful in utilizing for metaphor and suggestions. The attitude of the subject to the pain is assessed from behaviour of the subject with surrounding, interpersonal relationship with family members, environment and the coping mechanism.

Visceral Pain

There are various type of visceral pain receptors. Nociceptors receptors respond selectively to more than one modality, usually having high thresholds to

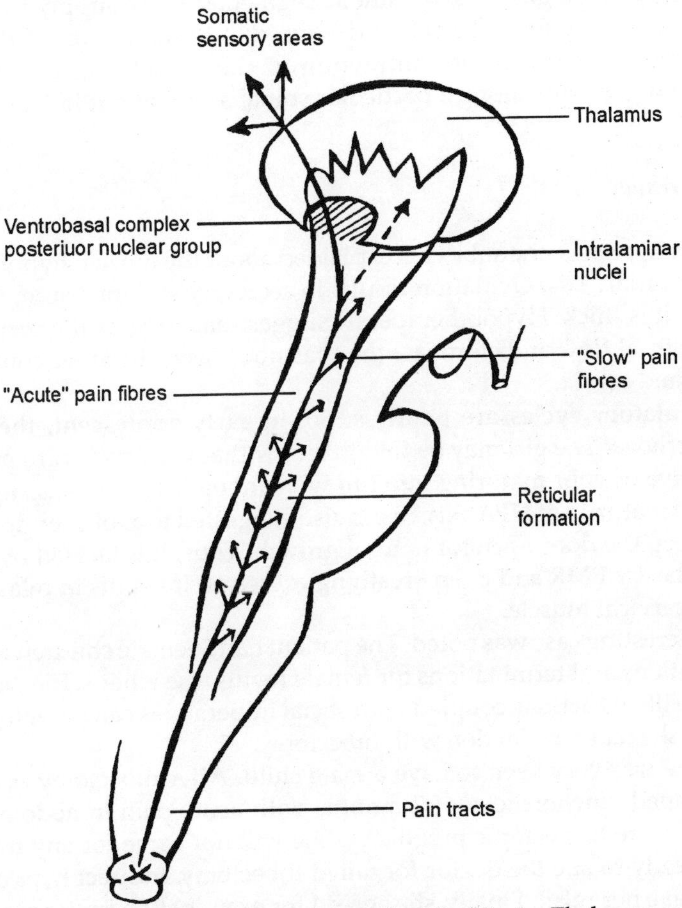

Fig. 14.2: Transmission of Pain Signals into the Hind Brain, Thalamus and Cortex

damaging stimuli. It responds to damaging stimuli, associated with irritation or pain. Nociceptors at the peripheral nerve endings are more sensitive to the substances like cytokines and the growth factors such as tumor necrosis factor and nerve growth factor. So, instead of analgesic substances antihyperalgesic substances may be more effective when considering drug therapy.

Interoceptors are receptors in the walls of the viscera, glands and vessels. Nerve terminals occur in all the layers of visceral walls. They are also in adventitia of blood vessels. Vagus, glossopharyngeal and other cranial nerves with hypogastric plexus and lumbar splachnic nerves control the pain sensation of viscera peripherally.

As mentioned above periaqeductal grey matter, with dorsal raphe nucleii, hypothalamus, amygdala and frontal somatosensory afferents have endogenous analgesic system. Substances secreted by them such as endorphin, enkephalin, and many more relieve pain.

As seen from above, viscera are supplied by both, autonomic central supply from vagus and ganglionic sympathetic segmental nerve supply from spinal cord regions. Therefore, the referred pain, due to distension of the organ, inflammation, or spasm or contraction of the muscles of the viscera is experienced generally along a particular spinal segment but its perception is central.

Dysmenorrhoea

In indirect hypnosis, the subject is explained about the normal hypothalamic-pitutary-ovarian axis. Ovulation results in secretory endometrium. So, when it is shed, it is thick. Hypnotherapeutic suggestions to relax the cervix allow easy menstrual flow and eliminate the spasmodic asynchronous contractions of uterus and cervix.

Anovulatory cycles are painless. So, in early adolescent, there is no dysmenorrhoea. The girl may be told that now that your cycles are painful, it is suggestive of your maturing into full womanhood. This acts as suggestion for normal maturity of HPA axis. She is also suggested to avoid cervical spasm so as to keep the door open for natural growth. Thus, it is tackled by making patient relax by PMR and deep breathing exercises. It results in relaxation of spasm of cervical muscle.

An interesting case was noted. The patient had 3 female children and 4 sex determinations and terminations for female foetus else where. The emotional load of the illegal actions coupled with social imperatives can be well gauged. Fifth time she had termination with tubectomy.

Yet, she was very keen to have a male child. After tubectomy operation, she developed amenorrhoea of 2 months with acute pain in abdomen. The symptoms were like ectopic pregnancy. She will not agree for any treatment and was ready to sue the doctor for failed tubectomy. Indirect hypnosis was done to make her relax. Finally, she agreed for examination under anesthesia.

Cervical dilatation was done and blood was drained. Patient went home with pain relief and later on had regular periods without pain.

Dysparunia

The detail history including the childhood sexual abuse, psychosocial background and any childhood trauma usually gives clue to the cause of dysparunia. The controversy of planning the child between the couple and also between the couple and other family members need to be discussed. Any doubts, misconceptions and fear are discussed at the first meaning.

The indirect suggestions are derived from the history. The conflict about using the contraceptives, or other conflicts like wanting to have the male child only are likely causes of dysparunia. The normal anatomy of introitus, hymen and vagina is explained. Capacity of vagina to distend like rubber balloon at the time of delivery is described. Levator spasm is demonstrated by vaginal examination where two opposite levators form a bridge and close the introitus. Same is explained by showing as to how the masseters in the angle of the mouth are capable of closing the mouth.

The hypnotic suggestions are tailor made. The heavy rain is used as a metaphor for foreplay before intercourse as it helps in secretion of Bartholin's glands during arousal. The wet land indicates the softness.

Obstetric Management of Pain

The pain during antenatal period is usually the discomfort due to distension of abdomen. It occurs gradually over 9 months. It accommodates about 10 lbs. During indirect hypnosis, the time progression is utilized to say that baby to be born is going to be healthy. And when the mother takes nourishment, she is equipping the baby to live life with all the attributes like intelligence, immunological support, and so on. When stretch is appreciated usually pain disappears. Carrying a baby in the carrier of uterus, caring to make it grow completely—physically, intellectually, immunologically for 9 months in the uterus as an incubator to be the most successful person in the world is the most pleasant thing in life. It is possible only for a woman to do it. This kind of prestige enhancement is enough to win the confidence and co-operation of most expectant mothers during antenatal period so that she is prepared for normal delivery.

It is noted world-wide that there is increase in the rate of Caesarian delivery. This is in spite of social and medical audit. Apart from the greed of the obstetricians, the main reason for the increase in the incidence is enhanced apprehension and fear of labour pain by the new generation of expectant mothers. Fear and apprehension cause spasm of the cervix through autonomic nervous system action. This retards dilatation causing inco-ordinate uterine action.

Delivery under Hypnosis

Antenatal exposure to hypnosis is very useful but is not a must. It is particularly easy to establish rapport with a woman in labour when she is assured that she is going to get additional help to relieve/alleviate her pain. There are two components to painless labour under hypnosis. She has to be relaxed between the contractions; this prevents incordinate uterine action. For pain relief, a suitable procedure is to induce glove and stocking anesthesia and transfer it to abdomen and perineum.

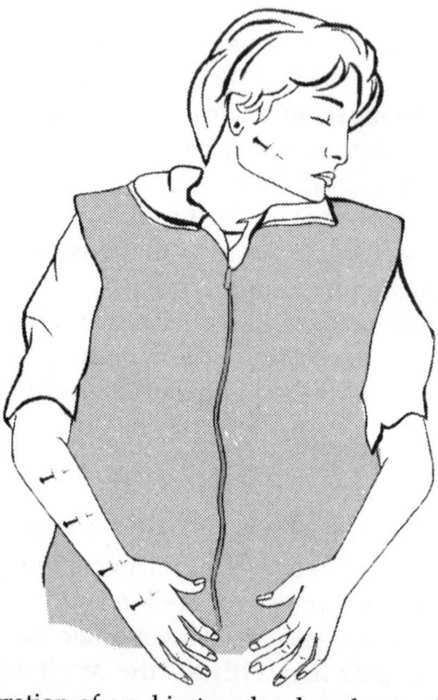

Fig. 14.3: An illustration of a subject under deep hypnotic trance showing hypnoanesthesia. Note the transfer of anesthesia to the cheek.

Summary

Summarising, studies of hypnotherapy suggest a benefit for various types of pain, including low back pain, surgery-related pain, cancer pain, dental procedure-related pain, burn pain, repetitive strain injury, temporomandibular joint disorders, sickle cell disease-related pain, irritable bowel syndrome, oral mucositis, tension headache and chronic pain. A 1995 consensus statement by the U.S. National Institutes of Health notes that, "Evidence supporting the effectiveness of hypnosis in alleviating chronic pain associated with cancer seems strong. with other data suggesting the effectiveness of hypnosis in other chronic pain conditions, which include irritable bowel syndrome, oral mucositis, temporomandibular disorders, and tension headaches."

Psychological Disorders and Psychiatric Conditions[2]

Trance phenomena have been utilized as part of religious and healing rituals in all ages and cultures since the earliest recorded history. The loss of control by the subject in the trance, the bizarre muscular movements, and the vivid imagery that is released have suggested "possession" by spirits and extramundane forces that have led observers to link hypnosis with mysticism and the paranormal. It is only recently that attempts have been made at scientific investigation of hypnosis in an effort to understand how it influences behaviour and particularly its therapeutic potentials. Modern uses of hypnosis embrace its employment of paradox, imagery evocation, double binds and variety of other interventions. Recently the dramatic innovative techniques of Milton Erickson have been analyzed (Rossi, 1980,[3] Zeig[4], 1985a and b) with the object of distilling from them strategies that can enhance the therapeutic process. Some new ideas have emerged from this contemporary work including: "neurolinguistic[5] programming" (Bandler & Grinder[6] 1975) through which an attempt is made to manipulate unique individual thought process in order to effectuate changes in behaviour and feelings.

Scientific studies have shown that employed by reasonably trained professionals, within the context of a structured therapeutic programme, with awareness of limits of its application, hypnosis can make a contribution as an adjunct to any of the manifold branches of psychotherapy, whether these be supportive, re-educative, or psychoanalytic.

Most professionals who are fearful of hypnosis as a therapeutic tool, or exaggerate its virtues, either have never experimented with it for a time sufficient to test the method or else are victims of superstition, prejudices or naïve magical expectancy. A number of spokesmen for hypnosis, some writing extensively, discredit it by over dramatizing the process, by exaggerating its powers, by participating in and publishing results of poorly conceived experiments, by engaging in naively organized therapeutic schemes, most elementary precepts of dynamic psychology, or by promulgating its presumed dangers for which there is little basis in fact (Wolberg[7], 1956).

Psychodynamics of Hypnotherapeutic Process

How hypnosis aids in securing therapeutic effects is not entirely clear, but we may postulate two important influences. First, hypnosis rapidly produces a remarkable rapport with the therapist, irrespective of the fact that this is probably linked to some anachronistic regressive dependency need. A strong impact is registered on the therapeutic working relationship. The placebo influence, a component of all therapies, is strongly enhanced. Suggestion, another universal component of all treatment processes, is so expanded in hypnosis that the patient responds sensitively and with dramatic readiness to both indirect, subtle persuasions by the therapist and to direct commands and injunctions that are not too anxiety provoking. The relationship with the therapist become endowed with noble, protective, and even magical qualities. The ultimate result of these combined forces can be substantive relief from a sense of mastery, which in themselves may restore adaptive defenses and produce a symptomatic cure.

Hypnosis as a Therapeutic Tool in Psychiatric Conditions

Hypnosis as a relaxing agency has been employed in physical and psychological disturbance that are characterized by stress and tension, since stress may have a damaging effect on all bodily functions. Its amelioration can be important for healing (Wolberg, 1957). Tension relief may, on the basis of suggestions during the trance state, be supplemented perhaps by self hypnosis (Wolberg, 1965) or by such techniques as autogenic training (Luthe[8], 1963; Luthe *et al.*[9] 1963).

Where the symptom does not bind too much anxiety or where its pleasure and masochistic values are not too intense, it may be possible to alleviate it by hypnotic suggestion without symptom substitution. Not only may the ensuing relief initiate a better adjustment, but also it may set off a chain reaction that, reverberating through the entire personality structure, influences its other dimensions. Suggestive hypnosis may also be of value in controlling the ruminations of chronic obsessive compulsive patients whose preoccupations immerse them in interminable misery by helping such victims to divert their thinking in anxiety and a better adaptation, With caution hypnosis may be adopted as a suggestive instrument in controlling certain habits such as overeating, excessive smoking, and insomnia. The phrasing of suggestions here is important.

Some therapists still use hypnosis like magic wand to dissipate in thin air symptoms that hamper the adjustment of the patient. While symptom removal by hypnosis is justified where the symptom blocks therapy, as in emergencies or where more extensive therapy cannot be applied, one must realize its limitations. For so long as we depend solely upon the authoritarian power with which the hypnotic situation automatically invests us, our therapeutic effectiveness will be no greater, and often will be less than miraculous healing.

The use of hypnosis in exploratory psychotherapy, such as in the insight approaches, is contingent upon the influence of hypnosis on unconscious resistance that in resolution helps the individual establish closer contact with repressed needs and conflicts. It may thus be possible to bring to the surface significant memories and repressed impulses that expedite the analytic process (Wolberg, 1964a; 1986).

Hypnosis is particularly useful in freeing verbalizations, in liberating transference and in helping the patient to recall dreams. Where anxiety blocks speech the mere induction of a trance may serve to release a verbal discharge. Moreover the provocation of transference feeling may bring to the surface painful emotions as well as fantasies that sometimes burst through with intense violence. Where free associations have been blocked for one reason or another, hypnosis may suffice to restore this form of communication. Hypnosis may serve also as a means of stimulating dreams in patients who are unable to remember them or who have "dried up" in their analytic productiveness.

In behaviour therapy hypnosis is useful in various ways. First it establishes in the mind of the patient the authority of the therapist who will act as the reinforcing agency. Under these circumstances positive counter-conditioning, aversive conditioning, extinction and other tactics will be catalyzed. Second, by promoting relaxation through hypnosis a positive stimulus is supplied that becomes affiliated with the conditioned stimulus and helps to extinguish it. Third, on the basis of suggestion the objectives of the therapist once explicitly defined may be more easily accepted. The patient is encouraged to behave in emotionally constructive ways in quest of reversing established patterns or correcting behavioural deficits. Thus in the method of desensitization through reciprocal inhibition, anxiety-provoking cues are presented in a climate of relaxation in progressively stronger form.

Factors Influencing the Outcome of Hypnotherapy

There is no way of predicting in advance the exact influence hypnosis may have on the patient or problems since each individual will respond uniquely to the phenomenon of hypnosis in lien with the special personal meanings. The mental set toward hypnosis, the motivations to be helped, the depth and quality of resistance, the preparation for induction, ideas about the therapist, the skill of the therapist as a hypnotist, the quality of the suggestions administered, the management of the patient's doubts and oppositional tendencies and the nature of the transference and counter-transference will all enter into the responsive Gestalt.

Potentially, hypnosis may catalyze every aspect of the therapeutic process. Whether or not a therapist will want to employ it will depend largely on how much confidence one has in hypnosis and how well one works with hypnotic techniques.

Hypnosis is an intense emotional experience that may affect both patient and therapist. In the trance a dynamic configuration of many kind of phenomena are constantly interacting in response to functional psychophysiological changes within the individual and the specific significance of the hypnotic interpersonal relationship. As attention is shifted from the external world toward the inner self there is an expansion of self-awareness and a lifting of repressions, with exposure of certain repudiated aspects of the psyche. A regressive kind of relationship develops between the subject and operator, the latter being promoted into the post of a kind of magical authoritative figure.

Hypnosis may also release powerful feeling in the therapist aspects of which in the form of counter transference may be inimical to the therapeutic objective. Particularly obstructive are omnipotent sadistic and sexual strivings. Only by experimenting with hypnosis can a therapist determine whether one is personally capable of employing is as a therapeutic adjunct. While one may be able to do good psychotherapy with the usual psychotherapeutic techniques attempts at hypnosis may alter one's manner toward the patient in ways that may prove antitherapeutic. Thus, a therapist may act aggressively toward patients perceived to be in a helpless state. Coordinately one may become suffused with feelings of grandiosity. Or one may as a projected Svengali figure find oneself sexually attracted to a patient whom one regards as passively seductive. Should these feelings arise in spite of measures to control them, it is best to pursue a pattern of caution and refrain from employing hypnosis in practice.

Hypnosis, then, is merely a device to facilitate the psychotherapeutic process rather than substitution for it. No problems need be anticipated in the induction of hypnosis and in the application of hypnotic and hypnoanalytic procedures, if the therapist masters at least one of the standard techniques, applies it confidently while constantly observing the reactions of the patient and of oneself. Protracted dependency reactions are no more common than in psychotherapy without hypnosis. It goes without saying that hypnosis is no substitute for careful training, extensive experience and technical competence. It will not make up for lacks in judgement or skill. However, a sophisticated psychotherapist who has learned how to utilize hypnosis has available to himself a most important adjunctive tool.

Therapeutic Applications

Many psychiatric inpatients may be incapable of sustained trance experiences. In general medical settings and in outpatient treatment, however, hypnosis can augment a variety of therapeutic strategies; the higher that a patient's hypnotizability is, the more likely a positive outcome will be. The clinician must remember however that a patient's hypnotizability per se does not make hypnosis an effective treatment for that person. Other important factors include motivation to change the presence of secondary gain and the transference and/or alliance with the therapist.

- ***Medical and Surgical Procedures***

Hypnosis is a powerful adjunct for patients undergoing variety of procedures. The relaxation and dissociation it provides decrease anxiety and discomfort. Its influence on the autonomic nervous system can produce selective bleeding. Hypnosis even if it is introduced only in the pre-anesthetic induction setting can establish positive expectation about surgical outcomes and can speed recovery. A recent controlled study demonstrated that formal hypnosis can diminish the procedure and recovery time (Lang[10] *et. al.*, 2000). Pediatricians may find that providing their healthy young patients with a "magic spot" which the patient controls and can apply as needed (e.g., for immunization, for suturing lacerations) to be useful.

- ***Medical Conditions***

Hypnosis has been applied with mixed success, to a broad variety of medical conditions. Unfortunately the results remain mostly anecdotal with few well-controlled trials in the literature. Nonetheless, because the risks of hypnosis are quite low (barring inadequate diagnostic evaluation and masking of important symptoms), clinicians may find the use of suggestion in hypnosis to be beneficial in many different settings (Pinnell and Covino[11], 2000). Among the conditions reported to respond to hypnosis are irritable bowel syndrome, asthma, migraine, warts and psoriasis. (*Note*: Each of these is an episodic condition in which exacerbations can be produced by stress).

- ***Psychosomatic Illnesses***

Some medical condition with large affective and stress related components, such as asthma, can be susceptible to intervention with hypnosis. The technique is similar to that used for anxiety. It consists of teaching the patient to master his or her somatic responses in the face of an atopic or emotional stress to prevent further decompensation.

- ***Anxiety***

Patients with recurring anxiety can be helped to interrupt the "snowballing" effect of their somatic and psychological tension. In such situations hypnosis can be used to disconnect the somatic symptoms from the subjective psychological distress. Patients are taught to use self hypnosis. In one self hypnosis exercise, for example the patients imagine themselves relaxed and floating in a comfortable chair while picturing their concerns on an imaginary split movie screen. On one half of the screen are seen the anxieties and problems; on the other half are the patient's own internal resources-stabilizing relationships, achievements and abilities.

- ***Panic Attacks***

Patients with panic attacks can be helped with hypnosis in several ways. One is the use of relaxation and the split screen technique. Patients are instructed to picture a feared situation on one side of the screen and means of coping with it, or other psychological resources, on the other, all the while maintaining the feeling of floating. The screen may also be used to estimate the real risk and to diffuse the confusion between probability and possibility that affects many patients with panic attacks or phobias. The enhanced control over the physical response that is obtained through hypnosis can help anxious and phobic patients master their physical symptoms instead of feeling frightened by them. The initial stimuli remain but the helplessness and immobilization are contained. The success of this particular technique is compromised when the anxious patient is unable to bind or contain the anxiety long enough to permit to mild anxiety. Hypnosis can also be used for the identification of triggers and for panic attacks and for desensitization to both the triggers and the panic experience itself. Hypnoanalytical work has the potential for uncovering and repairing unresolved conflicts that may be expressing themselves in panic attack.

- ***Simple Phobias***

These respond well to behaviour therapy, but they may also respond to hypnosis which in some instances, is less time consuming. Phobia patients can be taught to bring on a sense of relaxation and well being using the technique described elsewhere. For example, patients with flying or "floating with the plane" as if the plane were an extension of their own out bodies. For all simple phobias, the patient and therapist work out a series of steps involving exposure to the feared object or situation coupled with a self hypnotic state of relaxation. Again the goal is to contain the anxiety and to promote a sense of mastery.

Alternatively some clinicians find that phobias such as fear of flying can be approached by asking patients to visualize a successful outcome in the future e.g., walking off the plane at the planned destination and slowly playing their mental tape or imagery backward until they can see the entire sequence, e.g. from leaving their home to arriving at their destination as a series of successes. These same approaches can be helpful in patient who is anxious about a procedure such as surgery or, something they must accomplish such as a performance at a sporting event. For illustrative cases, see the Chapter on Transformation through trance.

- ***Obsessions and Compulsions***

A special case of anxiety control involves the alleviation of some the distress and anxiety that either alters the threshold and produces an increased frequency of obsessive threshold and compulsive action or results from attempts or an inability to resist them. The goal is to enhance the patient's sense of calmness and comfort thereby raising the threshold for the emergency of these unwanted experiences; one approach involves using hypnosis to place time boundaries around them. Once the patient with a compulsion to clean has been hypnotized, for example, he or she is asked to imagine spending 1 hour a day thoroughly cleaning the bathroom. After several sessions the patient would then the asked (while in a trance state) to describe the activities and feelings involved. Next, the therapist uses posthypnotic suggestion to give the patient the task of actually cleaning the bathroom in question within 1 hour limit. If this goal is met the patient is them helped to reduce the time (e.g. to 15 min per day).

Hypnosis can also be used to determine whether thoughts or contexts exit that lower the patient's threshold for the emergency of the obsessive thoughts and action. For patients with more severe symptoms and distress (e.g. those meeting the criteria for obsessive compulsive disorder) hypnosis rarely works as a primary treatment. It can have value as an adjunctive therapy in further reducing an unwanted behaviour (e.g. hair pulling in a patient who has had partial response to medication or behaviour therapy).

Obsessive compulsive symptom can be thoughts of as existing on a spectrum ranging from the most biologically determined to the most psychologically determined. Many patients with obsessive compulsive symptoms have dissociative difficulties as well (Frederick and Mcneal[12], 1999). At times hypnoanalytical work can help to resolve the psychopathologic underpinnings of obsessions and compulsions.

- ***Dissociative Disorders and Conversion Symptom***

Although hypnosis is considered by many to be extremely helpful in working with patients with dissociative disorders, the nature and treatment of these disorders has become a theoretical, forensic and political battleground in recent times (Brown *et al.*[13] 1997). Many patients with dissociative amnesia or fugue can be treated with simple hypnotic age regression. Highly hypnotizable people may be prone to conversion symptoms. They may be "willing" to give up or to eliminate these symptoms when the secondary loss has exceeded the gain. Hypnotic suggestion can be used to reduce, to exaggerate or, to transfer a symptom thereby showing the patients how to enhance control over that symptom. This should be done in the context and that does not interpret resistances. A nonhypnotizable patient is more likely to have hypochondriasis or a nonpsychogenic problem.

The diagnosis and treatment of trauma and dissociation is a rapidly developing field. The use of newer diagnostic tools has led many to believe that the incidence of serious dissociative disorders such as dissociative identity disorder is much higher than was previously believed. The diagnosis and treatment of dissociative identity disorder can be extremely complex. Although age regression and abreaction (recalling and reexperiencing or reliving suppressed or repressed events) of traumatic memory material can be used at times in the treatment of dissociative identity disorder and other serious dissociative condition, emphasis has shifted to phase-oriented treatment models in which the use of hypnosis for stabilization ego strengthening and mastery achieve prominence. Current standards of care require that hypnotically facilitated abreaction be conducted only in stabilized patients who have good ego strength and who have leaned how to exercise mastery over trauma material. The therapist must always use extreme caution in avoiding any suggestion to patients that trauma or abuse has occurred.

When working with the patient the therapist must be prepared to deal with emerging traumatic memory material, which may or may not be associated with accurate recall of actual traumatic events per se and the traumatic transference and counter transference associated with childhood trauma or abuse. Training in trauma and dissociation is now considered to be necessary for those who treat posttraumatic and dissociative disorder and additional advance education in hypnosis is essential for those who wish to use it for treating these populations especially for the victims of rape.

- ***Habits***

Hypnosis can facilitate a strategy of self affirmation in dealing with difficult problems such as smoking. Self-hypnosis is a widely used aid to smoking cessation. It is used in the context of the cognitive restructuring of the urge to smoke and it involves having the patients focus instead on a commitment to respect and protect his or her body. For example the patient is instructed during the trance to repeat "for my body, smoking is a poison. I need my body to live. I owe my body the respect and protection of not smoking. I am responsible for my body. I am a nonsmoker" Patients learn to stop smoking not by fighting the urge to smoke but rather by connecting this urge to broader interests in health and protection of the body. Some clinicians present the patient with a model in which smoking is seen as a conditioned response to external stimuli such as situation specific stress. Patients are then shown how to use hypnosis to extinguish that conditioned response by playing out in their trance how the presentation of the stimulus does not need to be followed by the evoked response. Hypnosis is used to illustrate to the patients the way that they relate to their bodies and how their bodies are dependent on them. Hypnosis is likely to be most successful when it is incorporated into a total treatment plan that includes group therapy and possibly the use of nicotine containing preparations (e.g., patches, gum) or the pro-dopaminergic agent, bupropion.

Similar approaches are used to help some patients who overeat especially those who overeat when anxious. Little success had been found for the use of hypnosis in the treatment of addiction to alcohol or other abusable substances. Hypnosis has also been applied to bruxism, nail bitting, gagging, tongue thrusting, enuresis and other habit disorders.

Spontaneous Hypnosis

A subgroup of patients may require training in how not to enter the trance mode. These extremely hypnotizable people are constantly being entranced by others are working to please them and are suspending their own critical judgement. Here the trance induction is used as a demonstration of how susceptible they are and they are taught how to control their own tendency to slip into trance states. Spontaneous hypnosis can also be observed to occur in houses of worship and in the emergency departments of hospitals.

Prof. Khurana, now diseased, here presents a classical and conservative comprehensive overview of hypnotherapy as a clinical tool. When seen as a tool in the armamentarium for the psychotherapist, the presentation gives us a panoramic view of its uses as an adjunct; with definitive curative therapeutic uses in a few conditions like fugue, phobia etc.

Teaching a diploma course at M.S. University, along with him and several others in the faculty, we have chiseled out a finely tuned strategy for hypnotherapy that is based on Ericksonian model, that is in consonance with Rossi's thesis of gene arousal and relies heavily on suggestions based on archetypal symbols relevant to Indian ethos. This has widened the ambit of our hypnotherapeutic field, so that apart from what he refers to as, "anecdotal success here and there", we have been having successful outcomes in a variety of conditions that range from what he has classically described to several other clinical conditions; say, success has been consistent with migraine, asthma, myofascial syndrome etc. What is noteworthy is the successful outcome in cervical rib syndrome, trigeminal neuralgia, prolapsed intervertibral disc, osteoarthritis of knees, infertility of unknown origin and such other conditions that are discussed later.

> For the sake of completion, we draw an exhaustive list of conditions, compiled by U.S. National Institute of Health. It lists the conditions where hypnotherapy has been tried with variable results.

Agoraphobia (fear of crowds), Alzheimer's disease, Amenorrhea, Anticoagulation (blood thinning), Arrhythmias (abnormal heart rhythms), Attention-deficit hyperactivity disorder, Bedwetting, Bleeding, Hysterical Blindness Blisters, Breast enhancement, Bruises, Cancer, Cancer chemotherapy, Cerebral palsy, Chronic diarrhea, Chronic dyspnea (shortness of breath), Chronic fatigue syndrome, Confidence building, Congenital ichthyosiform erythroderma (a skin disorder), Constipation, Conversion disorder (an anxiety disorder), Cystic fibrosis, Depression, Diabetes mellitus, Dissociative identity disorder, Eating disorders, Endurance, Enhanced concentration, Enhancement of immune system, Enhancement of memory, self-esteem, study skills, vision, Fear of flying, Gastritis, Peptic ulcer, Genital herpes, Gastroesophageal reflux, Gout, Graves' disease, Grief, Hay fever, Heart disease, Hemolytic anemia, High blood pressure, HIV/AIDS, Huntington's disease, hyperemesis gravidarum, hyperhydrosis, Hyperreflexic bladder, Increased strength, Infections, Infertility, Lactation stimulation, Law enforcement (recalling repressed memories), Life transition support, Maternal anxiety, Menopausal symptoms, Menstrual cramps, Migraine, Multiple sclerosis, Muscle spasm, Musculoskeletal disorders, Myasthenia gravis, Nail biting, Narcolepsy, Neurodermatitis, Panic disorder,

Parkinson's disease, Paruresis (psychogenic urinary retention), Pemphigus vulgaris (a skin disorder), Personality development, Phobias, Postpartum care, Post-traumatic stress disorder, Premenstrual syndrome, Pruritus (itchiness), Psychosomatic conditions, Raynaud's disease, Repressed memory recall, Restless leg syndrome, Saliva production control, Sleep terror disorder, Speech disorders, Stroke Systemic, lupus erythematosus, Thumb sucking, Tics, Tongue biting, Torticollis (neck spasms,) Trichotillomania (compulsive hair pulling), Tuberculosis, Ulcerative colitis, Vaginismus (involuntary spasm of vaginal muscles), Weight loss, Warts, Burn dressing, During radiation therapy, Rehabilitation of locomotor system, Grief and bereavement, Incontinence of urine, Encopresis (uncontrolled defecation), Psoriasis, Cardiac neurosis, Angina pectoris, Enhancement of Sports performance and in Dentistry.

Rather than rely on such arbitrary lists, the indication should be judged from the altered physiology that is implied in a patient. The rationale may then be derived as to what process from the entire gamut of hypnotic possibility can reverse the disease. For instance, it is known that irritable bowel syndrome is based on psychosomatic factors causing derangement of autonomic nervous system. And, hypnosis can set the autonomic nervous system back in balance. Same is the case with asthma. The skin derives from the same embryonic layer–ectoderm and reflects emotions. Therefore most skin conditions are amenable to hypnosis.

Emotions can alter the functions and even the structure of the skin. The course of some dermatological disorders can be modified favourably through hypnotherapy. Almost all modern textbooks on hypnosis cover dermatological disorders, e.g. condylomata acuminatum (Ewin, 1974), refractory dermatitis (Twerski and Naar, 1974), neurodermatitis (Lehman, 1978), blushing (Welsh, 1978), warts (Sheehan, 1978); (Johnson and Barber, 1978), and trichotillomania (Rowen, 1981; Galski, 1981).[14]

Hormonal balances in various diseases may not be possible to be restored to normal, but hypnosis may be employed as an adjunct. In autoimmune diseases, where there is hardly much to offer by the modern medicine, persistent hypnotherapy may produce such alleviation that life is restored to functional mode.

This method, based on scientific data and carried forward through logical positivism (in the absence of hard core scientific data) is best illustrated by the following discussion. There we go to provide extensions of hypnotherapeutic applications that are based on sound inductive logic. There after, the proof of the pudding will be in eating. We have found it very palatable. But let us review two instances from our practice critically. While the following instance is forward extension of a hypothesis, second example is how hypothesis translates into a breakthrough via research.

Forward extension of a hypothesis: Diseases of the Tissues of Mesenchymal Origin The connective tissue arises from the embryonic mesoderm.

> Apart from being tissue specific, it lies between the cells of all the organs of the body. Being in the nature of a matrix, it is scattered all over. Besides the fibrous tissue that may be present in any of the organs in the body, the entire muscle mass, bones and cartilages, all the fascia, tendons, tendon sheaths, synovial membranes and vessel walls are derived from the mesoderm. Moreover, many of the cells in the blood and lymph are derived from mesenchyme. And these cells permeate all the tissues except avascular tissue like cornea.

It is common understanding that the intercellular connective tissue has a structural role in maintaining contour and support. But the mesenchymal tissue also has a role in the defense, derived from the molecular components of the cells. These cells are fibroblasts, macrophages, plasma cells, mast cells, fat cells and pigment cells, in addition to the white blood corpuscles in the circulating blood.

The fibroblasts lay down the fibers which may be collagen, reticuliln or elastin type. They are concerned with the repair of the tissues. Other types of ground substances are several types of collagen, dermatan; laminins (of 18 different types), heparan and tenascin glucoprotein that guides the cell migrations.

Macrophages are phagocytic for bacteria as well as the damaged and dead tissue. They digest them through various lysosomes that they contain. Being part of the reticuloendothelial system, they have immunological role too. They are capable of migration in the tissues and fusion between themselves.

Lymphocytes and plasma cells are normally confined to the circulation and lymphoid tissue but permeate into connective tissue that is inflamed. They are immune competent cells.

Mast cells are rich source of histamine, serotonin and heparin.

Fat cells store fat, but that is not their sole function. They may be involved in the heat regulation. They also have specific receptors for hormones on their surface. Mobilization of the fat is both under the hormonal as well as nervous control through the release of noradrenalin.

Pigment cells are responsible for the formation of pigment in skin, iris and choroid. Their function is under the control of glucocorticoids.

The messenger molecules, particularly the mediators of stress systems affect the mesenchymal tissues. For instance, the glucocorticoids influence the activity of the fibroblasts, the fibrous tissue and chondroitin sulphate – the ground substance between the cells derived from fibroblasts, These actions are very wide ranging. They are described to some extent in the Chapters on Stress and Information substances.

Mechanism of the Pattern/Location of a Disease

There are conditions like collagen diseases that find generalized expression.

But the affliction of a tissue that is so wide spread is not be always in the generalized pattern all over the body. Why and how this could be so remains an enigma. The most simplistic explanation is to attribute a local manifestation to some mechanical cause. For instance, painful knee joints in old age are called osteoarthritis and the etiology is ascribed to wear and tear.

While this may indeed be so, the biological sciences of pattern formation and morphogenetic fields,[15] are indeed fascinating. The discussion involves space-time dimensions as well as development of "fields" that ranges from hard core scientific data to philosophical speculation. How the stem cells migrate to their ultimate location, what forces of intracellular changes make them to group together with some other cells, (if we were to call these "forces" autocrines,—the molecular information substances that a cell makes that in turn affects its "behaviour"), is still not clearly understood.

We have taken it for granted that oxygen is vital for the tissues. A cursory view of oxygen uptake by mitochondria gives the impression as if the gas molecules were talking to mitochondria. Since the messages are within the cell itself, by that restriction only, oxygen may not be called a messenger molecule. But when oxygen is involved in the form of hydrogen peroxide, the later does assume the character of a messenger molecule that has such wide ranging effects like angiogenesis and impervious nature of the cell wall of a fertilized ovum.

How the intercellular communication is brought about is too complex to be explained by the omnibus terms such as action of pericrines. The modulation of cell behaviour by hormones is well understood in the minutest details about the specific receptors and further molecular biological events. However, the localization of such actions is tissue specific, for instance the action of reproductive hormones on the reproductive organs.

Therefore, we have still to understand a great deal about the mechanism of affliction of a particular organ/region of mesenchymal origin.

Autoimmune Process

However, one fact is clear. The hypophyseal- pituary-adrenal axis has a pivotal role to play. This was unveiled by Hans Selye in 1936 in physiological terms, but the drama still goes on in therapeutics that began with the award of Nobel Prize jointly to Hench[16] and Kendall and Reichstein in 1950 following their demonstration of therapeutic effects of ACTH in rheumatoid arthritis.

The hormones of the adrenal cortex have such wide ranging effects that a detailed discussion is out of place here. The discussion in the chapter on stress will suffice: but a keen student of hypnotherapy should study the details in the textbooks of physiology[17] and pharmacology[18] so that, the complex pattern of physiology and pharmacology may be precisely understood. For the sake of wonder about the intricacy, a brief reference may be made about how a few molecules of the steroid hormone can bring about a cascade of molecular biological events through genes (Fig. 14.4). This is brought about by transmigration of steroid hormone molecule through the cell wall into the cytoplasm. Within the cell the hormone binds with its specific receptors. The hormone-receptor complex then tags on to the genetic DNA and causes it to replicate messenger RNA in abundance. This may change the behaviour.

Since thoughts, emotions and feelings generate messenger molecules, which in turn bring about a cascade of molecular biological events of the type depicted in the figure, it is plausible that similar events in the manipulation of the mind can bring about isomorphic events. This is the fundamental basis of hypnotherapy.

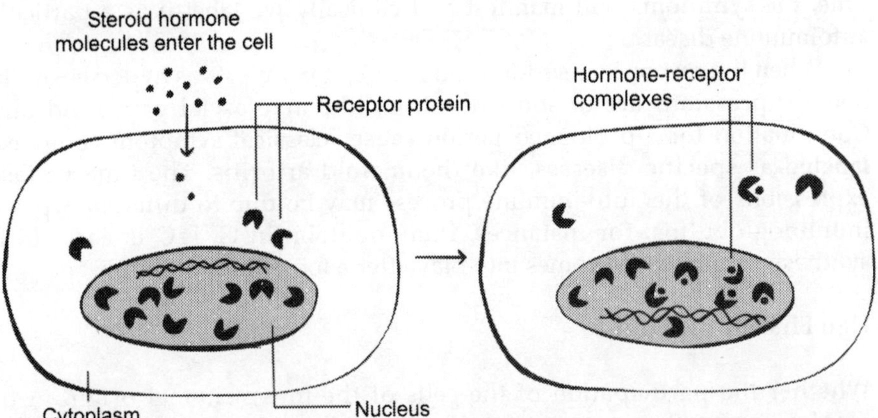

Steroid hormones diffuse across the plasma membrane and bind to specific reveptors within the cell. The hormone-receptor complex affects gene function by binding to chromatin in the nucleus

Fig. 14.4: Adopted from Molecular Biology of Gene, Watson *et al.*

It should also be evidently clear that the physiological secretion of these hormones are not at a constant rate; they pulsate as per the circadian and ultradian rhythms so as to maintain homeostasis that is state dependent to the external and internal environment.

In the formation of the ground substance and its maintenance, the role of Vitamin C and oxygenation (anoxia stifles the tissues, most important being the brain cells) is well established.

The ground substances,—collagen and like—have complex chemical structure of a large molecular weight that carries negative charge on it. It has high viscosity and is capable of binding water strongly. This is of relevance to our hypothesis that is enunciated below.

It is an enigma as to when and why and how the body silently starts derecognizing some tissues as non-self and begins to reject it[19]. As the proponents of mind-body continuum, we are convinced that it has psychodynamic origin. Any tissue that is not recognized as part of the self is, of course, treated as a foreign tissue and immune system starts a silent but sure process of rejecting it. The process involves decrease, degradation, destruction, isolation or ejection of the proteins that are now identified as non-self.

The entire process is a non-infective, inflammatory in nature. The cells, lymphocytes, basophils and eosinophils from the blood and tissue fibroblasts, mast cells, endothelial cells and resident macrophages in the local tissue, that actively participate, are all derived from mesenchyme. The autoimmune inflammatory process, though silent to begin with and therefore, asymptomatic, by the activation of these cells, in turn, activates stress system. At this point in time, the symptoms will manifest and clinically we label it as a particular autoimmune disease.

When the response is sudden and severe, it manifests as hypersensitivity. Some expressions are of short duration, like myofascial pain syndrome. Continuation for a prolonged period causes classical symptom complexes labeled as specific diseases, like rheumatoid arthritis. The time variable expressions of the auto-immune process may be due to different types of immunoglobulins; for instances, immunoglobulin G, IgG is early to be synthesized while IgM comes into play after a long time.

Hen First, or the Egg?

Whether the participation of the cells of the mesenchymal origin in the autoimmune inflammatory process causes the affliction of the tissues of mesemchymal origin; or autoimmune process against some of these tissues is the primary cause, is hard to tell. An autoimmune reaction towards a few anoxic muscle fibers at the trigger point by the fibroblasts and other locally occurring immune competent cells may precipitate an attack of myofascial syndrome, programmed through the psychodynamic neurolinguistic mechanism. The same process, somehow targeted at the collagen—which is a polysaccharide with a protein moiety—for a long period of time, manifests as one of the collagen diseases. Targeted at the small vessels all over the body, again for a prolonged period of time, the process manifests as vasculitis in lupus erythematosis.

At this juncture, it is important to visualize how different the process of homeostasis is from the rational, didactic, linear process of explaining the mechanism and its research investigations through the scientific methodology. Of necessity, when the action of a hormone, say cortisone, is explained or investigated, one variable is examined against a set of fixed parameters. It is like Newtonian physics: the cause and effects are directly measured. What happens in the organism is entirely different. Homeostasis is maintained by a vast array of innumerable interactions arising out of a single initial effect that may be visualized like the play of the pieces on a carom or billiard board; to be precise, it is governed by the laws of Chaotic physics. The result is predictable only up to a certain range[20] after a complex series of calculations and could be far beyond the expectation in terms of the magnitude.

Self and Non-self, Duality within the Self: Bodymind is One

What may trigger an autoimmune process is yet to be known. A smallest aberration in the protein component arising "accidentally" may activate the immune system or a sudden "derecognition" of certain cells transmutes them from "self" to "non-self". Emphasizing that the Bodymind is one entity, such an "accident" may be triggered psychodynamically. And the follow up response to restore homeostasis also has its psychodynamic initiation and propulsion.

Therefore, the pathogenesis of the clinical disease entities enumerated below, which are termed as syndromes because of ambiguity about their exact mechanism of origin, is difficult to be labeled as simply autoimmune, or stress mediated. It is also indeterminate whether the autoimmune inflammatory process may have begun initially to invoke the response of the stress system or whether the pulsatile nature of the activation of stress system was jolted into spurts and bursts. That may have knocked off the homeostatic balance causing the immune system to weaken and to false identification of "one's own flesh"[21] as "non-self". Whether the autoimmune response is towards some components of mesenchymal origin, such as dermis, fascia, synovial membrane, cartilage, laminin and so on or the clinical picture is due to the response of the immune component cells of the mesenchymal origin to some "auto antigen" is difficult to say.

The complex presentation appears to consist of both the components. The variable interaction between modulations of HPA-axis and immune mediated inflammation probably has a determinant role.

HPA Axis and Its Variable Response

An excessive HPA response does enhance resistance to autoimmune disease and conversely, a defective HPA-axis response can cause increased susceptibility to autoimmune disease. This is exemplified by the response of different strain of rats to stress. In Lewis rats hypothalamic CRH neurons respond poorly to neurotransmitters and the HPA-axis response to stress is decreased. The reverse is true for Fischer rats. It is yet to be proved that such isomorphism exists in humans. Considering that it is likely to exist, a distinctly different response form the individuals, based on their HPA-axis activity may categorize people into two type; at different phases in life.

That would mean[22] as follows (Table 14.1):

Table 14.1: Variable Response of HPA-axis

Increased HPA-axis activity	*Decreased HPA-axis activity*
Cushing syndrome	Adrenal Insufficiency
Melancholic Depression	Rheumatoid arthritis
Chronic Alcoholism	Atypical or seasonal depression
Chronic Stress	Chronic fatigue syndrome: fibromyalgia
Long term excessive exercise	Hypothyroidism
Last trimester of pregnancy	Post traumatic Stress Disorder
	Nicotine withdrawal
	After termination of treatment for Cushing Syndrome
	After glucocorticoid therapy
	Postpartum period
	After chronic stress
	Steroid resistant asthma
	Degenerative Osteoarthritis
	Systemic Lupus erythematosis
Fischer rat model: suppression of immune mediated interactions	Lewis rat model: activation of immune mediated reactions

Neuroimmunemodualtion[23]

Apart from the hormonal axis, there is concurrent neurological modulation as exemplified in the effects on the joints. Destruction of sensory innervation of joints whereby neurons responsible for secretion of substance P, somatostatin and such other tachykinins are destroyed, reduces the intensity of inflammatory arthritis. This indicates the role of nervous system in local release of neurotransmitters that can modify inflammatory process in synovial membrane, ligaments and cartilage. This is of particular relevance to osteoarthritis of knee as well as in various kind of dermatitis.

Hypothesis

Based on the influences of HPA-axis derived from chronic stress, the tissues of mesenchymal origin undergo inflammation. One gross feature of the inflammation is edema that causes swelling/rupture of the affected tissue. The swollen tissues, when encompassed by fixed, rigid surroundings get compressed producing clinical symptoms. Mechanical decompression by surgical means produces immediate relief.

The location of the lesion is determined neurolinguistically. Pathogenesis is psychodynamic as thoughts in form of suprathalamic stimuli → thalamus → when perceived with emotional content → hypothalamus and structures of the limbic system → activation and/or exhaustion of HPA axis; as well as neurological stimuli → effects on the tissues of mesenchymal origin.

The shorter the duration of the stressor, the relief of clinical symptoms is easier by hypnotherapy.

The Clinical Picture

Based on the above premise, we catalogue the following diseases/syndromes that may be amenable to treatment with hypnotherapy.

Diseases of nerves (The swelling of the nerves is due to the edema of the sheath of the nerve bundles).

1. Trigeminal Neuralgia
2. Facial Paresis/palsy
3. Brachial Plexus Syndrome/Cervical Rib Syndrome
4. Sciatica
5. Spinal nerve compression due to prolapsed intervertebral disc

Diseases of fascia/ligaments/fibrous tissue/synovial membrane:

1. Cervical Spondylitis
2. Frozen Shoulder
3. Tennis elbow
4. Carpal Tunnel Syndrome
5. Trigger finger
6. Duputryn's contracture (difficult to explain why not seen in India)
7. Rheumatoid arthritis
8. Osteoarthritis
9. Temporo-mandibular joint arthritis
10. Prolapsed intervertebral disc
11. Calcaneal Spur
12. Restless Leg Syndrome: Severe night cramps in the muscles of sole/ calf
13. Myofascial Pain Syndrome
14. Fibromyalgia

Diseases of Collagen: Collagen is lifeless in a living system. It has no cell, no cell apparatus, no chromosome and no genes. The influence over it can, therefore, be only indirect. This can be by the living cells, which generate it and/or by the immune competent cells which interact with it. The collagen diseases are:

1. Rheumatoid Arthritis
2. Systemic Lupus Erythematosus
3. Scelroderma
4. Polymyositis
5. Dermatomyositis
6. Sogrens Disease and Syndrome
7. Mixed Connective Tissue disease
8. Small vessel vasculitis

Auto immune diseases of tissues of mesenchymal origin elsewhere

1. Dermatitis of various non-infective types, psoriasis
2. Iridocyclitis
3. Acute and chronic glomerulomyelitis
4. Parkinson's Disease as well as Alzheimer's disease. The brain cells are being replaced by glial tissue in this condition. The mechanism of cell death seems to be anoxia. Whether it is glial proliferation that "strangulates and/or suffocates" the brain cells or it is secondary to the replacement of dead cells is difficult to say.

Relevance of Hypnotherapy

Hypnosis is an efficient de-stressor. Whenever a condition has arisen from the stress of a short duration, hypnotherapy will produce a gratifying outcome. The autoimmune process produces all the classical signs of inflammation. One of the dominant signs is edema of the inflamed tissue. The swelling so brought about increases the volume of the nervous/fibrous tissue. If this were to be passing from a rigid outlet, such as trigeminal nerve or a spinal nerve—the later is likely to be doubly increase in the size because of swelling of the fibrous components in the intervertebral disc—the neural tissue manifests signs of compression. These signs ameliorate when either the space is increased by surgical means or when the edema recedes when the inflammation becomes quiescent.

Acute on chronic or chronic stress management/coping requires a change of life style/behavioural change in the form of identification and response to stressor. In such situation, hypnotherapy will succeed provided it is carried out till such times as psycho-cybernetics bring about insight generation. That would also mean that the stressor is either eliminated or assimilated.

Hypnotherapy will certainly alleviate the stress associated with crippling collagen diseases. There can be no direct influence of the psyche on a non-living substance, particularly when the result is a product of false identity for several years. To change the long standing response of the immune system in collagen disorders psychodynamically is a tall order and is yet to be reported. But since the false identity could be due to deeply hidden forces in the unconscious mind, a protracted period of hypnotherapy may be justified, at least for clinical research. Isolated studies, like those from Simonton and Simonton[24] are an indicator of fertile hope. The nonreplicability of such trials points to the likelihood that finer nuances in psychodynamic manipulations may be missed.

How Hypothesis Translates into a Breakthrough via Research[25]

This is a brief account of our original research carried out in clinical settings. It was published as two original contributions in *J. Obst. Gyn. Ind.*, Vols. 52 and 53 in 2002-03.

The modern medicine has undergone a radical shift from Cartesian mechanistic view of the body. Mind body links are getting clear to understand mind body communication (Rossi, 1996) so that it is evident now that mind body is one. Each cell communicates with the other cell in various ways. The molecular biological basis of emotion is deciphered. Subsequently the division between the sciences of physiology, psychology, neuroscience, immunology and endocrinology is a historical artifact (Pert *et al.*, 1985). Thoughts are equated with floating particles in the blood stream (Reichlin, 1993). The information is transmitted non-contiguously by information substances (Schmitt 1984). This would mean that for most thoughts and particularly the thoughts with highly emotional contents, there is a corresponding physiological state that is encoded as memory by the body.

After the battery of investigations for infertility, have turned out normal, there is a big group of couples who remains unexplained. During the last decade or so, there have been many artificial reproductive techniques which have come forward. But it has really not given the definite results. Success rate in assisted reproduction is only about 15 per cent. From the feminist view, woman has now one more area where she is exploited in the service of science and species.

Linkage to stress as aetiopathlogy of reproductive failure is reported. The stress is of two different kinds, (i) the stress of barrenness and (ii) the stress that has caused the barrenness. The later component is not yet recognized widely and we are the first in the world literature to have published a large study (Vyas *et al.*, 2002, Vyas *et al.*, 2003). It is possible to explore the etiology in minds of such couples at the conscious, subconscious and unconscious psychic planes.

Femininity is synonymous with deep experiential feelings. When feelings connected with sexuality is concerned, man also is affected at all levels of consciousness.[26] This has been the basis of hypothesis that psychodynamic reverberations of negative emotional feelings result in stress. Chronic stress dislocates hormonal axis to cause reproductive failure.

We have been working over 40 years with unexplained reproductive failure. The observations are very revealing. It was maladjustments or negative feelings with husband, or with the family of either. There were tremendous negative feelings particularly to mother in law or society. When conscious about them, they were helpless/unable to cope with them. These were either repressed to subconscious or unconscious. The negative feelings were in the nature of conflict, fear, intense desire[27] or hyperanxiety.

- ***Conflicts***

The conflicts covered a wide range of personal, inter personal, social and cultural issues. Disparity of education, socio-economic strata and also the shift from a larger city to a smaller city were causes for maladjustment. Professional disparity, gender status considerations, discord for career expectations were points of conflict. A joint family was a common cause for conflict. Second marriage, hostility to either partner or to his\ her family were noticed often.

- ***Fear***

Fear of child bearing, caring, rearing, early abortion, family history of sterility, fear of pain, late age of marriage are seen to be operant at subconscious mind. Fear based on either history of or having suffered from ectopic pregnancy, previous traumatic delivery or having had a congenitally malformed child or previous Caesarian section, is also contributory. Apprehension that any of the partner's medical illness may be passed over to offspring weighed very heavily on the couple's mind.

- ***Hyperanxiety***

Agitation on any issue, need to have only male child, high ideal of looks, intelligence etc for the child to be born, were seen to be the negative feed back for conception.

- ***Intense Desire***

Hypnotherapists are familiar with the law of reverse effect. To have a baby as soon as possible generated enough stress to destabilize the reproductive axis.

Mechanism of Causation

Fertilization of an ovum by a sperm is a molecular biochemical event, based on many known and unknown biochemical factors. The infertile couples are known to be under various levels and kinds of psychological stress. We postulate a different paradigm where by the stress arising out of a difficult relationship or vitiated perception of any of the facets of child bearing is seen as the cause of unexplained reproductive failure. We hint at the mind body continuum where by molecular biological events are seen arising from the ideas, thoughts, and emotions. The negative feelings undergo transduction to result in such molecular biochemical events that the conception is thwarted, resulting in reproductive failure.

At laparoscopic examination under general anesthesia, we have seen white, string like tubes that will not allow any dye to flow through. Repetition after intravenous administration of atropine and taking the patient under deep anesthesia made the tubes to relax and open out. This demonstrates the role of autonomic nervous system.

It is platitude to say that hormones are the key factors in reproduction. The chronic stress has its effect on the function of the endocrine glands. It is usual for the menstrual cycle to be irregular during bereavement and such other emotional turmoil. It may also become anovulatory or there may be irregular ovulation. While single readings of the hormones were found normal in our studies, the hormone levels may fluctuate during exacerbation of stress to abnormal levels causing failure in fertilization and nidation. In male, impotence and low sperm count are frequently seen as a consequence to stress.

The third tier of operation is immunological. The "hostile factors in the cervical mucus have been identified as immunoglobulin IgG, IgA and rarely IgM (Sood *et al.*, 1987). The prognostic value of their presence in the cervical mucus is established (Shulman 1988). The exact mechanism of transduction of psychodynamic factors to immune response remains to be worked out.

During the early period of our practice (1959-1978), we were guided only by the standard therapeutic norms and were confused when we encountered unexplained reproductive failure. Every clinician matures in her practice. This happens not only because of better dexterity. It is also on account of the generation of insight. Following the changing paradigm of the body mind relationship, in 1979 we came to believe that psychodynamic factors might be causative in such cases.

Hypnotherapy

It was client oriented to suit the individual need. The therapy comprised of various methods, like non-directive psychotherapy, rational emotive psychotherapy, guided imagery as well as hypnotherapy. Initially through indirect hypnosis and later, if needed with direct strategic hypnotherapeutic intervention, the couples relaxed and generated insight. Insight generation made them understand their life situations better, that reversed the abnormal psycho cybernetics.

Case Study 1

A middle aged lady was bed-ridden with the diagnosis of prolapsed intervertebral disc at the lumbar region. When I went to see her at her home, it was a typical middle class Indian family. Four generations were staying together in a small house. Additionally, the elder brother of the husband, a schizophrenic, also lived with them. The husband was a busy medical practitioner. The son, elder of the two children was appearing at standard 12th examination which was crucial for his career. Her NMR was done. She was fixed for surgery next week.

A hypnotherapeutic session for 90 minutes was given and recorded. The imagery involved her children who metamorphosed from the young ones to care for into guardian angels carrying for her. The recorded session was heard twice in a day.

Her surgery was postponed since the pain ameliorated. After two weeks she was ambulant and surgery was cancelled.

Case Study 2

A middle aged lady, with a highly logical and didactic mind-set was having "dermatitis and itching" since 20 years. This began after her marriage. She has been treated by several dermatologists. When she came, she had bruises and abrasions over both her forearms.

Following hypnotherapy for 90 minutes, the signs of inflammation disappeared. Only the marks of subcutaneous hematoma remained. (Another person undergoing a concurrent session for stammering was made to walk in somnambulistic state to her, open his eyes and see what has happened. His stammering was corrected to a major extent post trance).

Case Study 3

A lady of 60 years of age, with both her children married and son abroad, was diagnosed as having osteoarthritis of both knee joints clinically and radiologically. She was advised bilateral knee replacement. She was seen by 3 orthopedic surgeons who had the same opinion. They opted to try naturopathy and hypnotherapy.

She was a religious lady with *Lakshmi* worship in her home. She was given hypnotherapy utilizing the quality of maintenance of *Lakshmi*). She lost a couple of kgs. In a month time with naturopathy. The pain was absent. The gait returned to normal. After three years since then, she is completely symptom free and is living abroad now with her son.

Case Study 4

A lady in her early sixties, wife of a retired army personnel, had Restless Leg Syndrome diagnosed since last six years. She had severe hostility to her husband and was open to say so in his presence. She was on heavy doses of cortisone. She could barely sleep for a couple of hours at night.

She came for hypnotherapy two years back. She had been a meditator and had spiritual connections with some famous *gurus*. This was utilized. Following 4 sessions, each at the weekly interval, she had remarkable improvement in her symptoms. She was advised to continue to listen to the recorded cassette of the sessions.

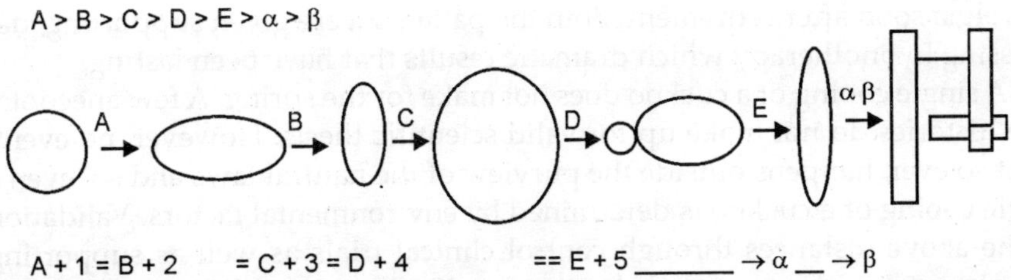

Fig. 14.5: Shift and Transformation of paradigm through hypnotherapeutic sessions

She developed a great deal of transference. She stopped all the medication including cortisone abruptly on her own. She fell unconscious after a couple of days in her house. She returned to her pre-hypnosis state after recovery.

She had problems with her aged mother for about an year. Barely able to manage herself, she came back for hypnotherapy again. After repeating the therapy, she is now free from her restless leg syndrome, is able to sleep and is weaned of cortisone.

Case Study 5

A professional middle aged lady, with two young children, living in a joint family of four generations, was additionally looking after her sister in law suffering from pancreatic cancer. At about the same time, her father had suffered from myocardial infarction and had to undergo bypass surgery.

She developed bilateral symptoms of Cervical Rib Syndrome. There was vascular insufficiency in the finger tips. She underwent the rib removal on one side and was advised surgery next month on the contralateral side.

Following indirect hypnotherapy, she had insight about her stressful state. She cancelled surgery not the next side when the vascular symptoms abated. She is well five years later.

Case Study 6

A lady aged 39 years, developed symptoms of Cervical Rib Syndrome following the death of her sister. The symptoms disappeared following indirect hypnotherapy and she is well four years later.

Case Study 7

Contributed by Dr. Chandrahas Rawal.

Following my training in hypnotherapy, I happen to treat two cases of trigeminal neuralgia that came to my dental practice. The neuralgia has surfaced in both of them after a period of stress. One patient had started getting milder symptoms prior to his retirement and the pain surfaced in classical trigeminal neuralgia soon after retirement. Both the patients were given supporting, de-stressing hypnotherapy which dramatic results that have been lasting.

A single cooing of a cuckoo does not make for the spring. A few anecdotal case histories do not make up for valid scientific thesis. However, no event, what so ever, happens outside the purview of the natural laws and so, even a single cooing of a cuckoo is determined by environmental factors. Validation of the above instances through control clinical trials as well as supporting experimental evidence can only be the scientifically accepted when established from several studies. Then also, the variable of the hypnotherapeutic skill will be hard to standardize. Till that happens, is it fair to deny the random benefit of a non-invasive therapy to those who have a chance to avoid major surgery? And, without knowing exactly what exactly is the etiopathology of Myofascial Pain Syndrome, we have treated numerous cases of through hypnotherapy.

Applications in Plastic Surgery

In late 1980s, there was a case report in Plastic and Reconstructive Surgery of a leg submerged in molten metal at 400°C: salvaged by hypnotherpy in USA.[28] That bolstered our interest in its advanced study and applications. Applications in plastic surgery may be learnt in a short time.[29] To enumerate the applications:

- Establishment of rapport
- Evaluation of cosmetic surgery clients
- Acute burns[30]
- For burn dressing and minor operations, hypnoanaesthesia[31]

Hypnoanaesthesia does not require empty stomach. So, burns patients who require frequent dressings, when dressed under hypnosis, do not suffer lack of nutrition. Nutrition is most needed to heal. This way it can be a life saving application in major burns.

- For better take and spread of the graft; though not scientifically documented, we have found that it does happen.
- For maintenance of position for flap surgery.[32]

Cautions and Contraindications

Hypnosis should never be attempted under threat or coercion. The therapist should explain briefly the nature of hypnosis and should emphasize that trance is a nature state into which all enter on a daily basis, that all hypnosis is really self hypnosis, that the patient will remain aware of what is happening, and that he or she is free to break the trance state at any time. The purpose of the hypnotic intervention should be explained clearly and the nature of the induction procedure should be briefly reviewed. The clinician must remember that hypnosis is only a technique and clinicians should never attempt to so anything with hypnosis that they are not trained to do without hypnosis. Even with some of the patients noted in the next three subsections, hypnosis can sometimes be used successfully to ease the discomfort associated with specific interventions such as dental phobias, preoperative preparation or obstetric and gynecologic procedures.

(a) Severe Depression

Many hypnotic techniques can help with the mitigation and resolution of depression. Hypnosis can be used to augment both psychodynamic and or object relations oriented psychotherapy and cognitive behavioural approaches (Yapko,[33] 1996) hypnotically facilitated ego strengthening can be "of unparalleled value "with suicidal patient when conducted by therapist well trained in therapeutic hypnosis (Brown and Fromm,[34] 1986; Frederick and McNeal,[35] 1999). However, the inexperienced should approach depressed patients with extreme caution. Persons who are severely depressed and suicidal may have their hopes for a magical cure raised and then dashed by an unsuccessful induction as one more failure in life; and if he or she is suicidal already, this experience could be used as an excuse for a suicide attempt. Careful assessment of level of depression, expectation and suicidal tendencies is critical.

(b) Paranoid Thinking of Psychotic Proportion

At one time hypnosis was thought to be contraindicated with psychotic and borderline patients because it activates archaic preoedipal transferences, thus producing a state of regression. Later work (Baker[36], 1981-1994; Fredrick and McNeal, 1999; Murray-Jobsis,[37] 1985-1991) showed that hypnosis can be a premier tool for developmental repair with such patients when it is used by those who are highly trained in this area. The regression is actually "a regression in the service of the ego" and hypnosis can be used with psychotic patients for relaxation and stabilization and as a significant medium for transitional experiences, boundary formation and strengthening, affect containment, impulse regulation, the correction of cognitive defects and other aspects of developmental repair (Fredrick and McNeal, 1999). However certain cautions must be exercised. A person who had developed a projective framework of thinking for example is not likely to appreciate the subtleties of hypnosis or self hypnosis as distinct from mind control. He or she may attribute great powers to the therapist and may get quite angry at what seems to be a loss of control. This does not need to be the case, however, and paranoid persons may discover to their surprise that they achieve even greater control with hypnosis. Paranoid persons should not be approached by inexperienced. Most paranoid persons will make the therapist's decision to use hypnosis an unnecessary one by simply refusing to participate.

(c) Patients with History Suggestive of Abuse; Attempting to use Hypnosis to Find out "What Really Happened"

This issue often arises with patients who have a history suggestive of abuse. These patients are often problematic for the casual hypnotherapist and the concerns noted earlier are important considerations especially the realization that although material accessed through hypnosis may bear some relationship to historical reality, it may also be untrue, distorted or even symbolic of the patient's conflicts.

Recent clinical and legal cases have focused on the issue of patients coming to believe that certain events occurred when they in fact had not. The use of hypnosis when sexual abuse may be involved or suspected creates some legal exposure for the therapist. Many hypnotherapists require an informed consent from patients with whom they work.

Whatever justification is advocated in terms of physiology and molecular biology, for hypnotherapy to be accepted as a rational definitive alternative therapy in the practice of modern clinical medicine, rather than a useful psychotherapeutic adjunct, several controlled clinical trials from different centers have to be forthcoming. This is a distant vision as of yet.

Notes

1. Harvard Medical School, *Family Health Guide,* 2003.
2. This section is a contribution by late Dr. Anand B. Khorana M.D., D.P.M., M.R.C. Psych. (London). F.A. P.A.
3. Rossi, E. (ed.): Collected papers of Milton H. Erickson. New York, Halsted Press, 1980. Schultz JA.
4. Zeig, J.K., *Eriksonian Psychotherapy,* Vol. 1, New York, Brunraner/Mazel, 1985. Zeig, J.K. : Experiencing Milton H. Erickson, New York, Brunnes/Mazel, 1985.
5. Utilization of the programme involves identification the personality characteristic of the subject in accordance with a particular sense perception that is prominent, say, some subjects use auditory, visual or kinesthetic verbalization in their talk. Depending upon the high lighted sensory choice, the suggestions are so tailor made as to emphasize the use of language.
6. Bandler, R., Grinder, J., *The Structure of Magic: A Book about Language and Therapy,* Vol. l. Palo Alto, CA, Science and Behaviour Books, 1975.
7. Wolberg, L.R., *Hypnoanalysist,* New York, Grune & Stratton, 1945, I964(a).
8. Wolberg, L.R., Current practices in hypnotherapy, in Fromm-Reichmann F/Morano J.L. (eds): *Progress in Psychotherapy,* Vol. 2.
9. Wolberg, L.R., *Short-term Psychotherapy* Orlando, F.L., Grune & Stratton, 1965. Wolberg, L.R., *Hypnoanalysis,* in Kutash I.L., Wolf A. (eds.): *Psychotherapists Casebook,* San Francisco, Jossey-Bass, 1986, p. 311.
8. Luthe, W., Autogenic Training: Method, research and application in medicine. *Am-J. Psychother* 17:174-195, 1963.

Edwin D.M.: Emergency room hypnosis for the burned patient. *Am J Clin Hypnosis* 1983; 26:5-8.

9. Luthe, W., Jus A., Geissman P., Autogenic State and Autogenic Shift: Psychophysiologic and neurophysiologic aspects. *Acta Psychother,* 11:1-13, 1963.
10. Lang, E.V., Benotsch, E.G., Fick, L.J., *et al.* Adjunctive non-pharmacological analgesia for invasive medical procedures: a randomized trial. Lancet 2000; 355:1486-1490.
11. Pinnell, C.M., Covino, N.A., Empirical findings on the use of hypnosis in medicine: a critical review. *Int J Clin Exp Hypnosis,* 2000; 48:170-194.
12. Frederick, C., Mc. Neal S. Inner strengths: contemporary psychotherapy and hypnosis for ego-strengthening. Mahwah, NJ: Lawrence Erlbaum Associates, 1999.
13. Brown, D.P., Scheflin, A.W., Hammond, D.C., *Memory, Trauma, Treatment and the Law.* New York: W.W. Norton, 1997.
14. Johnson and Barber, T.X. (1978). Hypnosis, suggestion, and psychosomatic phenomena, *American Journal of Clinical Hypnosis,* 21,1; pp. 13-27.; Ewin, D.M. (1974). Condylomata accuminatum: Successful treatment of four cases by hypnosis. *American Journal of Clinical Hypnosis,* 17, 2; pp. 73-78.; Galski, T.J. (1981). The adjunctive use of hypnosis in the treatment of trichotillomania: A case report. *American Journal of Clinical Hypnosis,* 23, 3; pp. 198-201.; Johnson, R.F.Q. & Barber, T.X. (1978). Hypnosis, suggestions, and warts: an experimental investigation implicating the importance of "believed-in efficacy". *American Journal of Clinical Hypnosis,* 20,3; pp. 165-174.; Lehman, R.E. (1978). Brief hypnotherapy of neurodermatitis: A case with four-year follow-up. *American Journal of Clinical Hypnosis,* 21,1; pp. 48-51.; Rowen, R. (1981). Hypnotic age regression in the treatment of a self-destructive habit: trichotillomania. *American Journal of Clinical Hypnosis.* 23,3; pp. 195-197; Sheehan, D.V. (1978). Influence of psychosocial factors on wart remission. *American Journal of Clinical Hypnosis,* 20,3; 160-164; Twerski, A.J. & Naar, R. (1974). Hypnotherapy in a case of refractory dermatitis. *American Journal of Clinical hypnosis,* 16,3; pp. 202-205; Welsh, D.K. (1978). Hypnotic control of blushing: A case study. *American Journal of Clinical Hypnosis,* 20,3; pp. 213-216.
15. Williams, P.L., Bannister, Lawrence and others. *Gray's Anatomy,* London, 1995 75-91.
16. Hench had observed temporary remission during pregnancy in arthritic patients as early as 1929.
17. Guyton.
18. Goodman, L.S. and Gilman, A., *The Pharmacological Basis of Therapeutics.* New York, 1970, pp. 1472-1506.
19. Nobel Prize in Chemistry, 2004.
20. Prediction of weather is based on physics of chaos. It can precisely be foretold only up to four days.
21. Self identity is evident in transplant surgery of all organs.
    Harvested and freeze preserved skin behaves in interesting pattern over a period of time. It maintains its self identity for about three weeks; used for resurfacing in the same subject, it behaves as autograft. After a period of three weeks to six months, it is still live tissue. But it has lost its self-specificity. Applied to the donor, it will behave as a homograft.
22. Ciirousos G.P. The Hypothalamic-Pituitary-Adrenal axis and Immune-mediated Inflammation, *N.Eng. Jour. Med.,* 332; 1351-1361, 1995.

23. Reichlin S., Neuroendocrine-immune interactions, *The New Eng. Jour. Med.*, 329; 1246-1253, 1993.
24. Simonton and Simonton, *Getting Well Again*, New York, 1984.
25. Dastidar, S.G., JIMA 97 734, 1999. ; Domar AD. Seibel MM. Benson H. Fertil & Steril S 246, 1990; Edelmann RJ. Connolly. Brit J. Med. Psychology 5 209, 1986.; Jeker L. Micione G, Ruspa M. Zeeb M. CampanaJ Intern J. Fertil. 33:411, 1988. ; Kroger W.S. Clinical and experimental hypnosis. First edition, 1963, 41, JB Lippincott & O Philadelphia.; Pert CB. Ruff MR. Weber R.J. Herkenham M.J. Immunol. 135: 820-826, 1985.; Pines D. *Intern. J. Psycho Analysis*, 71: 561, 1990. ; Reichlin S. The New *Eng. Jour. of Med.*, 329: 12* 1993.; Rossi EL. Biosystems 38:199, 1996.; Schmitt FD. Neuroscience. 13: 991, 1984.; Shulman S. in: lizuka R. and Semm K ed. Transactions of VI World Congress on Human Reproduction, Japan: Elsevier. 93-95, 1988.; Sood M. Gupta P. Saha K.J. Obstet. Gynecol. Ind. 37: 331, 1987.; Vartiainen H. *Acta Obstet. Gynecol.* Scand. 69:671 1990.; Vyas Rajni, Gita Adwanikar, Hathi Leena, Vyas Bhaskar and Parikh Ratubhai, *J. Obst. Gyn. Ind.* 52; 35-38; 2002.; Vyas Rajni, Adwanikar Gita, Hathi Leena. *J. Obstet Gynecol Ind.* 53; 359-362, 2003; Wasser S.K. *Am. J. Obstet. Gynecol.* 180:272, 1999; Wright J. Allard M. Lecours A. *Intern. J. Fertil.* 34 126, 1989.
26. A sharebroker described it very nicely. His sperm count was directly related to the index of sharemarket.
27. Let us pay tribute to George Bernard Shaw, "There are two tragedies in human life; one is to get the heart's desire and other is not to get it."
28. Kenneth, R. *et al. Hypnosis in Plastic Surgery*, PRS 76; 140-46, 1985.
29. Esdaile, J., *Hypnosis in Medicine and Surgery*, Julian Press, 1957.
30. Wakerman, R.J. *et al.*, Hypnosis in Burns, *Am. J. Cl. Hyp.* 21; 3, 1978.
31. Hopayian, K., Hypnoanaesthesia, *Anaesthesia*, 39:1139, 1984.
32. Kelsey, D. *et al.*, Maintainance of posture by hypnotic suggestions, *Br. J. Pl. Surg* 34; 478, 1981.
33. Yapko, M.D., A brief therapy approach in the use of hypnosis in treating depression. In: Lynn, S., Kirsh, I., Rhue, J., eds. *Casebook of Clinical Hypnosis*. Washington, D.C.: American Psychological Association, 1996; 75-79.
34. Brown, D., Fromm, E., *Hypnotherapy and Hypnoanalysis*. Hillsdale, NJ: Lawrence Erlbaum Associates, 1986.
35. Frederick, C., MCNeal, S., *Inner strengths: contemporary psychotherapy and hypnosis for ego-strengthening*, Mahwah, NJ: Lawrence Erlbaum Associates, 1999.
36. Baker, E.L., An hypnotherapeutic approach to enhance object relatedness in psychotic patients. *Int J Clin Exp Hypnosis*, 1981; 29;136-147.
    Baker, E.L., Resistance in hypnotherapy of primitive states: its meaning and management. *Int J Clin Exp Hypnosis*, 1983; 31:82-89.
    Baker EL. The therapist as transitional object in intensive hypnotherapy. Presented at the Annual Meeting of the American Society of Clinical Hypnosis, March 16, 1994, Philadelphia, Pennsylvania, 1994.
37. Murray-Jobsis, J., An exploratory study of hypnotic capacity of schizophrenic and borderline patients in a clinical setting. *Am J Clin Hypnosis*, 1991; 33: 150-160.
    Murray-Jobsis, J., Ego building. In: Hammond D.C., ed. Handbook of hypnotic suggestions and metaphors, New York, WW Norton, 1990: 136-139.
    Murray-Jobsis, J., Exploring the schizophrenic experience with the use of hypnosis. *Am J Clin Hypnosis*, 1985; 29; 34-42.

15
Practice Set-up

Hypnotherapy is an orphan in India, so far. Therefore, there is hardly any institutional practice. Psychiatrists are just waking up to its immense potential in their arena. But then, modern psychiatry is rightly not institutionalized: it is office practice. So, hypnotherapy practice is better discussed as relevant to solo office practice.

A practitioner in hypnotherapy is as much an expert as any other therapist. However, some of his/her needs are special. His office should be spacious, with the facility for the paradigm shift in the arrangements. We recommend a minimum space of 150 sq. ft as office cum therapy room; exclusive of reception. When dealing with subjects with phobia and panic attacks, this of paramount importance. In such other conditions too, e.g. paranoid subjects, it is recommended that no compromise with spaciousness be made: it is better to refuse rather than end up confused and failed.

Eventually groups will generate as practice advances. Group therapy needs a minimum 100 sq. ft. of space per participant: more the better. There should be enough space between the participants, so that, therapist and other facilitators can move in between.

Most other specialists do their consultations closed doors. Privacy of the client is precious; it is the duty of the therapist. However, we recommend a partially open door[1]! If an anteroom is interspaced between the therapy room and reception, open door would still ensure privacy and, is a subconscious metaphoric assurance to the client that he can any time walk out or opt out of therapy.

Consulting Rooms

Besides being spacious, the rooms are tidy and neat. Simplicity and elegance should go together. Whatever honours have accrued to the therapist may be displayed without being ostentatious. Expectancy, wonder and astonishment are conducive to induction and therapy. Displays such as authoritative books, paintings, curtains and idols are taken as metaphor by the visitors and, initially they derive some meaning about the personality to encounter and the process to ensue.

Hypnotherapy is a calm, cool, comfortable and cozy experience. Ambience should be such as to enhance it. The colour scheme should be so selected: our recommendation is faint cerulean blue or azure blue. Though this is a matter of individual choice, it may be remembered that red and its hues are excitatory while blue and its allied shades are cooling. Gaudy colours reflect poor choice and are avoided. The furniture is comfortable and elegant.

Since Freud conducted his sessions with the subject lying down on a couch, it has become a general practice for most therapists to use a couch. Our choice is a cozy reclining chair with arm rests. While conducting group therapy and at workshops, often this is not available. At workshops in India, even when subjects are made to recline on comfortable chairs, it is usual that during the trance they make themselves more comfortable by sliding down to the floor. Expecting such a situation, the floor may be carpeted.[2] For ladies, clean sheets to cover themselves are made available.

Hypnotherapy Sessions

If the therapist has some open hours for consultations, first visit should be confined to history taking and rapport building. The therapy should be by appointments. Often, in several conditions positive results accrue even after a single session or two. If the subject drops out then, there may be a likely recurrence or relapse later: this gives bad name to the therapist and the process both. All clients should be explicitly told that even when they feel almost cured, repetition and reinforcement is necessary for the sustained result.

We recommend a minimum of four sessions spaced once a week. The interval is subject to convenience. All clients are given recorded cassettes of the sessions that they have undergone and, are advised to listen to them before/ while going to sleep. Even when they go to sleep while listening, recoding shuts itself of when finished. But the subconscious mind listens to the record and it works.

For prolonged illnesses like auto immune diseases, positive results take time. Assessment of the therapy is to be made after eight sessions (arbitrary number). If the rapport is well established and subject has undergone deep trance-experience of Fourth state of consciousness, at least some improvement should be noticeable. Then the therapy may be timed till it improves the client further. If the rapport is dwindling and belief of the client is shaken, it may be advisable to terminate therapy.

Attire and Attitude

Plain and simple is professional. Entire demeanor should be simple and placid: the client is to be won over by refined manners and not by flamboyancy. The therapist is in parent situation as per transactional analysis mode: but soon reverts back to "I am okay – you are okay"; adult-adult mode no sooner the therapy is terminated. Convention protocols and etiquette of welcome and good bye are fundamental to rapport.

Records

As of today, there is not a single case of litigation against a hypnotherapist in India: physical violence is reported against "trainers" and gurus. Litigation is not uncommon in the West and may be imported soon. Properly maintained records have academic value and, are a good insurance against litigation.

Appointments and Fees

Following history taking, first therapy session may be immediately on next day. Subsequent sessions are spaced weekly for chronic conditions, but may be scheduled as needed for acute conditions, e.g. in post operative patients, burns, cardiac conditions etc. The first session is of 90 minutes.[3] Subsequent session should be a minimum of 20 minutes.[4]

Fees should be explicitly quoted and understood by the client. Usually, it is drugless therapy and people often do not understand that here talk is the real work. Charity for the underprivileged has always a place in most human situations: hypnotherapy may be one exception. A free lunch, how so ever well served, does not taste as good when not paid for. This is particularly so for hypnosis. Apart from the usual transference, free sessions enhance it further. Therapist runs the risk of being misunderstood as a nonprofessional when he waives the fees. Alternately, the client is left with the burden of gratitude that generates undue transference.

The therapist may set-up what ever fees he chooses to charge a particular client; when the session is paid for, it sets the professional protocol in communication! This is the best way to avoid being a Guru! Hypnotherapists beware!Indian Society of Clinical Hypnosis recommends fees to its members from time to time. However, it is professional prerogative for each therapist to decide what his/her fees are. At times, clients have agreed to pay very high fees with full understanding and, have been grateful to the therapist for results obtained. Thus, fees are a non-issue.

When immediately benefited, clients are inclined to drop out mid way. They may relapse. Collecting fees for the therapy of a said condition for minimum prescribed sessions is one way to ensure that appointments are kept.

Missed Appointments may be a Message

It is said that in India, only Governors and the President are in time! The Indian mind-set is not tuned to be on time. Apart from that it is not easy for a commoner to be on time. All the same, it does amount to waste of time for the therapist and such instances are irritants and a common cause of frayed interpersonal relationships.

Failed appointments are irksome: they are a global phenomenon and best example of lose-lose interaction situation. Client does not benefit: therapist wastes time. Charging for the failed appointment may be considered as punitive that is counterproductive to rapport. It is best to understand the dynamics. Whether the failure was a willful neglect and the client wanted to terminate therapy or there was indeed an impasse or a covert denial to get well. Consider the case of insomniac who fails to turn up for an appointment in the morning. In brief, what cannot be cured has to be endured.

From the psychotherapeutic mode, a missed appointment may be a message – a Freudian slip. It may reflect the subject's resistance or denial to get well.

Overstay at Sessions

Combined with the pleasant state in hypnosis, transference commonly makes the subject in trance to overstay the allotted time. The therapist has judiciously pre-decided the time needed. The next appointment is as important. And laxity about the therapist's availability can send a wrong message. The additional time spent does not mean additional therapeutic work. The hypnotherapeutic work is done by the subject for a variable time for indefinite time. After asking the subject to wake up, if the subject remains in trance, the therapist may move on to the next appointment in another room. If there is a space constraint, the subject should be firmly told to wake up, since the work is to go on for long time regardless of the presence in the therapy rooms. Kripa Thakur in his Canadian set up used money as a wake up tool. When the subject did not comply with the above protocol, he would tell his clients that should they continue to be in session, it is going to cost them more. His subjects never failed this Wake Up call! We find this hard to put to practice in Indian situation.

Termination of Therapy

With the well deserved motivation by the client and specifically articulated goals, the therapy should terminate as either successful, amelioration or failure within a reasonable time. Only a majority of successes should ensure the continuation of the therapist in practice; he should be inclined to enrichment through sharing with the peers and learning from the advanced teachers. A successful case terminates in the last session with a specific delegation of credit for the success to the client: it is a candid admission that the work was done by the subject and, the therapist was only a facilitator. Failure may be owned up as limitation of any scientific practice without attributing the blame to the subject: though that indeed may be the cause, since the subject may just be pretending to follow the instructions in the session and may not have done the home work of listening to the recorded sessions.

Notes

1. For those therapists who are familiar to J. Krishnamuti's teachings, this will sound as a familiar metaphor. For those not familiar, we recommend to read him since his teachings are metaphorical and useful in therapeutic strategy.
2. We have faced some embarrassment when a high profile eminent, senior citizen lady did so.
3. While Milton Erickson fixed this duration arbitrarily, it is likely to have a relation to circadian rhythms and gene expression (Rossi).
4. Ernest Rossi, *20 minutes break*, 1998, London.

16
Hypnotherapy Clinic

This is an example of how you can prepare a client/patient case history.

Client/Patient Case History[1]

Reg. No:
Date:

Identification

Name
Address:
(R)
(O)
Age:
Marital status
Sex-male/female
Occupation
Nationality
Religion
Family
Educational qualifications

Telephone:
Mobile:
Email:
Language/s

Presenting Symptom

- History of present illness: Time and mode of onset, description of symptoms, details of previous medical or other treatment.

Past Medical History

- Previous illnesses, operations, accidents and treatment.
- In a woman, menstrual history, pregnancies, confinements or miscarriages.

Family History

- Description of father, mother, sister and brothers, family relationships, past and present, attitudes and feelings towards each other.

Childhood History

- Childhood illnesses, particularly bed-wetting and sleep-walking, educational history, reactions to various schools and other children.

Psycho-sexual History

- Teenage knowledge of sexual matters, and how acquired, habits (masturbation, etc.), past and present emotional matters, marriages (if any), marital and extra marital relationships or difficulties. financial status.

Psychiatric Illness

- Neurosis or epilepsy in parents, close relations or members of the family. h/o depression, schizophrenia,

Present State of Mind

- Depression, anxiety, phobias, insomnia, lack of concentration or interest, memory, suicidal thoughts, fear of insanity

Psychiatric Interview

- Purposeful interaction between the therapist and patient:
  (1) Gathering information to assess the patient's condition and
  (2) Establishing a therapeutic doctor-patient relationship with rapport.
- In the interview the patient usually reveals intimate, private and potentially painful aspects of his/her life to the doctor.
- Patient may be highly motivated to unconsciously motivated to unwilling to disclose.
- The psychiatric interview may also be complicated by the fact that not all psychiatric patients have voluntarily sought the doctor's help and their willingness or ability to cooperate may be impaired for this reason.

The psychiatrist's relationship with the patient strongly influences what the patient does and does not say therefore their training involves the specific and sophisticated techniques of listening, observation and interpretation.

- Management of time-30 min to 1 hr
  Psychotic and medically ill-Brief
  Emergency Rooms-Longer
  2nd Visit–Varies
- Doctor's Office
- Seating arrangements, initially and with paradigm shift
- Note-taking
- Subsequent interviews

Specific Interviewing Situations

Differences linked to diagnosis
Depressed and potentially suicidal patients
Violent patients
Delusional patients and interviewing relatives
Forensic interviews

Psychiatric History

- Chief complaints according to the patient
- Chief complaints according to the informant
- History of present illness
- Previous Illnesses—Past Psychiatric and medical Illness
- Past Personal History—Prenatal and Post natal Illness
  Early Childhood
  Middle Childhood
  Late Childhood
  Adulthood

Psychosexual History and Family History

- Dream, Fantasies and values

Mental Status Examination

- MSE is a part of clinical assessment—Examiner's observation and impression of the patient at the time of interview
- Change from time to time

1. General Description
   Appearance–Posture, Poise, Clothing and Grooming
   Behaviour–Psychomotor activity—Retardation or agitation
   Attitude—co-operative, unco-op, friendly, attentive, hostile, seductive
2. Mood and Affect

Mood–Patients perception
Affect–Psychiatrist interpretation
Appropriateness—unappropriateness and appropriate

3. Speech
Quantity, rate of production and quality
Pressure and speed
4. Perceptual Disturbances
Hallucinations and illusions—Auditory, Visual, olfactory, tactile
Hypnagogic and hypnopompic
Depersonalization and Derealization
5. Thought
Thought process—Derailment, Flight of ideas, Racing thoughts, Tangentiality,
Circumstantiality, Word salad, Neologism, Clang association, Punning, Thought blocking, Vague thought
Content of Thought—Delusions, Paranoia, Preoccupation, Obessions and compulsions, Phobias, Suicidal and homicidal ideas, ideas of reference and influence, Poverty of content
6. Sensorium and congnition
Alertness and level of consciousness,
Orientation – Time, place, person and self
Memory – Remote, recent past, recent and memory
Concentration – Impaired and intact
— Abstract Thinking –Ability to deal with the concepts
— Fund of information and Intelligence –
Organic mental impairment
— Vocabulary and general fund of knowledge
7. Impulse control
Sexual, aggressive, Social appropriate behaviour, Potentially danger to self and others
8. Judgement and Insight—
Judgement—Social Test
Insight –
Grade 1 – Complete denial of illness
Grade 2 – Slight awareness of being sick, needing help but at the same time denying it
Grade 3 – Awareness of being sick but blaming it on others, on external factors or on organic factors
Grade 4 – Awareness that illness is due to something unknown in the patient
Grade 5 – Intellectual insight – Admission that the patient is ill and that symptoms and failures in the social judgment are due to the patient's own particular irrational feelings or disturbances without applying that knowledge in future

Grade 6—Emotional Insight—Same as above with applying that knowledge to prevent future illness.

Emotional Responses

Ego defenses

Denial	[ ]
Displacement	[ ]
Regression	[ ]
Repression	[ ]
Rationalization	[ ]
Reaction formation	[ ]
Compensation	[ ]
Projection	[ ]

Attitudes

Self
World
Future

Personality Inventory [ ]

Indecisive, boastful, lacking in perseverance, reserved, lacking in self confidence, feeling inferiority,
Or relaxed, calm, mature, competitive, bright, warm, sociable, adventurous, enthusiastic, conscientious, confident, assertive

Psychiatric Report

Addresses the critical questions of further diagnostic studies that must be performed
Adds the summary of both positive and negative findings
Makes a tentative Multiaxial Diagnosis
Gives the prognosis
Gives a psychodynamic formulation
Gives a set of management recommendations

Further Diagnostic Studies

Physical examination
Additional Psychiatric diagnostic interviews
Interviews with family members, friends or neighbours

Psychological, Neurological or laboratory test

Summary of Positive and Negative Findings

Mental symptoms, Historical data (family History), medical and laboratory findings, Psychological and neurological test results

Tentative Diagnosis

On basis of DSM IV/DSM V (Multiaxial Evaluation Report Form)

AXIS I:	Clinical Disorders
	Other/conditions that may be a focus of Clinical Attention
AXIS II:	Personality Disorders
	Mental Retardation
AXIS III:	General Medical Conditions
AXIS IV:	Psychosocial and Environmental stressors
	Problems with support group
	Problems with social environment
	Problems with Education
	Problems with Occupation
	Problems with Housing
	Problems with Finance
	Problems with access to health care services
	Problems with interaction with the legal system/crime
	Problems with psychosocial/environmental
AXIS V:	Global Assessment

Occupational history: Ambitions as a child, history of various occupations after leaving school, reasons for changes, present employment, and reactions to work – mates and environment.

Stress inventory

Traumatic events: Fire—being hostage—witnessing gory crime—rape
Recent life events: Family—death of spouse-divorce and marriage
Personal life: Change in residence—change in the eating habits—personal injury
Work: Trouble with boss—retirements
Financial matter: Mortgage—major changes in financial condition.
Hassles: Happening in daily life—preparing children for school—looking after home work—care of family—attending emergency.
Psychological stress: Frustration—conflict—pressure

Prognosis

Immediate and future course and extent and outcome of illness
Bad and good prognostic factors
Psychodynamic Formulation
Psychological make up, Primary and secondary gains, major defense mechanisms, genetic

Recommendations

Psychiatric Treatment—Target symptom
Psychotherapies
Length of treatment

Hypnotherapy Management

Explanation

Mind body relationship in context of the patient's Problem.

Conscious/Unconscious mind.
Thinking feeling-behaviour relationship.
Stress Reactions.
Coping mechanisms.
Decomposition upon repeated exposure to stress.
Hypnosis—Misbelieves, daily trance experiences, Present status, Self hypnosis and cue.

Induction and Deepening of Hypnosis

Eye fixation
Progressive relaxation
Deep breathing
Counting
Arm heaviness
Arm levitation
Imagery
Hands moving together
Cloud gazing
Any other

Ego strengthening suggestions

Ideomotor signaling

Finger movement
Head nodding/shaking
Any other

Direct suggestions for symptom amelioration

Symptom substitution
Symptom transformation
Assertiveness

Strategy

Positive imagery such as
Red balloon
Black board
Helmet image
Ice Cube melting
Sunrise
Flowering
Germination of a seed
Flowing river

Any other

incorporation of archetypal symbols (depending upon patient's life experiences, interests and values)
Time distortion
Age regression and cognitive restructuring
Age progression and mental rehearsal
Response substitution

Post hypnotic Suggestions

Training of self hypnosis and positive autosuggestion

Group Therapy
Family Counseling

Other Treatment Modalities used

Medication
Ayurvedic

Homeopathy
Naturopathy
Yoga/Meditation
Acupuncture
Any other

Note

1. Inputs by Dr. Jatin Nayak and Dr. Venkat Iyer.

17

Communication in Hypnotherapeutic Session

Emphasis on being positive such as:

> *Yada bhavah, tad bhavana;*
> *Yada bhavana, tad bhavatu.*
> (as may be your mood, so will be your affect;
> as will be your deep affect, so will it happen.)

Positive Suggestions in Hypnotherapeutic Session

Positive psychology is said to be a new concept. In fact, philosophically, it is old wine in a new bottle. Since time immemorial, blessings and prayers were emphatically positive. *Rishis* of *Rig Veda* prayed so that good thoughts may come to them from all the sides. Patanjali, a master positive psychologist, first laid out the preparations for spiritual progress by defining what to do and what to avoid. Only thereafter the meditation follows through the steps of focalisation on positive creative visualisation of one's choice; be it a symbol of a deity, of aesthetic beauty, a musical chant or simply a brief *sutra.* Besides this royal road to spirituality (*Raja Yoga*), our tradition developed intricate – and at times, intriguing – mystical techniques that came to be called *tantra.* The masculine principle came to be best illustrated in its singularity in *Vigyana Bhairava;* the multiple feminine manifestations as in *Panchastavi* and other masterpieces, symbolising the best of charm and grace combined with artistic elegance of the environment made one realise the Divine at ultimate destination, *Samadhi. Samadhi,* though apparently experienced as a state of Void, was positively full since it had the portent and potential to generate immense creativity. Even the road map was charted as to how *Ichchha-shakti* created and guided *Kriya-sakti* to accomplish the goal.

Science speaks a different language, yet it is about to find the truth of what was seen through the Third Eye of intuition. It is only now that with the cutting edge research through molecular biology and genomics, we come to understand the molecules of stress as well as the healing pathways in genomics and stem cell regeneration that reverse the effects of the former. They indeed are the floating particles in the blood stream—not virtual but actual—that are generated by thinking processes—let us call it mind. We are about to know how to carve a certain future for ourselves and be the creator of our destiny through positive thoughts that generate positive actions through changes in the circuitry of neurones, transformations of programmes in the Unconscious and, as seen in the process of hypnosis, by mirror imaging of the neurons as well as brain plasticity.

We therefore understand that human being stands alone in animal kingdom by the function of speech. The versatile nature of human speech has made expression of complex thoughts possible and that has played fundamental role in human progress. Communication is a basic instinct of life. It is a social process, which is fundamental and vital to human happiness as it allows an individual to express thoughts, feelings and ideas.

Any process that leads to an exchange of information is communication. It may be both, verbal and nonverbal. It can be highly stylized as a technique or may be simple or terse; but the aim is that of an attitude directed towards the sharing of information for a purpose. It is through communication that we establish, maintain, explain or alter the relationship. Thus communication is "who says what to whom through which channel and to what effect." The communication brought about by senses other than speech is termed as non verbal. It is also called body language. This has been paraphrased succinctly to interpret various expressions on the face, demeanor and gestures.[1]

Milton Erickson has stressed importance of regarding hypnosis as a continuous process of communication. Considering that the activation of ultradian cycle (that can reverberate for long time) is brought about in hypnosis and the dispersion of information substances, secreted as a consequence there of, can permeate through the extra cellular fluid for an indefinite time, the simple statement assumes profound significance.

Neurolinguistic Traits; Neurolinguistic Programming (NLP)[2, 3]

While the subject is narrating his/her story to the therapist, he may note the dominant sense/motor modality of expression. For effective communication the mind is engaged through various sensory inputs like eyes, ears, nose, tongue and skin (touch). In most persons, the inter-phase between thoughts, brain and speech finds a route via a dominant sensory motor medium. Neurolinguistic programming is based on this premise. Let us be more explicit and categorize:

- *Olfactory*: "There is some thing fishy"; "I smell a rat"; "It was so nice as if the whole place was filled with perfume".
- *Auditory*: "It happened with a bang"; "Your voice is sweet music to my ears"; "The ticking of the clock was like a hammer on my head".

- *Gustatory*: "You are as sweet as honey"; "How juicy!"; "Add some spice to the story!"
- *Visual*: "Not even in my wildest dream could I see myself as a prime minister!"; "I see, I see"; "I have a vision of the future where life is filled with colours so splendid!"
- *Tactile*: "I am touched by your kindness"; "You have a finger in each pie"; "Those words pierced through my heart".
- *Kinesthetic*: "He landed high on the summit of success"; "I darted my way like a bullet"; "I was so pressed with the situation that I could not move my little finger".

Indulging in such fine nuances is not a must for effective therapy. However, the therapist may do well to develop a habit of observation and suitably design the strategy as per the dominant expression.

Metaphors: The Language of Hypnosis

And there is a complex form of conveyance through symbols. It can be said that all communication is actually symbolic since there is no inherent semantic content to any language. Mind tries to make the sense of the world around by comparison. It identifies the objects by similarities and contradiction. And in the different state of consciousness that hypnosis is, the boundary zone between real and surreal is obscured: it may even be obliterated. Thus, stories have a tremendous impact to deliver the message. So do the metaphors since stories when told in hypnoidal state become metaphorical. Through veiled disguise of a seemingly interesting metaphor, the subject can be made to intrinsically juxtapose his/her situation so as to generate insight. Zen parables are classic examples. Let us illustrate:

- *To a subject who gets into disputes and quarrels*: A Zen master asked his pupil, let us hear the sound of clapping with one hand.
- *To a subject who has landed himself into an impasse*: A person found a hapless chicken. He put it into a flask and fed it regularly. Now, the chicken has grown into a hen. It wants to get out. He wants it out too; but without breaking the flask. How can he do it?
- *To a subject of phobia*: Two students of a Zen school saw the flag fluttering on the temple staff. One said, "The flag is fluttering": Other argued, "The wind is causing the flag to flutter." They went to the Zen Master to settle their dispute. What would Zen Master say?

Indian Names[4, 5, 6, 7]

While most therapists are at a loss to devise the metaphors suited to their patients, it is lost to them that Indian names have a wide variety of connotations.

They are ideal metaphors. We like to play frequently with the vast repertoire that is available through this medium. It will be simplistic to emphasize that one's own name has neurolinguistic connections that will suit the natural sensibility of the individual for ego strengthening. Of course, the same applies to a lesser extent to the names from other sub-continents. But to be explicit, let us see some examples from India:

- Yogesh is a master of yoga. He is also a master amongst yogis-practitioners of yoga.
- Chandarana stands for the glorious moon.
- Bhaskar is the bright sun.
- Vyas is a Maharshi (seer) with enormous literary talent.

Pantheon of Gods and Goddesses

This is culture specific but the appeal is universal. The Indian lore has epics full of sub-stories. The wisdom of the *Upanishads* is conveyed through stories and perennial questions. The study of Greek mythology, Shakespeare or John Keats may have faded: but there are still Anthonies, Henries, Juliets and Sophias. They come alive in the lost paradise of the subjects since they have archetypal connotations: when utilized, apart from rapport building, they yield rich dividends in therapeutic results. That one should only try to realize full potential.

Archetypal Symbols in Indian Ethos: Utilization in Hypnotherapy

We have seen that the state of hypnosis is distinctly different from the ordinary three states that we are aware of in every day life. One of its distinctively different characteristic is heightened suggestibility that effaces the distinction between the real and surreal. A surreal painting yields to various explorations by the viewers according to their own sensibilities. In the same fashion, the metaphors and allegories used in hypnotic mode reveal themselves according to the contents of the unconscious mind of the subject. This is the crux of the transformation that is achieved through hypnotherapeutic mode. It will make sense to the computer literate audience to simplify as a single and swift operation of a transformation of the data of a particular programme to other programme, say data from the files of power point from the slides to the text format in Word. Or more precisely, the bits on the chips may store memory in the Word format or in the form of a painting or music.

All cultures have understood the operation of the archetypal symbols even before Jung formally enunciated their meaning. The national flags and such other symbols were utilized by the mankind since antiquity. Though it still remains an enigma as to what is the basis of their expression, we see their operations in the incidental hypnoidal state as well as in the dreams. Most of the literature and poetry is portent with much more meaning than the words can convey because of their metaphors and allegories. The archetypal symbols belonging to the entire human race or a particular culture have perpetuated themselves over the millennia by some unfathomable mechanism. What we know for sure is the certainty of their impact. This impact is profound in hypnotherapeutic mode so as to bring about a therapeutic change.

Archetypal Symbols in Dreams

It is difficult to say whether dreams are just condensation of various memories or there is an element of precognition or telepathy. Freud described it as royal road to unconscious mind. Adler described it as individual key to understand life style and choices available to a person in social situation. Jung expressed it as self confrontation. But to all of them symbols were with specific metaphysical references. To us, they are not only attempts by unconscious mind at wish fulfillment but also a method of problem solving. And, they are certainly symbolic of stress and discomfort, such as missing a train, writing an examination etc.

Dream starts as condensation of thoughts that gets encapsulated in a single format. There is displacement of time, space and personalities. There is intense symbolization. This can transgress to neologism-coining of new words. All of this may progress to secondary elaboration. That can be based on fulfillment of cherished and yet, unfulfilled desires, expression of repressed fears and conflicts as well as completion of a psychodynamic drive. Such a completion has a constructive role in the sense of completing a loop or answering a telephone call that has been repeatedly ringing.

All cultures from ancient times ascribed such roles to dreams. Freud put a theoretical construct to their interpretation when he published, The interpretations of dreams[8] in 1900 A.D. And it paved a way for psychoanalysis. The analysis rested heavily on the interpretation of certain recurring symbols in different individuals. This also raised the question as to what is the origin of this commonality. This led Jung[9] to postulate the theory of memory of the

Freudian Interpretation of Symbols

Symbol	*Interpretation*
1. Finger, nose, numbers-1,0, 3	Male sex organ
2. Bag, pocket, window, pot, box, chest, lake, boat, cupboard, drawer, cabbage, rose	Female sex organs.
3. Telephonic talk, writing a letter	Coitus
4. Any mutilation	Castration
5. Cane	Phallus; support
6. Jumping water; fountain	Fountain of life,
7. Umbrella, necktie, key, pen, rifle, rope, any long object such as snake, rat with a tail, horse	Male sex organ.
8. Shadow	Part of the personality to be rejected.

herd, memory of the species as well as the theoretical construct of collective unconscious.[10] However, the relevance of such symbolism is evident at the personal, societal, cultural, national and global scales. As for the psychologists belonging to any of the schools, there is no hesitation in accepting archetypal symbols as dynamic, demiurgic forces in the unconscious mind.

This is for an illustration. It is out of place to make an exhaustive list since that can fill a volume.[11] While the dream contents yield to arguable psychoanalytical understanding, what is of more relevance is that the dreams can be manipulated in such a way as to incorporate the archetypal symbols that may promote healing/therapeutic cure.[12]

Indian civilization is more than 5000 years old. The first line of the most ancient *Veda, Rig Veda* begins with a symbolic statement, *"agnimide purohitam"*. The *rishi* has put *agni,* the fire as the foremost. And thereafter, there are several symbolic *mantras* and rituals that involve fire to connote that it is primordial source of energy. More ancient a symbol, more efficacious it may turn out to be.

Having illustrated the point, the archetypal symbols in Indian tradition are in the forms of sound and image as well as in the form of rituals that have compounded inputs involving all the senses. We shall restrict our enumeration to only some of mantras and visual symbols.

Archetypal Symbolic Sound	*Connotation/Utilization*
A. *Vedic Mantras*	
Gayatri mantra	Invocation of sun, connoting provider of energy, protector, one who dispels darkness of ignorance, produces brilliance of intellect. Utilized generally where the energy levels are low, say depression to low Immune levels
Shanti Mantra	Connotes peace within and everywhere. Utilized for hyperactive conditions like mania, stress, post traumatic stress syndrome.
Om[13]	Innumerable connotations with three components carrying various different aspects, some of them are: (i) return to the primordial source, detachment; (ii) the voice that is the greatest assenting Word[14] Utilized for de afferentiation, say, anxiety neurosis and such other neurotic compensation
Archetypal Symbolic Sound	Connotation/utilization
Tantric Mantra	
Complex monosyllabic or cryptic Sanskrit words, apparently meaningless. There is mystery about them and they are not to be chanted/discussed publicly.	"It is the sound-body of a power charged with intense vibrations of the spiritual personality of the creator or the seer of the mantra. The *mantra* is an ever living embodiment of the Truth and Power of the creator rishi."[15]
Sutras	
They are composed of more than one word, are necessarily short and terse. They occur in *Vedas, Upanishads, Gita and Yoga Sutras*; viz.	Elicitation of numerous *siddhis*

(Contd.)

Archetypal Symbolic Sound	*Connotation/Utilization*
Ritumbhara Pragya	To impact intellect to be always full of discriminative wisdom.
Jyotismati	Everlighted mind
Kurma nadi	Development of patience
maitri, karuna, mudita and upeksha	Development of friendliness, compassion, appreciation of virtue and indifference to shortcomings of others
B. Buddhist Mantra	
Om mani padme hum[16, 17]	Development of adamantine and beautiful mind
C. Jain Mantra	
Naukara Mantra	Invocation of intangible protective forces that are capable of everything
Archetypal Symbol in Form	Connotation
A. Pantheon of Hindu Gods[18]	
Ganapati	Wisdom, steady and stable mind, attainment of affluence and subtle powers. Auspiciousness.
Sun	Strength, energy and illumination
Saraswati	Mother, knowledge, aesthetics, creativity, purity
Lakshmi	Maintenance of affluence and values, ethical and spiritual
Durga	Destruction of evil; false values Utilization: Teaching psychobiology of genes: twenty arms of Durga connote twenty intermediate active genes![19]
Maha Shakti[20] (i) Maheswari (ii) Mahakali (iii) Mahalakshmi (iv) Maha Saraswati	Feminine empowerment Utilization for any feminine suffering for ego-enhancement, assertion
Asta Laskshmi	
(i) Dhanya Lakshmi	Controller and giver of food: utilization for eating disorders
(ii) Dhana Lakshmi	Material wealth; utilization for all kind of fears and phobias
(iii) Santana Lakshmi	Goddess of fertility; utilization for Infertility of unknown origin
Archetypal Symbol in Form	Connotation
(iv) Vidya Lakshmi (v) Vijaya Lakshmi (vi) Dhairya Lakshmi (vii) Gaja Lakshmi (viii) Adi Lakshmi	Connotation and utilization is in the similar fashion.
8. Symbols in Epics[21] e.g. Savitri[22]	
Satyavan	Divine truth in the grip of ignorance
Savitri	Divine Word, daughter of sun
Ashwapati	*Tapasya*, spiritual endeavour. Utilization: Emanations of living and conscious Forces with whom we can enter into concrete dialogue (Sri Aurobindo)
B. Buddhist tradition:	
Vajrayana[23]	
Amitabha Buddha	Vajrasattva Buddha
Amoghasiddhi Buddha	
Akshobhya Buddha	
Ratnasambhava Buddha	

Archetypal Symbolic Sound	*Connotation/Utilization*
Tara	Embodiment of Feminine Forces; Utilization for feminine empowerment
JAIN TRADITION	
Vipassyana as:	
Kayanupassana	Observation of body with observer outside; utilization in somatiform disorders
Vedananupassyana	Observation of pain; utilization for pain relief
Archetypal symbol in form	Connotation
Chittanupassyana	Observation of mentation as an outsider;
Dhammanupassyana	Utilization in neurosis, Stress, personality disorders
	Connotation and Utilization in similar fashion
Tirthankaras; 24 forms	Connotation and Utilization in similar fashion
Padmavati Devi	
Archetypal Symbols in Tantric form	Self-restructuring
	Utilization for re-educative and reconstructive psychotherapy, say drug addictions
Creation of a temple	Union of ascent and descent
Srichakra	In the descending order from crown of the head to the level of coccyx
Chakras in the body[24]	Each has distinctive features
Sahasrara Chakra	
Agya Chakra	
Vishuddha Chakra	
Anahata Chakra	
Manipura Chakra	
Swadhishthana Chakra	
Muladhara Chakra	
Kundalini	
Mandalas; Kalachakra	Invocation of *Tirthankaras* through *Naukara Mantra*; Prabhavati
Jain Tantrik Practices	Devi as the source of energy; virtues assigned to various *Tirthankaras*

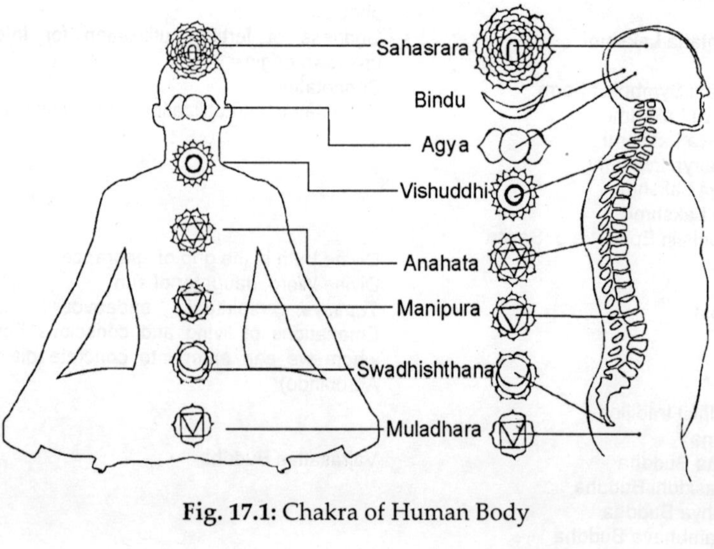

Fig. 17.1: Chakra of Human Body

The Following is Narrated as an Illustration for a Hindu Lady

A lady aged 28, scientist by education, was married since five years was having unexplained reproductive failure. She was having irregular, anovulatory menstrual cycles. She has been treated for one year by assisted reproduction techniques. Larger doses of follicular stimulating hormones as well as luteinizing hormones failed to produce ovulation/fertilization for 12 cycles when she approached us.

Her name literally translated as the goddess Saraswati. Over a period of six months, the following psychodynamic programme of hypnotherapeutic manipulation was given:

River Saraswati has dried up; but recent satellite pictures that appeared in the news papers have shown that it is flowing subterrestrially.

There have been good rains and the river has surfaced. It is flowing across the banks

The field have been ploughed and flowers have been sown.

The plants have made a beautiful garden and there are buds of roses.

There is a temple built in the center. It is the temple of Saraswati. Description of the form in all its details.

She is going to the garden with her husband, riding on a scooter.

They seek the blessings of the Goddess of creativity.

They go around the garden; she sees two buds opening into two flowers,

Watch the children play.

There is a mother with a baby in her arms.

Her husband clicks a picture. Develops it. Yes, it is she herself.

They arrive home, there is difficulty opening the door, Dr. Rajni helps her to unlock.

She opens the door wide, opens the side windows of the bedroom, hang the picture at the foot end of the bed,

Make love

Love is creativity and creativity abounds.

She has ovulated normally on the fourteenth day from both the ovaries.

Suggestions for fertilization are given, as,

A prince charming and a princess cute are arriving. The red carpet is laid out. She is standing at the end of the carpet to welcome the honoured guests.

Till the time of writing, she is now menstruating regularly. However, she has failed to conceive but is ovulating regularly. We have decided to have a break at trying. This is in consonance of the law of reverse effect.

A subtle incorporation of the relevant symbol, appropriate to the subject's sensibility has far reaching effect in the outcome of the therapy.

Thus, in therapy session, begin with the reinforcement of understanding that in the hypnotic state, there is heightened suggestibility, uncritical acceptance of a suggestion and a lasting imprint that is in accordance with the stated goal in therapy. Our subject approaches us for a discomforting symptom or a disorder in their psychosomatic environment. Most of them have already tried to avoid consciously not to do what causes their symptoms, but without success.

In planning the strategies keep the physiological Basis of Curative Response that ensues from a positive suggestion.

It is as follows:

Duality causes waste of mental energy; trying to decipher how to and *how not to* means two tasks for the brain.

Cognitive perception in Brain: Do Not *Do This;* is perceived as two different suggestions in hypnosis.

State dependent memory: Hypnosis can *re-live* the memory. Living in positive situation creates happiness and joy. Emotionally that can be further engrafted.

Milton Erickson's sessions were typically persistent with emphasis on positive reinforcement. This may be with play of language so as to be gently persuasive double blind. Erickson utilized the impact of a negative suggestion at the concluding part of the session.

This gets interpreted as a further reinforcement of positive suggestions by utilizing the law of paradox. Erickson took to creative heights when each session was so structured as to whirl around creative visualisations of positive symbols through metaphors. Most effective metaphors are derived from archetypal symbols.

Archetypal symbols in all cultures are a vast repertoire of positive psychodynamic metaphors. They contribute enormously to create state dependent archetypal memories so as to generate a ground state of positive change.

Archetypal symbols from Greek and Roman Mythology

- *Aphrodite*—The goddess of love, beauty and desire. Her symbol is the rose. Her sacred animal is the dove.
- *Apollo*—Associated with light, truth and the sun. The god of music, healing, prophecies, and poetry.
- *Hercules*—God of Strength
- *Roman god Janus*—had two faces which looked both backwards and forward.
- *Achilles*—Weakness in his heels

Non-specific Positive suggestions

- *Sea*—Depth, Vastness, unconscious mind
- *Garden*—Pleasant environment—Beauty, colours, smell in flower
- *Trees*—Bears fruits, regeneration, rejuvenation, reward for effort

Communication: three elements and two way traffic

(1) The Source (Therapist) → (2) The Message (Suggestion) → (3) The Destination (Client)

Some therapists believe that the change is brought about primarily through the use of hypnosis and the modulation of language is more a need of the therapist. This is just not true: hypnosis like any other placebo will be therapeutic in about 50 per cent of the cases. But the failures, apart from the wrong selection of the cases, are due to inept handling of the communication. A therapist selects a certain message and gives a special treatment for transmission over the selected channel particularly tailored for a client. In hypnotic state, the explicit or implicit interpretation undergoes transduction. This is mediated through profound physiological processes that bring about desired therapeutic change. In this regard, the communication in hypnosis is like the strokes of a surgeon's knife. All surgeons perform surgery: deft and dexterous surgeons do it in a better way. In hypnotherapeutic session, strategic communication raises aspiration of the individual, it can project future in the present, reactivate and vivify the past and can cause its selective ablation, can raise external and internal awareness, reinforce existing belief and also motivate through promise of self-gratification or reward.

It should be kept in mind that if a message challenges attitudes, values and beliefs of the subject in a direct confrontation, it may get rejected or distorted or misinterpreted.

The therapy session may have any one of following outcome:

- *Win-Win:* Through successful outcome of the treatment, the therapist wins by job satisfaction, prestige enhancement and good relationship. The client/patient wins the cure/amelioration of the condition and value for the time, effort and money. In this "I am okay, You are okay"[25] situation, what ever transference was generated during the therapy is consumed in the service of transformation and ends with the therapy.
- *Win -lose:* The therapist wins his fees; may attribute the failure to various factors with the subject: the subject loses time, effort and money because of unsuccessful outcome of therapy. He/she may remain hankering for the therapist's support in spite of his short comings.
- *Lose-win:* The therapist tends to lose his time, prestige and even fees when dealing with subjects who pride themselves in defeating the therapist. For their neurotic compensation, they cling to their symptoms and even refuse to be hypnotized. Such subjects win by getting what they implicitly want, to retain their neurosis.
- *Lose-lose:* The therapist has not been able to pin point a diagnosis nor has he been able to set up a goal. He is shooting in the dark and administrating blunderbuss hypnotherapy that has not yielded even "feel good" factor common to hypnosis. Earning the fees is a poor

reward for the waste of professionalism. The subject loses money and gets frustration.

Milton Erickson's passive, permissive technique is highly successful for many reasons; one of them being the use of double bind phrases/strategies that he deftly employed. This requires subtlety and craft of the language. But that evolves with practice. Let us see some examples of double bind situations that result in win-win situations:

- *Pascal's wager* is a classic. If God were to exist as the Omnipotent, Omnipresent force that can do immense harm to those who are non-believers in Him, it will be a safe bet to believe in Him. If He does, He will not harm you; if He does not, it does not matter!
- *Alexander Solzhenitsyn's hero* in The First Circle: Why worry about death? So long as you exist, it is not there: when it comes, you are not there
- *A rich law college student* loaned to his friend the study expenses on the condition that he will return the amount when he wins the first law case. He turned politician instead, did not practice law and did not return the money. The friend sued him and the politician engaged himself as the defending lawyer arguing that he has not to return the loan. Does he have to pay when he loses/wins the case?
- *Let us toss* Heads I win, tails you lose!

These are just illustrations to demonstrate how double binds can be used to facilitate the therapy. In fact such usage itself is a double bind; when the therapist wins by its application, the therapist's win is in service of the client! Some double binds that are constantly handy to apply on difficult to induce clients:

- You have spent considerable time, effort and money to undergo hypnosis. Now, if you choose not to have the best value in terms of the best experience of your life, I shall honour your choice: even when it means that you will be a loser!
- The use of positive aspect cannot be overemphasized. Milton Erickson termed it as the use of "yes set". Through its use, therapist transforms the negative mindset to a positive one. This may then become a habit for life time. This is best illustrated by a story that former President of India, Abdul Kalam said:

Kalams Story

"I remember my dad teaching me the power of language at a very young age. Not only did my dad understand that specific words affect our mental pictures, but he understood words are a powerful programming factor in lifelong success.

One particularly interesting event occurred when I was eight. As a kid, I was always climbing trees, poles, and literally hanging around upside down from the rafters of our lake house. So, it came to no surprise for my dad to find me at the top of a 30-foot tree swinging back and forth. My little eight-year-old brain didn't realize the tree could break or I could get hurt. I just thought it was fun to be up so high.

My older cousin, Tammy, was also in the same tree. She was hanging on the first big limb, about ten feet below me. Tammy's mother also noticed us at the exact time my dad did. About that time a huge gust of wind came over the tree. I could hear the leaves start to rattle and the tree begin to sway. I remember my dad's voice over the wind yell, "Bart, Hold on tightly." So I did. The next thing I know, I heard Tammy screaming at the top of her lungs, laying flat on the ground. She had fallen out of the tree. I scampered down the tree to safety. My dad later told me why she fell and I did not. Apparently, when Tammy's mother felt the gust of wind, she yelled out, "Tammy, don't fall!" And Tammy did fall.

My dad then explained to me that the mind has a very difficult time processing a negative image. In fact, people who rely on internal pictures cannot see a negative at all. In order for Tammy to process the command of not falling, her nine-year-old brain had to first imagine falling, then try to tell the brain not to do what it just imagined. Whereas, my eight-year-old brain instantly had an internal image of me hanging on tightly.

This concept is especially useful when you are attempting to break a habit or set a goal. You can't visualize not doing something. The only way to properly visualize not doing something is to actually find a word for what you want to do and visualize that. For example, when I was thirteen years old, I played for my junior high school football team. I tried so hard to be good, but I just couldn't get it together at that age. I remember hearing the words run through my head as I was running out for a pass, "Don't drop it!" Naturally, I dropped the ball.

My coaches were not skilled enough to teach us proper "self-talk." They just thought some kids could catch and others couldn't. I'll never make it pro, but I'm now a pretty good Sunday afternoon football player, because all my internal dialogue is positive and encourages me to win. I wish my dad had coached me playing football instead of just climbing trees. I might have had a longer football career.

Here is a very easy demonstration to teach your kids and your friends the power of a toxic vocabulary. Ask them to hold a pen or pencil. Hand it to them. Now, follow my instructions carefully. Say to them, "Okay, try to drop the pencil." Observe what they do.

Most people release their hands and watch the pencil hit the floor. You respond, "You weren't paying attention. I said TRY to drop the pencil. Now please do it again." Most people then pick up the pencil and pretend to be in excruciating pain while their hand tries but fails to drop the pencil.

The Point is Made

If you tell your brain you will "give it a try," you are actually telling your brain to fail. I have a "no try" rule in my house and with everyone I interact with. Either people will do it or they won't. Either they will be at the party or they won't. I'm brutal when people attempt to lie to me by using the word try. Do they think I don't know they are really telegraphing to the world they have no intention of doing it but they want me to give them brownie points for pretended effort? You will never hear the words "I'll try" come out of my mouth unless I'm teaching this concept in a seminar.

If you "try" and do something, your unconscious mind has permission not to succeed. If I truly can't make a decision I will tell the truth. "Sorry John. I'm not sure if I will be at your party or not. I've got an outstanding commitment. If that falls through, I will be here. Otherwise, I will not. Thanks for the invite."

People respect honesty. So remove the word "try" from your vocabulary.

My dad also told me that psychologists claim it takes seventeen positive statements to offset one negative statement. I have no idea if it is true, but the logic holds true. It might take up to seventeen compliments to offset the emotional damage of one harsh criticism.

These are concepts that are especially useful when raising children.

Ask yourself how many compliments you give yourself daily versus how many criticisms. Heck, I know you are talking to yourself all day long. We all have internal voices that give us direction.

So, are you giving yourself the 17:1 ratio or are you shortchanging yourself with toxic self-talk like, "I'm fat. Nobody will like me. I'll try this diet. I'm not good enough. I'm so stupid. I'm broke, etc."

If our parents can set a lifetime of programming with one wrong statement, imagine the kind of programming you are doing on a daily basis with your own internal dialogue.

Here is a list of Toxic Vocabulary words.

Notice when you or Other People Use them

- *But*: Negates any words that are stated before it.
- *Try:* Presupposes failure.
- *If:* Presupposes that you may not.
- *Might:* It does nothing definite. It leaves options for your listener.
- *Would Have:* Past tense that draws attention to things that didn't actually happen.
- *Should Have*: Past tense that draws attention to things that didn't actually happen (and implies guilt.)

- *Could Have*: Past tense that draws attention to things that didn't actually happen but the person tries to take credit as if it did happen.
- *Can't/Don't:* These words force the listener to focus on exactly the opposite of what you want. This is a classic mistake that parents and coaches make without knowing the damage of this linguistic error.

Examples

Toxic phrase: "Don't drop the ball!"
Likely result: Drops the ball.
Better language: "Catch the ball!"
Toxic phrase: "You shouldn't watch so much television."
Likely result: Watches more television.
Better language: "I read too much television makes people stupid. You might find yourself turning that TV off and picking up one of those books more often!"

Exercise

Take a moment to write down all the phrases you use on a daily basis or any Toxic self-talk that you have noticed yourself using. Write these phrases down so you will begin to catch yourself as they occur and change them.

However, Erickson did make a selective use of negative that served as double bind, by phrases such as:

- And you will like to co-operate, will you not?
- You do want to experience hypnosis, do you not?
- You would not want to displease me, would you?
- You want to be helped, why not let that happen?
- You can try, cann't you?
- You do not wish to challenge me, Do you? And let me make one thing clear. I value your esteem. Rather than winning by hypnotizing you against your challenge/resistance, I may rather accept defeat and not try to help you.

Value based Assessment and Suggestions

The patients approach a therapist to seek amelioration/cure of their situation: they are not going to a court of law! Even in a court of law, the complainant is seldom punished. They do not want recrimination for themselves. Even if they were to feel at the remotest corner of their subconscious mind that they were wrong in conducting themselves some where, the grievance would be that the punishment is far too harsh. Least that a patient would like to hear from a therapist is a reprimand based on morals or ethics. Therapist must steer clear of any value based advice: otherwise it is most likely to end up in lose-lose situation.

See what happened to a highly intelligent man who joined politics to win and joined the race along with an intelligent candidate. The intelligent fellow lost to the stupid guy and he was left in the company of an intelligent man feeling stupid that he is on the losing side!

The values of the therapist may be as per his personal preference to a particular school of psychology/code of ethics. This is his personal tool. It is for his preferred way to interpret and understand the personality of the subject. But when he is serving the client, his paramount value is what works in the service of the client: he utilizes all the beliefs of the client, sense and nonsense and all the incidental occurrences during the session in the service of the client towards his/her cure. Let us pay homage to Freud with a parody about psychoanalysis[26]:

A mother went to a Freudian psychoanalyst with her daughter with the complaint that her daughter is obsessed with sexual thoughts. The therapist decided to employ ink-blot test for psychoanalysis. He showed the first bolt to the girl. She showed surprise. Another blot. More surprise, she frowned at him. Next, and the girl started giggling. With the next one, she burst out laughing, looked at her mother and exclaimed, "Look mummy, what a dirty mind this man has. He is coming out with dirty pictures all the time!"

Traffic Rules

- *Credibility*–Communication starts with a climate of belief and this climate is built by previous performance of the practitioner (prestige factor). Confidence and high regards for the therapist by the patient plays important role.
- *Context*–The context must confirm and not contradict the goal.
- *Content*–Making the subject feel good is a common context for all sessions. Contents have to be so related. The message must have a meaning for the patient and it should be compatible with his/her value system. The message must aim at positive aspect all the time. Consider this as for illustrations:
  - A half empty glass is never empty: it is half full!
  - A village elderman had one son. How nice it was for him to have to look after only one child! The boy grew up and as a young man, asked for a horse from his father. The father bought him a horse. The villagers exclaimed as how gorgeous he looks on a mounted horse. One day the horse escaped to the jungle. The villagers bemoaned the loss but the elderman said now he has less expenses to bear on feeding the horse. After some days, the horse returned from the woods, but he was accompanied by a mare! Villagers

congratulated the elder man on being lucky!. One day, the young man fell down the mare while training her and broke his leg. He had to be bed-ridden. How good that there were so many well wishers and they came to ask about him! Suddenly, a war broke out and the king's men came and recruited all the young man for the army. The young man with the broken leg was spared!

- *Clarity*–The message should be in simple words or terms.
- *Confusion*–The use of confusion is a highly skilled method. In fact, it enhances the depth of the trance and at the same time, because of permissive approach by the therapist, is better accepted. The subtle skill is required to use double bind phrases. This is better avoided by the beginners.
- *Continuity and consistency*—Communication that results in the desired change can be an unending process. It requires repetition. Repetition with variation contributes to both factual and attitude learning.
- *Channel*—Established channels of communication should be used, channels that receiver uses and respects. Speaking in clients language, i.e. "use the currency of the country where you are" approach should be used.
- *Capability of the client*—Communication should be at level of the client, i.e. with child it should be in the form of a story. The stories when employed should be in the forms of metaphor.

Communication in a Hypnotherapeutic Session

A hypnotherapeutic session consists of everything the client will experience, including the reception area.

Clinical Setup and Décor of Reception Area

The earliest or first communication that client receives about therapist is from the "prestige factor" of therapist which is communicated by some other person who has referred. This starts building an image of the therapist. This gets endorsed at an early phase at the time a telephone call is made for an appointment. The receptionist interaction plays important role. This should be welcoming, warm, sympathetic and soft.

The set-up of the reception and the clinic is the first indirect message that the client receives. The reception area should have pleasant, warm and soothing décor in the form of colour of walls. The pictures on the wall should preferably be scenes bringing you close to the nature. There may be flowers or bouquet in the corner or the central table. The receptionist should be with pleasing personality. Playing soft music in the background may enhance the friendly environment of the décor.

In-office Rapport

The office is the meeting place of therapist with the client where direct and indirect communication takes place simultaneously, direct communication in the form of verbal and indirect in the form of body language, gestures, postures and environmental feel by the client. Here the first impression is built with the look of therapist where therapist needs to be in professional poise with confidence, welcoming the client with courtesy due to his/her status. On the other hand, the therapist starts receiving messages before the first word is spoken. This is by observing the demeanor of the client, noting the accompanying persons (or noting that none is accompanying) and other features that are generally written large in the form of body language.

After a formal welcome, the first sentence by the therapist is, *"Yes, what can I do for you?"* The use of the phrase, *"so, what is your problem?"* is avoided: often the client retorts to such an question by saying, *"it is for you to find out!"*

The interaction with patient can be in the form of passive and active listening. Passive listening can be with making eye contact and listening intently to what client is saying without making statements of your own except *"Go ahead, I am listening"*. However sounds may be made such as *"Mmm-Hmm"*, *"I see"*, *Okay"*, *"Right"*.

Usage of metaphors by the patient can provide important cues. When the patient says *"It's a headache"* meaning thereby that he is facing a difficult to solve situation. Sometimes patient uses phrases like *"Pain in the neck"* or *"Backache"* and *"Heavy burden on my shoulders"*. Commonly, a frozen shoulder(s) is a symptom of failure to maneuver some intricate situation. They provide clues to pathogenesis.

Active listening can be in the form of listening for content and feelings. Active listening for content can be enhanced by saying *"Tell me more about that."* Or, *"Help me understand that better, please!"* This encourages the client to speak more about his/her complaint.

Active listening for feeling is most important as it deals with the emotional part. All emotional decisions are made in relationship to values. Active listening is initiated by utilizing phrases like *"You feel."*, *"You are...."*, Such phrases let the other person know that you are in touch in with what he/she is feeling. Tell the patient *"I can understand what you are feeling...."* The goal in listening with feelings is to

SYMPATHIZE → ANALYZE → SYNTHESIZE.

This is put to a severe test when a subject undergoes catharsis. On the other hand, the therapist should watch out to avoid burn out for himself.

The usual protocol of having a female attendant standing by is strictly to be followed. This is regardless of the sex of the therapist. The room door is better left partly open: it is metaphorical message to the subject that he/she may exit out of the session at any time.

Finally, before the induction of trance, tacit understanding is established that the subject may say, yes, by the movement of index finger of the right hand and no, by the movement of the index finger of the left hand.[27]

The pre-induction communication is over when the client is explained about what hypnosis is and what it is not by eliminating the mis-concepts. Client's active participation and involvement during the procedure should be discussed and explained before starting induction. Formal consent should be signed in. Consent to touch, explaining its relevance to activation of certain genes, if necessary should always be taken.

Communication during Trance Induction

When the session begins, a change in sitting arrangements is an indirect suggestion that there is now a paradigm shift. The distance between therapist and subject should be discreet: not too close and not to near. There should be enough space around the hypnotized subject: we recommend at least 150 sq.ft. in therapy: the same amount of space will make a group session more expanding. Should there be a space constraint, a minimum space that we recommend is about 100 sq.ft. per subject in a group session. The space for the observers is not that important. They are made to sit separately. The fact that it is usual for the observers to become participants unknowingly adds extra responsibility for the therapist. No hypnotized subject should be left out of site, unattended, since he/she is comparable to a patient under anesthesia.

The use of language for the induction may be

- Positive and confident.
- May be authoritative (Direct communication) or permissive as per the style of therapist.
- Monotonous at the base line: with ups and downs when the therapist desires emphasis. There are pauses when the speech becomes slurred or appears to fade away. The sentences may be broken and may deliberately left incomplete. There is repetition. For instance:

Now…. that we have agreed… yes, we…have…agreed to so work…yes, we are now engaged in…useful…creative, work…yes, this most pleasant experience is a new creation…by you…of your own…. potential talent…. I am indeed, yes indeed, privileged…. privileged to have discovered your immense human potential….that for you…. in your service, we are now…. engaged in the activity, a joyous pursuit…. to co-create…. a new dimension of your well being!

Confusing (vide supra)

Let us illustrate with an example as to how the use of alliteration as a figure of speech can cause wonder leading to confusion by play of words with different connotations. This was taught as a method of induction and Y. Chandarana surprised and "hypnotized" peers and teachers with the following at the farewell function. This is how it was worded:

Dear colleagues.... We joined the college for Clinical hypnosis with curiosity, choice or with clarity about hypnosis or to clear confusion and to change the common concept seen in community.

Confirming our convincing career commercially we gained confidence in close association and with cooperation of our most clever and capable coach who at his command created a convincing communication through confusion constantly and carefully but cautiously and consciously inducing hypnotic trance which conveyed and confirmed our conviction about hypnosis.

Our concealed, conflicting concepts collapsed completely, calling our competitive comments in company of co-existing colleagues. Our current teacher taught us correct conditioning of mind casually, conveniently without cheating and condemning but by converting our old belief to change and channelizing our cravings to conquer the summits of success in community and country to be a better hypnotherapist and good citizen of tomorrow.

Let us commence with clench fist technique in contrast to the form of our curriculum or consequently combining and considering collectively the currency of the country approach we compromised and conclude one of the methods of hypnosis.

I confess at my cognitive and affect level to express at connation level of salute that I conceived this idea of conclusive hypnotic communication conveyed by our beloved teacher for the sure cure of psychosomatic problems in every corner of the country.

The indirect language like above can be used along with the body language of touch to the client with prior permission or consent_in conscious state to make patient feel that some manipulation is done to create a state of relaxation.

Communication in Trance

In trance, the mind has to be engaged through its various sensory inputs like ears, eyes, nose, tongue, and skin (*touch sensation*). For example when you take a patient in garden (in trance stage) from the place where he/she is, through a busy road in a vehicle (*kinetic*) of his/her choice, with sounds of various vehicles on the road (*auditory*) and on reaching the garden, he/she is made to experience the smell of wet soil and fragrance of flowers (*olfactory*). With gentle breeze and cool wind passing around (*touch*) while walking, (*kinesthetic*) seeing the birds and people around (*visual*) and along with the people eating some tasty food (*taste*). The panoramic perspective of garden evokes the feelings of peace, pleasure and happiness of a serene and sublime nature (*aesthetic*) that is a natural due for the subject (*ego strengthening*). The key words like please, good and thank you used as often as possible. The positive response of patient, ascertained through ideomotor signals is reinforced using similar words.

Communication should be at the intellectual level of the client. While treating a child it should be in the world of cartoons and animals. For any age, story telling in direct or indirect way is always better and care should be taken to involve in it the emotional component of the story.

With currency of country approach wherein if a patient believes in some God or Goddess or Deities, the blessings may be invoked during trance state as it works in our country where most people have firm beliefs about their spiritual lineage. The basic beliefs of the individual are not violated but made use of. The ideomotor signals in the form of yes and no movements of the finger can convert a session into an exploration of all the layers of mind so that the session may turn out to be hypnoanalysis. Such a session almost turns out to be a communion in consciousness.[28]

This is advanced technique that requires supervised practice to start with. It is also possible to communicate verbally in deep trance. Demonstration of other subjects in deep trance states, with demonstrable phenomena like arm levitation, hypnoanethesia and somnabulism can also work as communication in therapeutic session.

So in trance it is important to project or picture his/her personal, protective preferences with powerful praise, administered patiently, preferably peacefully, purposefully, persistently and permanently for positive result. Summarizing,

VERBALIZE → EMOTIONALIZE→MATERIALIZE TRANSFORMATION

Posthypnotic Suggestions

Freud went to learn hypnosis from Bernheim. As a post hypnotic suggestion, it was told to the client that at the end of the session, he will get up from his chair and straight go to the corner where his umbrella was kept and pick it up. The subject did so no sooner his trance ended. The importance of this was lost to even Freud and some how he did not patronize hypnotherapy[29]. The relevance of the matter is that post hypnotic suggestions are as much important as therapeutic strategy. The cues provided at this level work very effectively, such as:

- At your next appointment, as soon as you will sit down in this chair, you will put yourself in deep trance.
- As soon as you perceive the built up of anger within yourself, you will take three deep breaths. That will relax you and make you retain your poise.

- As soon as you feel anxious/nervous to face audience, you shall put your left hand in left side pocket of your trouser and touch index finger to the thumb. Your confidence will surge!

A standard nonspecific post hypnotic suggestion is assurance of optimum hopeful future. It may be suggested as desired outcome with time progression.

At the conclusion of the therapy, before the discharge, suggestions should be given that the result is well deserved and a natural due. This the patient has earned for his/herself. While the therapist is privileged to have been a facilitator, perhaps he is no more needed. This will help eliminate residual transference.

Hypnosis with Deaf

Though it may appear formidable, through non-verbal communication, hypnosis can be easily induced. Such occasions are rare. But pantomime practice with the subjects with normal hearing will be helpful.

Notes

1. Rankin J.A. *Body Language: First Impressions*, Bangalore, 2003.
2. O'Connor J. and Seymour J. *Training with NLP*, San Franscisco, 1994.
3. Neuro-linguistic programming (or NLP) is a interpersonal communication model initially co-created by Richard Bandler and linguist John Grinder in the 1970s. It is claimed that it draws from aspects of neurology ("neuro-"), linguistics and computer science ("programming").
   Tension exists between several divergent groups within NLP. NLP has often been promoted as an art and science of effective communication and "the study of the structure of subjective experience". Others have tended to define NLP as a methodology for effective communication or modeling excellence as it was originally created.
   NLP has enjoyed little support within the psychological profession following research reviewed in the *Journal of Counseling Psychology* in the early 1980s. This led some skeptics and psychologists to dismiss NLP as a pseudoscientific or New Age form of psychotherapy. A recent survey of mental health professionals rated NLP as having questionable validity as a psychotherapeutic technique. While there has been some efforts within NLP to improve its practice, recent research is spread thinly across various disciplines and the field remains splintered.
   Our perspective of this is that all psychotherapeutical intervantion are neurolinguistic. The words are symbols and take creative meaning on reflection and pondering. NLP in practice does function in the ground of hypnosis. Since most important parameter of hypnosis is that it is altered state of consciouness, it alters the perception of linguistic semantics: words become metaphors and metaphors transform as reality. We recommend hypnotherapists to learn NLP.
4. Maneka Gandhi, *The Penguin Book of HIndu Names for the Girls*, New Delhi, 2004.
5. Maneka Gandhi, *The Penguin Book of Hindu Names for Boys*, New Delhi, 2004.

6. Maneka Gandhi and Ozair Hussain, *The Complete Book of Muslim and Parsi Names,* New Delhi, 2004.
7. *Umashankar Joshi, Prachina (Gujarati),* Bombay, 1950.
8. Sigmund Freud, *The Interpretation of Dreams,* Ware, 1997.
9. Carl Jung, *Psychology and Religion,* New Heaven 1938, p. 63.
10. The scientific foundations in terms of neurological parameters are still to be established.
11. Pamela Ball, *10,000 Dreams Interpreted,* New Delhi, 2000.
12. Ernest Rossi, Sleep, Dream, Hypnosis and Healing: Behavioural State-Related Gene Expression and Psychotherapy, *Sleep and Hypnosis,* 1:141-157;1999.
13. Swami Suddhabodhananad Saraswati, *Om Based Meditation,* Commentary on Pancikaranam by Adi Sankaracharya, Mumbai, 1998.
14. Sri Aurobindo, *Savitri,* Pondicherry,1990, p. 310.
15. Kapali Shastri, T.V., *Further Lights—Vedas and the Tantras,* Pondicherry, 1951, pp. 132ff.
16. The Dalai Lama, *Kindness, Clarity, and Insight,* Ed. Jeffrey Hopkins and Elizabeth Napper, 1985, pp. 116-117.
17. Vyas Bhaskar and Vyas Rajni, *Space—Time—Consciousness,* The Fifth Dimension, Delhi, 2004, pp. 220-228.
18. Nathan, R.S., *Symbolism in Hinduism,* Bombay, 1989.
19. Ernest Rossi *4th National Congress of Society of Clinical and Applied Hypnosis,* Bangalore, 1999.
20. Bhaskar Vyas, *A Philosopher's Journey, Reflections on the Times and Values* of Rohit Mehta, Vallabh VIdyanagar, 1998, pp. 103-04.
21. Savitri is a modern epic by Sri Aurobindo. In this context a case history is illustrative:

    A middle aged lady, chartered accountant, was found to have tuberculosis of pituitary gland following exploration for a pituary tumor. She has developed quite come de-personalization following the removal of caseous material. She developed allergies to all the five antituberculosis drugs and would not tolerate them. She rapidly lost ground.

    Though not a religious person, she was a follower of Sri Aurobindo. She has been to Pondicherry several times. She would not agree to hypnotherapy but could be engaged in talking about the epic Savitri. Utilizing indirect hypnosis, it was impressed upon her that the poet in his introduction to the epic emphasizes that the characters can come alive and can be engaged in a dialogue. And she was made to experience the presence of three madonnas described in the epic while she went to the Ashram at Pondicheery in hypnosis. Following four sessions, her allergies disappeared. The endocrinologist could complete her therapy.

    This was about 12 years ago. She is well and professionally engaged. She has no memory of her therapy.
22. Sri Aurobindo, *Savitri: A Legend and A symbol,* Pondicherry, 1990.
23. John Blofeld, *The Way of Power,* London, 1970, pp. 103-112.
24. C.W. Leadbeater, *The Chakras: A monograph,* Adyar, Chennai, 1927.
25. Erik Burne, *I am okay, You are okay,* New York, 1976.
26. Through out the book, we wish this approach to be maintained. We are not Freudian, and yet, on the basis that psychoanalysis helps to explain so much of neurotic behaviour and decompensation, a chapter on Freud is thought important.

27. Interesting cross over are observed in the trance while eliciting this kind of ideomotor signals. Sometimes, other than the prefixed finger moves; at times the whole of the hand, or all five fingers move. This indicates a deep trance: so does no movement at all in an otherwise deeply hypnotized subject.
28. To quote Patanjali: *pratyayasya para-citta-jnanam*. It translates as, By communing with the thought-expression of the other, one can understand how his mind functions. III, 19.
29. We believe, had he done so, the future of the civilization would have been different.

18
Induction Techniques

There are innumerable techniques for induction. Apart from what one can absorb from the West, Indian tradition of *tantra* and Buddhist Vajrayana describe innumerable techniques for meditation that may as well be used for induction of hypnosis. It is therefore, impossible to explore all of them. We shall describe a few that are easy to practice and learn. Before we do that, let us reiterate some fundamentals that we have already established so far.

Hypnosis is easy to induce. Hypnotherapy requires in depth understanding. As surgery cannot be learnt by reading books on operative techniques, so is the case with hypnotherapy.

The objective is to bring the patient to a hyper suggestible, altered state of consciousness. Toward this end the operator executes a number of maneuvers, the most common one being a state of muscular relaxation and the fixation of attention. Important rules are:

1. Engage the attention of the patient by assigning a task, (muscle relaxation, hand clasp, levitation). The description follows.
2. Approach the induction with a confident manner. Any faltering or lack of confidence in vocal expression influences the patient negatively. Adopt a persuasive, calm, reassuring tone of voice, droning suggestions rhythmically and monotonously.
3. Employ repetition in suggestions to focus the patient attention.
4. Excite the imagination of the patient by building word pictures so that the patient practically lives and feels what is suggested. Emotional situations have to be relived.
5. In children engage their attention by asking them to imagine watching a television screen and observing their favourite programmes.
6. We have already emphasized to use positive rather than negative suggestions. For example where pain is to be deadened do not say "you will have no pain." Say, *"The sensation will change so that instead of feeling what you have been feeling it will feel dull, numb, and tolerable."* If a hypodermic injection is to be given, do not say, *"This will not hurt,"* but *"rather—this will be like a tiny mosquito bite."*

7. Should the patient at any time open the eyes and insist that he or she is not hypnotized, put your fingers on the eyelids to shut them and say, "That doesn't matter, I just want you to relax...." Or, "they are your own eyes, you can keep them open or you can keep them closed; but when you keep them closed, you will feel so much better relaxed." Then continue with suggestions.
8. Almost universally, patients after the first induction, even those who have been deeply hypnotized, may insist they were not in a trance. Reply with "Of course you weren't asleep or anesthetized. You were in a state of relaxation and this is all that is necessary. You may go deeper next time but it really doesn't matter. Or, explain that hypnosis is one of the states of consciousness; consciousness means that you are aware." Give the patient a printed copy of material describing some phenomena of hypnosis.
9. Some operators find it important to tell the patient that all that will be achieved in the first session is not hypnosis but a state of relaxation that will help the patient quiet the symptoms: "If you fall asleep, that is fine; if you feel completely awake, that too is fine. The effect will still be there." To some people the word "hypnosis" has many unfortunate connotations. It often embraces expectations of an immediate miracle cure. When the patient fails to go into the depth of trance he or she expected to achieve with the "hypnotic" induction, one may become upset, feel hopeless, and lose confidence in the therapist.
10. Through out the session and duration of therapy, one has to keep the psycho cybernetic rules of suggestions in mind. They are:
    - *Law of concentrated focalized attention*: What ever is said repectitively, is likely to be believed. The proof is evident in marketing; people buy what they repeatedly hear to be the best. So, the suggestions revolve and revert back to one single message.
    - *Law of reverse effect*: Trying hard makes the subject resist even more: let the process be smooth, effortless and gentle. If you cannot hypnotize easily, better to suggest: "It is up to you to relax and follow my suggestions or to resist. You need help and have asked for it and I am here to do my best: but it can be done with your explicit cooperation. You have invested your time and money by way of my fees.... If you so choose, we may try some other time."
    - *Imagination supersedes will*. To make effort by strong "will power" negates the first law. In Classical Indian tradition, two kinds of mental energies are described: creative power of wish and formative power of will. Subconscious wishes and imagination so evokes the creative power that it autonomously propels the actions in the desired direction. Formative power of will materializes the desired results.

- *Law of dominant effect.* If there are two contradictory processes going on in the psyche, one that is more profound will be perceived and the other will be subdued. A person with chronic pain may be made to experience anesthesia and, then a profoundly joyful experience be substituted with the suggestion that it will continue as post hypnotic effect too.
- *Carrot principle.* Rather than pushing from behind, lure from the front. Goals have been defined while taking the history. During the session, gentle reiteration of the goals that are natural dues of the subject keeps the psychodynamic movement in that direction.
- *Law of trance reinforcement.* When a person in trance comes out partially and views some phenomena of hypnosis on display, say hand levitation, needle passed through his skin, ideomotor signals etc. the trance is deepened. To see other subjects in trance in a group induces hypnosis in the viewer also. Pendulum is very useful for induction as well as reinforcement.
- *Principle of utilization.* All that happens during hypnosis is to be utilized in the service of deepening the trance. For instance, swallowing commonly occurs during induction and during sessions. Then, the suggestion is to say that as you have swallowed that saliva, you are going in to deeper trance. When the subject coughs, to suggest that you have coughed out your irritations.

Induction techniques may be employed depending upon what the therapist is trained with. In brief, all techniques revolve around the following steps:

1. Promoting motivations that will lead to hypnosis by associating the desire to get well with cooperation in the hypnotic process.
2. Removing misconceptions and fears about hypnosis by explanation and clarification.
3. Introducing a suggestibility test, like the hand clasp test to demonstrate that the patient can follow directions.
4. Giving the patient a short preparatory talk to the effect that the patient will not really go to sleep even though sleep suggestions will help one relax and that one will not be asked embarrassing questions or forced to do anything one does not want to do.

Hand Clasp Method

One of the easiest ways of inducing hypnosis is by means of the suggestibility test of the hand clasp. To do this the patient is made comfortable in an armchair and asked to relax the body progressively, starting with the muscles in the forehead, then the face, neck, shoulders, arms, back, thighs and legs. Following this the patient is enjoined to clasp hands, about a foot or so away from the eyes.

With eyes fixed on the hands, they are clasped together more and more firmly as the therapist counts from one to five stating that then, it will be difficult or impossible to separate the hands. After the patient has cooperated with this suggestion, the patient is to stare at the hands while the eyes begin to feel tired and the eyelids get heavy. The eyelids progressively will get heavier and heavier until the eyelids feel like lead. The eyes will soon close and a pleasant sense of relaxation will sweep over the patient. These suggestions are repeated over and over in a monotonous cadence and in a firm, reassuring tone until the eyes close. The hands are then unclasped with or without the help of the therapist.

Progressive Muscular Relaxation Technique

It involves deep relaxation of the muscles of body in a definite sequence, which does not require imagination, willpower or suggestion.

Physiological Principle of PMR

The deep muscle relaxation technique is based on the premise that the body responds to anxiety-provoking thoughts and events with muscle tension. This physiological tension in turn, increases the subjective experience of anxiety.

Deep muscle relaxation reduces physiological tension and is incompatible with anxiety. The habit of responding with one blocks the habit of responding with the other. It is aptly stated that in a relaxed body, a tense mind cannot exist Progressive relaxation of the muscles of body reduces pulse rate and blood pressure as well as decreasing perspiration and respiratory rates. At the psychological level deep muscle relaxation, when successfully mastered, reduces the feelings of anxiety and psychological stress.

Some believe this method as a better one in the treatment of muscular tension, anxiety, insomnia, depression, fatigue, irritable bowel disease, muscle spasms, neck and back pains, high blood pressure, mild phobias and stuttering.

Recommended Practice

In order to successfully master deep muscle relaxation for self hypnosis, it is recommended to practice the technique for one to two weeks, two 20 minutes sessions per day.

Four major muscle groups are covered during the technique:

1. Hands, Forearms and biceps.
2. Head, face, throat and shoulders, including concentration on forehead, cheeks, nose, eyes, jaws, lips, tongue and neck. Considerable attention is devoted to the head, because from the emotional point of view, the most important muscles in the body are situated in an around this region.

3. Chest, stomach and lower back.
4. Thighs, buttocks, calves and feet.

Progressive relaxation can be practiced best lying down in a bed in *Shavasana* (the dead body posture) or in a chair with head supported. Each muscle or muscle group is tensed from five to seven seconds and subsequently relaxed for twenty to thirty seconds. This procedure is repeated at least once. If an area remains tense, you can practice up to five times. The following relaxing expressions will prove to be useful to use when getting rid of tension:

- Let go of the tension
- Throw away the tension – you are feeling calm and rested.
- Relax and smooth out the muscles.
- Let the tension dissolve away.

During the procedure it is important to keep the eyes closed and focus attention on just one muscle group at a time.

Procedure

Get in a comfortable position and relax. Now, clench your right fist, tighter and tighter, studying the tension as you do so. Keep it clenched and notice the tension in your fist, hand and forearm. Now relax. Feel the looseness in your right hand, and notice the contrast with the tension. Repeat this procedure with your right fist again and mark the difference between tension and relaxation. Repeat the entire procedure with your left fist, then both fists at once.

Now, bend your elbows and tense your biceps. Tense them as hard as you can and observe the feeling of tightness. Relax, straighten out your arms. Let the relaxation develop and feel the difference. Repeat this once again.

Now, focus your attention on your head. Wrinkle your forehead as tight as you can. Then relax and smooth it out. Let your entire forehead and scalp become smooth and at rest. Now frown and notice the strain spreading throughout your forehead. Let go. Allow your brows to become smooth again. Close your eyes tightly now. Look for the tension.

Relax your eyes. Let them remain closed gently and comfortably. Now clench your jaw, bite hard, notice the tension throughout your jaw. Relax your jaw. When the jaw is relaxed, your lips will be slightly parted. Experience the difference between tension and relaxation. Now press your tongue against the roof of your mouth. Feel the ache in the back of your mouth. Relax. Press your lips now; purse them into an "O". Relax your lips. Notice that your forehead, scalp, eyes, jaw, tongue and lips are all relaxed.

Press your head back as far as it can comfortably go and observe the tension in your neck. Roll it first to the right, then to the left and feel the changing locus of stress. Straighten your head, and then bring it forward. Press your chin against your chest. Feel the tension in your throat and the back of your neck. Relax. Allow you to return to a comfortable position. Let the relaxation deepen. Now, shrug your shoulders. Keep the tension as you hunch your head down between your shoulders. Relax the shoulders. Allow them to drop back and feel the relaxation spreading through your neck, throat and shoulders.... Pure relaxation.... going deeper and deeper.

Allow your entire body to relax. Feel the comfort and the heaviness. Now breathe in and fill your lungs completely. Hold your breath. Notice the tension. Now exhale, let your chest become loose. Continue relaxing, letting your breath course freely and gently. Repeat this several times, experiencing the tension draining from your body as you exhale. Tighten your abdominal muscles and hold. Note the tension, then relax. Now, draw a deep breath in and allow your abdomen to move out, freely and slowly. Hold, and relax. Next push the air out gently through the abdomen and watch your abdomen going in slowly. Repeat this several times. Feel the contrast between tension and relaxation as you breathe in and out. Now arch your back without straining. Keep the rest of the body as relaxed as possible. Focus on the tension in your lower back. Then relax, deeper and deeper.

Next, tighten your buttocks and thighs; flex your thighs by pressing down your heels as hard as you can. Relax and feel the difference. Now, curl your toes downward, making your calves tense. Note the tension. Relax. Then bend your toes upwards, creating tension in your shins. Relax again.

Feel the relaxation throughout your lower body as the relaxation deepens. Relax your feet, ankles, calves, shins, knees, thighs and buttocks. Let go of the tension in both the legs. Let the relaxation spread to your stomach, lower back and chest. Let go more and more. Experience the relaxation deepening in your shoulders, arms and hands.... Deeper and deeper.... Notice the feeling of looseness and relaxation in your neck, jaws and all your facial muscles.

Quick Procedure

This procedure achieves deep muscle relaxation quickly. It shortens the procedure by simultaneously tensing and relaxing many muscles at one time so that deep muscle relaxation can be achieved in a very brief period. Each muscle group is tensed for five to seven seconds and relaxed from 20 to 30 seconds. Every time it is important to notice the contrast between the sensations of tension and relaxation.

1. Curl fists, tightening biceps, and forearms. Relax.
2. Wrinkle up forehead. At the same time, press your head as far back as possible, roll it clockwise in a complete circle, reverse. Now wrinkle up the muscles of your face; frowning, eyes squinted, lips pursed, tongue pressing the roof of the mouth and shoulders hunched. Relax.

3. Arch back as you take a deep breath into the chest. Hold. Relax. Take a deep breath, pressing out the stomach. Hold. Relax.
4. Pull your feet and toes back towards face, tightening shins. Hold. Relax. Curl toes, simultaneously tightening calves, thighs and buttocks. Relax.

Special Considerations

1. It is only a matter of practice to achieve deep muscle relaxation. Initially it takes about 20 minutes of work to bring only partial relaxation, but with regular practice, eventually, it will be possible to relax the whole body in a few moments.
2. After complete relaxation it is helpful to scan different muscle or muscle groups in to the body and pay particular attention to those muscles which may be partially relaxed, a certain number of muscle fibers will still be contracted. It is the act of relaxing these additional fibers that will bring about the desired emotional effect. It is helpful to say during the relaxation phase, *"Let go more and more"*.
3. Caution should be taken in tensing the neck and back. Excessive tightening may result in muscle injury. Over tightening of the toes or feet can result in muscle cramping.

Eye Fixation Technique

Test the hypnotic suggestibility by asking the subject to look up and see the roll of the eye ball. When there is a lag of the eye ball so as to show the white of the sclera between the upper lid and the eye ball, the subject is highly suggestibile.

Ask the subject to: Look at a spot on the ceiling or a picture hung at a higher level... focalize and gaze steadily.... Wink if you have to; but you feel relaxed without winking... That helps you to take a deep breath and as you do that, you can now let go your tension ... and see how relief from tension causes relaxation all over the body...so that your eyelids are now getting tired and...they want to close...they are indeed getting very...very heavy and it is getting impossible for them to remain open...let them close...and relax completely.

A Hypnotherapy Session My Way: Bhaskar Vyas

My method of therapy is passive and permissive. Even when I am incorporating a therapeutic suggestion, I ascertain the implicit willingness to accept by ideomotor signal. I have evolved my own method; however, my peers and students label it as Eriksonian. I do not set a prescribed number of sessions but I always explain that reinforcement is necessary and should be asked for when needed. Sometimes the subject derives benefit from a single session but a word of caution is always given that follow up is must to avoid recurrence.

The first session, and preferably the second one too, are of at least 90 minutes duration. That way I am strictly Eriksonian about the time frame. This is subsequently expounded by Cheek and Rossi[1] and further explored by Rossi.[2]

Psychodynamic principles viz. The principles of reinforcement, law of reverse effect and the law of dominant effect[3, 4] are utilized often with a double blind so as to ensure compliance.

A standard session is structured as:

1. History taking, medical check up, rapport building/follow up of the previous session after the first session.
2. Diagnosis/Provisional diagnosis is written down. Goal is set and written down.
3. Change of paradigm by shifting the positions.
4. Induction.
5. Ego strengthening.
6. Deepening.
7. Elicitation of ideomotor signal.
8. Therapeutic suggestions.
9. Termination of the trance.
10. Post hypnotic suggestions.
11. Alerting the subject.
12. Review of the session/fixing next appointment.
13. The last session terminates the treatment. Ejection of the therapist and transference are covertly executed.

- *Change of Paradigm*

It helps in induction to change the positions. Usually in clinical set up, the therapist sits across a table opposite to the patient. Hypnotherapy is a change of paradigm from the ordinary awake rational logical state to a state of hypersuggestibility and such other parameters.

This is implied when the subject is asked to lie down, or change into an easy chair or to a couch. I prefer an easy chair where the subject can recline. I sit on the right side/left side of the subject after verifying whether the person is right handed or left handed.

Permission to touch is obtained. I employ what was described as stroking by the earlier generation of hypnotherapists often times in a session. An empathetic touch can promote healing through the activation of IEGs.[5]

- *Method of Induction*

For the first session, I use a quick technique for induction that relies heavily on confusion. I take the hand of the subject in my hands and appear to be making athetoid movements at the wrist, elbow and shoulder of the subject. He relaxes. Then I use rotational movements of the neck and, when that is found to be relaxed, I give a tap on the vortex.[6] This is combined with vague, non articulate communication. In a few minutes only, trance is induced. For the subsequent sessions, confusion is further utilized by using a different method. For this, the use of an improvised pendulum and demonstration of an electromagnetic field between two hands—resulting in hand clap—are my favourite methods. Post hypnotic suggestion is given that you are a fast learner and next time you come for therapy, no sooner you sit in this chair, you shall so well relax that you will put yourself in a trance. At the subsequent sessions, I utilize this to say, now that you are comfortably seated, relax and put yourself in trance.

Regardless of the method of induction, suggestions for deep breathing and relaxation are incorporated.

Coin Induction Method

It is rare to come across resistance to induction in subjects who have willingly come for therapy and have paid for it. In case it is there, I utilize coin induction method as follows:

I have here some coins of the same denomination. I am told by the bankers that their weight varies according to the date of issue. Yet I am at a loss to find out which is the odd piece that is heaviest. Could you please help me? (After some shuffling of the coins)…Yes, I think now I have got it… Thank you…And I was also told that the odd piece has some mystique about it…It can change its weight…. Would you like to verify it?….The physicists tell me that when you look at it, it gathers some subatomic particles that increase its weight….Hold it in your palm with the arm straight at the level of the heart and just stare at it…More intense you look, the more particles are absorbed it….So just stare, try to avoid blinking….and as you are staring intently, you find that it gets heavy…heavier and heavier….so that at some point… your hand is no more able to hold it….it starts shaking….and the coin is so heavy now…that it falls down….What potential have you got!. Very nice….let your eyes close…they have done lot of work…but should you like them to be open….fine, that is the way we have come over here…but probably you may like to be more comfortable now….so you be more comfortable with eyes closed, deep breathing and relax…relax all over.

- ***Ego Strenghtening***

There is a general rejection of the word ego in the Indian psyche (See the Chapter on Indian Psyche). It is a cultural bias and it is not implied that the Indians are any way less ego-centric. Therefore, I avoid the use of word, ego, even when I am dealing with subjects who are well versed with psychology. I pick up from a trivial matter, like how very nice of you to come on time and build up from there. If the person is highly educated, he is complimented for being so intelligent and making my work easy; if otherwise, it is so nice to work with subjects who have studied less and understood more that they are not argumentative all the time.

There is no subject that cannot be complimented for some of the qualities like dress, simplicity, innocence, refinement, etiquette and even absurdities can be complimented as the traits of geniuses.

- ***Methods of Deepening***

The usual methods of deepening that I use are:

1. With every deep breath, you are relaxing more and more.
2. As you are listening to my voice, you are going into a deeper and deeper state of trance.
3. Your eyelids are deeply relaxed. They are very heavy. You try to open them and find that you can not open them.... Yes, try to open them.... How difficult it is to open them!... And as you find you cannot open them, you go into a deeper and more peaceful state of enjoyable trance.
4. Every gesture that the subject makes, like swallowing the saliva, is utilized as: As you have swallowed that saliva, it goes down your gullet and as it goes down, you are getting down and down into a deeper state of trance.
5. Arm levitation and catalepsy of the arm.
6. Surgical anesthesia: using glove and stocking anesthesia induction and insertion of a hypodermic needle.
7. Following hypnotic phenomena are frequently utilized as may be appropriate to the subject's symptoms.
8. Time dilatation and distortion, to and fro undulation of moment of time. My most frequently used method is age regression (See the Chapter on Age regression).
9. Space transmigration to a comfort chamber, sea shore, mountain peaks.
10. Journey through Space-time dimension.
11. Goal setting by age progression.

- ***Ideomotor Signalling***

While some of the phenomena mentioned above are ideosensory and may be utilized all through out the trance, the therapist derives inferences from the ideomotor signals by the subject. Their importance cannot be overemphasized. Before the beginning of the session, the subject is told that the "right hand" is Yes hand and left is "No hand". No sooner the person is in trance, he is taken

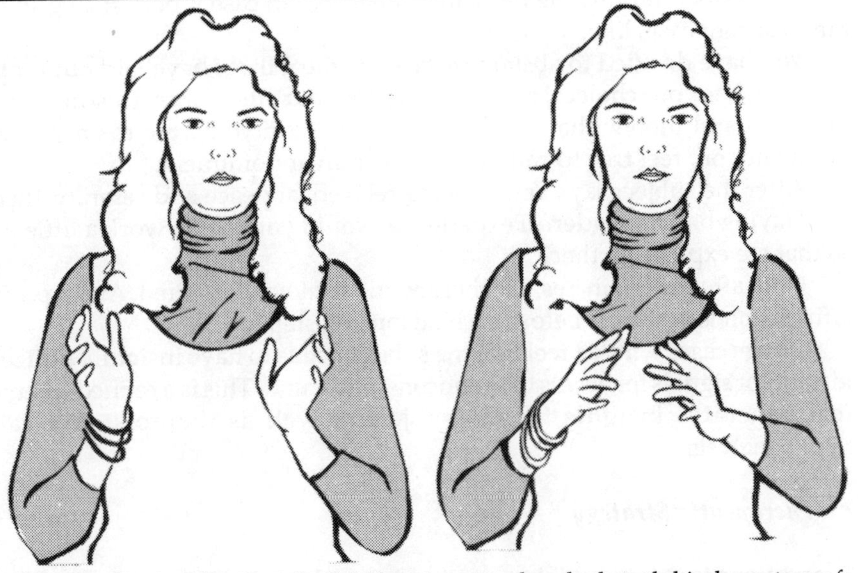

Fig. 18.1: Demonstration of a field between two hands though kind courtesy of ernest and Kathryn Rossi

Field between the Two Hands Technique

Ask the subject to sit comfortably and hold the hands straight at the shoulder level about 14 inches apart. Ask him to oscillate the hands a few inches towards each other and as he does that, perceive that with every move towards each other, it is gradually getting difficult to draw them apart. They move closer and closer with each oscillation so that they come to clasp each other eventually. It is difficult to separate them now. Apply some force to unclasp them and still they remain stuck. Suggest that as the therapist separates them, they do so easily and fall in the lap. Trance ensues.

forward to do therapeutic work through eliciting ideomotor signals to the questions such as:

As you have relaxed, with each deep breath you are feeling an increasing feeling of peace, quietude and serenity. If you are feeling so, move the index finger of the right hand. Generally the answer is movement of Yes hand.

- ***Resistance to Induction***

In case there is resistance, the dialogue will proceed somewhat like:

> It is my privilege to make you experience one of the finest moments.... That is the fundamental attribute of all mankind.... It is your prerogative whether to let yourself have this experience or not.... As only you can decide whether to allow yourself the pleasure of a nice meal that is laid out....or go fasting. Would you like to deprive yourself of a fine treat?

Generally after this the resistance melts, but in case it persists, I give up a rare resistant case, like;

You have decided to abstain from a fine meal that I have laid out for you. Any way, it is your choice; I am privileged for your attendance. I also appreciate the effort and money that you have spent. Should you were to change your mind later on, feel free to call up and make an appointment.

After the subject says Yes, to being relaxed, at peace and serenity, then,

Having had a wonderful experience, would you like to work a little more so that we explore further?

Only after a certain Yes, the therapeutic strategy is applied. And a positive affirmation is obtained before each advancing step.

In rare cases where I feel that the subject needs to have insight, I utilize the ideomotor signals for access to the unconscious mind. This is a refined technique that generates insights for the subject as well as therapist. We call it hypnoanalysis.

- ***Therapeutic Strategy***

Suggestions involve metaphors and archetypal symbols; their acceptability is verified utilizing ideomotor signals. The method is entirely permissive. The speech and the direction is tailored as elaborated in the Chapter on Communication in Hypnotherapy. Double bind is frequently necessary in case of resistance.

I avoid command hypnotherapy, though it is said to work. I believe most of the controversy about the efficacy and primary/adjuvant use of hypnosis is because of variation in technique at this stage. I like to innovate and structure the suggestions for each case.

- ***Termination of Trance***

After having reached a set goal in the session, verified by ideomotor signal/or the subject chooses to do further work at subsequent session, I terminate the session over a period of at least five minutes as:

It has been a very pleasant privilege for me to have this communion in consciousness...In the process I have been fortunate to witness some of the refined sensibilities in your wonderful personality... Now, we shall count from 10 to 1, and with the count of 1, you shall wake up completely and come back to my rooms...Ten, nine, eight, seven, six...I have learnt a few things that will help me to help other patients more effectively...You have a beautiful mind...five, four, three, two and one... and the time now is (the date and time of the session).... We shall endeavour to make it more beautiful.... This experience is your creation and it stays with you.

- ***Post Hypnotic Suggestions***

Unlike some therapists who give post hypnotic suggestions before termination of the trance, I prefer to utilize the post hypnotic, hypnoidal state for that purpose. Here the permissive technique gives a certain leeway to commands such as:

You have a high hypnotic talent. I congratulate you on your ability. Every time you will listen to the recorded cassette, you will relive the same wonderful experience that you just now had. And so I am sure, you will listen to the recorded cassette at least one before going to sleep.

And every time you will listen to the cassette, your creativity shall be so aroused that the work you have so successfully done now will be recreated and, even more easy will be the execution.

When you come for the next appointment, no sooner you sit in this chair, you will experience profound relaxation and go into deep trance. It shall go deeper as you start listening to my voice.

When I find the subject in grossly hypnoidal state, post session, I put him into trance again and reinforce the suggestions. This is described as Vogt's fractionation technique and is very effective therapeutically.

- ***Alerting the Subject***

Counting from 10 to 1.... you are now alert and wide awake... Stretch your arms.... Have a drink...Alert and wide awake! (I make sure that the subject is under full control before leaving the rooms and driving).

- ***Summary of the Session***

I ask the subject to describe the session and prod him to speak. The interruption is necessary only to encourage and to clear out any doubts. Quite often the subject comes out with elementary objections like, I was never asleep; I was listening to every thing that you spoke; I never wanted to wake and you disturbed me by waking me up. Such expressions are utilized positively to build up further expectations for the next session.

- ***Management of Catharsis***

Though some therapists prefer to terminate the session when catharsis occurs, I believe that leaves the therapeutic work unfinished. I quietly give reassurance. When it prolongs, I ask the subject to convey ideodynamically whether he/she will like to continue or terminate the trance. The usual response is to continue. Eventually when the subject settles down he/she has shed lot of burden.

- ***Therapy in Group Sessions***

I started to do group sessions in the management of infertility couples. Here, the subjects are likely to be of the same age groups and are suggestible/likely to respond to the same metaphors and archetypal symbols.

At the teaching class as well as at workshops, I do employ group sessions with more than one subject with diverse conditions–though this is being frowned upon by some of my colleagues. It works in my hands and saves time. It facilitates therapy too. To illustrate:

Two patients in their middle age were simultaneously hypnotized by quick induction technique and put into deep trance. One of them was a lady having itching all over the body since 22 years. She had abrasions and blotches on her forearm. An abscess was developing at one place. The other subject had stammering since he remembered.

After about 45 minutes of trance and age regression beyond 23 years, the signs of inflammation started to fade on the forearm of the lady. The man was at this time, made to stand up and walk somnambulistic to see the change in the condition of the fore arms of the lady. He was put in his chair and suggested that what she has been able to do, he can also do to his stammering.

Both of them recovered.

A Hypnotherapy Session My Way: Rajni Vyas

I use indirect hypnosis most of the time as an adjunct in my obstetric and gynecology practice. I have found it most rewarding in the treatment of unexplained reproductive failure.

Indirect hypnosis[7] is passive and covert. Formal induction is absent. Rapport is established. Thereafter, it delves on six key concepts. The session progresses in the form of a dialogue, while the therapist tacitly keeps on:

(1) *Observing the body language of the subject*: Observation of the subject begins from the time of entry. It is useful to know the accompanying person, expression on their faces, verbal and non-verbal communication and language as well as the tone of speech.

(2) *Suggestibility and rigidity are monitored*: During the course of history taking, some conclusion is tentatively made about the personality type, cognitive structure and behaviour pattern. The attitude of the subject is judged as parallel or at cross roads to the relationships, as well as regards to aggression, assertion, detachment, rigidity, non concern or compliance. Whatever that is observed is utilized in the therapeutic strategy. Correlation of symptoms with the observations made may provide a clue to successful therapy. Procedure involves, apart from the routine clinical observation, utilization of data concerning the psychodynamics. The language of the patient is used

so as to utilize the emotions and moods so as to suit the personality of the subject.

(3) *Neurolinguistic pattern is deciphered* and therapist decides to use the same currency; say, for a religious person, invoking the grace of favourite deities, for a rational scientific person to talk scientific terms about mind-body continuum, for the believer in preordained destiny, to indicate that your coming to therapy is also so ordained that now you are going to be well etc.

(4) *Utilization of patient's situation* as a symptom path to cure.

(5) *Eventual hypnoidal or hypnotic state*

(6) *Multiple level communication* where complex interpolation of archetypal symbols or reliving of past and expectancy of future are utilized as an integral whole is the service of the client, e.g. conceiving and then, carry on the pregnancy for nine months, in a carrier that is uterus, caring for full nine months to carry up to the labour, so that, you have a good obstetrics career; then to continue to carry on till the child is of 3-5 years so as to care towards its independent existence; that is lots to care for but that carrying just happens. That will carry up to care of your old age. This way multiple level of communication is used to induce hypnoidal state.

Over a study period extending over 25 years, along with my colleagues, we have established that unresolved psychodynamic conflicts are the prime cause, operating as dynamic demiurgic forces from the unconscious mind of the woman/couple. No sooner rapport is established, the history reveals the sources of psychodynamic tension. I utilize re-educative and reconstructive psychotherapy for change in perception and better adaptation. Simultaneously, as the couple reports every month in their follow up, I start using indirect hypnosis.

By the time I utilize indirect hypnosis, the couple has followed up with me a few weeks. So there is trust, confidence and rapport. There is a harmonious relationship between the doctor, team and couple. This is most essential for the success.

One of the most important contribution to the therapeutic success, I believe, is rapport. That is built because of nature of my work that extends over a sufficiently long period.

Alteration of the tense, randomly oscillating from past, present and future is useful. Interplay of thoughts and imageries are also applied in the same way. This may be interspersed with therapeutic suggestions and physiological explanations. This also incorporates demonstration under microscope of spermatozoa and the alterations in them following contact with cervical mucus.

Symbols contribute most significantly to indirect hypnosis. Symbols may be selected from the cultural or environmental background or from the dream contents. Stories ranging from *Panchatantra, Anderson Tales* or science fiction constitute an invariable part of the session. It should be mentioned that science has come to be almost equated with God since there is no area in the life of any body any where now that science has not influenced people significantly. Symbols from general understanding about science, like $E = mc^2$; black hole, satellite, electromagnetic effects of a remote control, space travel may work out well in scientifically oriented subjects.

Only when indirect hypnosis did not succeed, I have employed direct hypnotherapy.

Notes

1. David Cheek and Ernest Rossi, *Mind Body Therapy*, 1992.
2. Rossi, E., *The Psychobiology of Gene*, 2000.
3. Kroger, W.S., *Clinical and Experimental Hypnosis*, Philadelphia, 1963, pp. 41-42.
4. Wester, W.C., *Clinical Hypnosis: A Case Management Approach*, 1987, pp. 8-9.
5. Ernest Rossi, *Psychobiology of Gene Expression*, 2004.
6. This I have learnt from traditional *Gurus*. Their interpretation is that it is a tap on the *Sahasrara Chakra*. I do not know. But it helps profoundly in quick induction.
7. Williams, J. Adrian, Indirect Hypnotic Approaches, in Webster Williams, *Clinical Hypnosis: A Case Management Approach*, Ohio, 1987.

19
Group Hypnosis

Therapy is ideally conducted on 1:1 basis between therapist and patient, respecting confidentiality and clinical situation. On the other hand hypnosis has several nonspecific benefits to a state of general well being and common, personal aspirations. Poetically speaking every moth craves to be a butterfly and butterfly wants to be a star. Creativity is built in human genes; its expression is dependent on both "soil and the seed". It is natural right of every human being to self-actualize his potential as defined by Abraham Maslow; not only for achieving what is one's natural due, but also for defining destiny.

Self-hypnosis is a great help. It is easy to learn than meditation and, it can lead to altruistic meditation; since this is a universal attribute and ubiquitous need. There is thus a need to teach self-hypnosis in a group of large number of a normal, healthy individuals who desire to do better, and aim at excellence.

Such a group can be taught self-hypnosis; the base line being common positive motivation and clear goals. The group may vary from a few to a few hundred people at time.

Milton Erickson planned his therapy session for duration of 90 minutes. His results in therapy are matched by only a few today. This is generally attributed to creative genius of Erickson. This might indeed be so, however, we believe, one of the main reasons may be the duration of the session. Ernest Rossi attributes this to the creative cycle described by him and circadian rhythm. A session of 90 minutes has constraint of time; we therefore, utilise group hypnosis as a time saving tool for teaching self hypnosis for memory enhancement, excellence in studies for school and college going students and unfolding of creativity. The motivation and goal in such a group match. Therefore, there is no conflict of consciousness between the participants in the group. On the other hand, there is a definite evidence of "Hawthorne effect.[1]" This effect is a known psychological phenomenon.

Moreover, we have utilised group session hypnosis for treatment of infertile couples with unexplained reproductive failure (vide *supra*), for the therapy of dysmenorrhoea in student nurses and for a teaching demonstration at workshops. The participants at the workshops would differ with their problems, but they benefit by the indirect hypnosis in a group since the group gets hypnoidal as a whole: the induction is time saving.

There is a distinct evidence of transpersonal "diffusion" of hypnotic effect in a group. It is a clear validation of Kan Wilber's postulates of transpersonal psychology.

The format we follow: ideal size of group is less than fifty: on the other hand there is no limits to the number. Guru's and politicians hypnotize huge crowd. The motivation and the goal in the session should be identical for most participants. More often than not, they vary. Therefore, after a brief introduction to the topic, a division is asked. The group is divided into two with freedom to choose to be an experiencer or observer.

The formal session begins with the selection of a volunteer from the group willing to experience.

- ***Ask for a Volunteer***

Out of those who raise their hands, select the one that is showing sign of high hypnotic suggestibility, such as–

1. Already in a hypnoidal state, showing body language of earnestness, eagerness and wonder, sitting on the edge of chair or almost gotten up from it with some flush on the cheeks, palpebral fissure of eyes wide; almost showing a rim of sclera on the top.
2. Look into the eyes of the subject for dilatation of pupil.
3. Look for the rolling of the eye ball sign.

- ***Get the subject in Yes Set by Establishing rapport***

The other volunteers who raised their hands are assured of the same experience by asking them to sit in the front row (shift of paradigm), but focus on a single volunteer initially. The session progresses with utilisation of phenomenon of transference, postulations of transpersonal psychology and recently established scientific fact that there is parallel firing of neurons.[2]

- ***Proceed Further***

Say: Just as the reflection in a mirror is dependent on the attributes of there being a reflecting surface, as well as an object being reflected; our session is dependent on us both. For elucidating the point more clearly, let us now take resort to a dialogue by a monk of the Madhyamaka School, with Buddha. We shall simple call them Participant and Therapist here. The story goes on as:

Therapist: Participant, when you wish to see fine features of your face, what do you do?

Participant: I take up a vessel full of refined oil, or clean water, or I look into a crystal or to a mirror.

Therapist: Dear Participant, do you think what you see in any of these four objects has already been in existence there?

Participant: No.

So is it to be regarded altogether as non-entity?

No.

Is it to be regarded as being within any of them?

No!

Is it to be regarded as outside of them?

No.

Then what is the image? Where does it come from?

To this Participant replied: As the oil, water, crystal and mirror are clear, transparent and free of from muddiness and dust, the image is reflected in them. The image does not come out of the object, nor does it get into them from outside, nor it is there by itself, nor it is artificially constructed. The image comes from nowhere, vanishes always no where; it is no subject to birth and death; it has no fixed abode.

To this Therapist said: so it is, as you said, Dear Participant. When objects are pure and clean, the image is clearly reflected in them. So, it is with Bodhisattvas. When he meditates with singleness of thought, he sees them; having appeared to him they stay with him; staying with him they explain things to him he wishes to understand. Being thus enlightened by them, he is delighted; he now reflects: whence do these Bodhisattva-therapists come from? And whither does this body of mind vanish? When he thus reflects, he sees that all the enlightenment comes from nowhere and go out to nowhere. So, it is with your own body, it has no definite path by which it comes, and how can there be any returning to anywhere?

The story illustrates the point that there is no intrinsic reality to the physical self though we do experience various qualities within this reflection. Interpolation of high Buddhist postulates creates some confusion: but the participant is in "yes" set; so confusion facilitates hypnosis.

It is usual for participants to experience different depths of hypnosis, some will require individual attention and facilitation with stroking while those who may experience deep trance will need helped to be in a comfortable and easy position and may need to lie down while the session is conducted by a single therapist, a few facilitators are needed.

The size of the room should be to accommodate to the number of participants; a minimum of 100 square feet space per person is recommended. Between the participants there should be space to move for the facilitators. After the introduction and the division of the group, the lights are made dim, the subjects are advised to remove shoes and spectacles, they may be seated on reclining chairs or may be allowed to put their legs up on another chair or sit on floor with back supported by the wall; or may lie down comfortably. The ladies should cover themselves.

The session begins with the therapist using Progressive Muscular Relaxation (PMR), deep breathing and breath watching. Ego strengthening is utilized complimenting the group as well as individual. It is useful for the participants to use a badge bearing their names. Addressing participants, at random, by their names facilitates the process.

The therapist moves around the participants who have opted to experience; giving them strokes by touching the forearm or shoulder is very productive. A gentle tap on the forehead between the two eyebrows at times produces instantaneous hypnosis. The facilitators also move around to facilitate individual participant.

Therapist in the meanwhile has kept an eye on the group of the observers. Some of them, through the transpersonal experience, get hypnoidal. The therapist moves across to them and encourages then to join by words like, "you have made a choice and you can also choose to change your choice. There is freedom to choose and there is absolute freedom to change the choice, change your choice if you may and let us experience the vast sea of collective consciousness".

When a gentle stroking is applied with this indirect inclusive approach more than 90 per cent of group experiences medium to deep trance and is amenable to receive appropriate suggestions.

The strategy undergoes bifurcation at this point for helping the students with the studies as well as memory enhancement. The session is outlined in chapter-17, including a metaphoric suggestion like cleaning a black board with disjointed diagrams and script; and then, beginning to write a new script. This is very useful. The therapist may utilize alternative metaphors based on archetypal symbols such as, "*all the ripples in a pond full of sparkling clear water expand and fade away... now there is silent water... yes the water is silent, and... ready to listen and... as you lean over the pond to listen to the sound of silence... you see your calm, cool, composed self... a face full of confidence and cheer... and... in the voice of silence that you have seen...*"

For those who want to expand their creative potential, the subsequent sessions utilize the metaphors of subtle and yet relentless rising of a sun; imperceptive and yet definitive, unfolding of a sprouting flower bud and, opening of the third eye of creativity that Shiva displays explicitly; and... it is implicit gift of nature to each and every human being in the form of insight... and, variable function of right brain! (This kind of apparent disjointedness of science and the poetic narration helps to deepen the trance. Poetic metaphor as well as scientific fact stick together in the heightened state of suggestibility).

In subsequent sessions the same script is utilised with replacement of the word "you" by the first person singular "I". The subject may record the self-hypnosis script. Listen for at least 20 minute a day or recite in a self hypnosis-meditative session in mind before going to sleep.

Therapy of patients with an identical diagnosis like dysmenorrhoea, IBS, and unexplained reproductive failure as well as chronic pain have been successfully carried out by us.

Maitri Shah, a professor at a medical college hospital treats a large number of student nurses having dysmenorrhoea with group hypnosis session; thus saving time for individual session for those that are left out with the situation after being treated in a group. She has published her results.

The study was conducted in the Department of Obstetrics and Gynaecoology, SSGH, Baroda (India) for a period of one and half year from July 2009 to December 2010. It was a randomized controlled trial.

116 nursing students were given questionnaires regarding their menstrual history. All the students of Group 1 (Hypnotherapy) had statistically significant decrease on Visual Analogue Scale (VAS) for Pain scores during first three months when hypnotherapy sessions were given. The effect was evaluated for another three months and it was found to be persistent even after stopping the therapy. There was significant decrease in pain in Group 2 (Drug therapy) for the first two months. The decrease was more in Group 1 (Hypnotherapy) for the next four cycles. Once the therapy was stopped, effect was persistent in Group 1 which was not seen in Group 2 (Drug therapy).

With hypnotherapy, there was significant improvement in the pain scores on VAS which was even persistent after six months. On Description of Pain Scale, pain was reduced significantly with hypnotherapy but the effect was not maintained over a period of six months. Hypnotherapy was also effective in relieving the symptoms associated with dysmenorrhoea (nausea/vomiting, diarrhoea, headache/dizziness) with persistent effect.

The study indicates that hypnosis treatment even in a group with dysmenorrhoea has positive effects, and that the effect persists over time.

Rajni Vyas utilises the following strategy in group therapy for unexplained reproductive failure.

Once upon a time we all were in a village; in such a small village in such a small compact entity, everybody knows everybody and streets are few and straight...The present day civilization is urban oriented... village is simple; cities are complex; so are the people... A city can as well be a mega city or even a metro, the people are same... but ways are different... there is so much of interlinking connections between streets and drive ways and... at various junctions the blinking of traffic lights... at times it is likely to mislead us to the wrong path... and yet you have paired up, two of you have decided to stick together... there is a great partnership in your comradeship and, you have fallen in love... with each other... to co create a newer dimension in creativity that you wish to capture in your camera... you therefore decide to ride on a motorbike and your friend is giving you a joy ride... a motorbike ride is joyful, though bumpy and vast openness, the gusty flow of wind and the rapid flow of the speed is so exhilarating....while accelerating... that you take a deep breath, inhale fresh, air draw it into your nostril so that your nostrils are now wide open, your eyes have widened and your pupils dilate... and all the openings in your body open up now, relax now and relax further and all the openings in your body open up... and you now arrive at the garden in the city.

The Eden garden. The Eden garden is everywhere... The garden where Adam and Eve once upon a time played together, they play even now and every now and then make love... to make the human species...

Now, you have entered the water walks of the garden, you see the lush grains long flowing of the water ways at times silently and at times you hear the rustling sound of flowing water... there are beautiful flowers bet on all your sights and flowers of various shapes of violet, indigo, blue, yellow, orange, red and even black and white are seen everywhere... and there are tall trees, with erect trunks moving to and fro with gentle breaths... the gentle breath touches you all over the body and this romantic touch, the hair in their follicles stands up... falling with hand in hand you arrive at a spot where there is children's park, you see several children at a play, a boy and a girl and girls and boys, you see them gliding, you see them playing pee ca boo! And... you see them gliding, you see some of them on swing and you see there is a women appearing beautiful, lovely, calmly, smiling women approaching you... is she Madona?... or she is a fiery or kind or an angel? Is she the wife of Sun god; Cassandra[3] or is she *Rati;* wife of *Kamadeva,* the god of love, several such questions will pop up in your mind... but as she approaches you nearer and nearer she is carrying ... a smiling baby boy Krishna or is she a girl, the eternal girl within you, that everyone knows as Durga (the mother of divine creation and destruction).

The question subsides as you see the child smiling at you and you take out your camera... and click the picture of smiling child.

You have pocketed your camera, the camera in your hip pocket is safe and sure with the baby and along with your partner you now go in your motorbike sauntering, leisurely with joy and surety, once again you ride the motorbike and with a gingerly drive come back to your home.

Standing before the door of your home, you see the lock. You want to open it but get nervous and fidgety as you look for the key. Where you see your doctor arrives. Dr. Rajni has a master key. The master key can open up all and any kind of locks with a gentle and swift move Dr. Rajni opens up the lock. You open the door and move in.

With arm in arm you enter in the bedroom and put on the lights. You are filled with surprise and joy... at the foot end of the bed, your partner has fixed the picture of the baby that you saw in the garden! Basking in the wonder, excitement and joy, you open up both the windows on each side of bedroom... a fine fragrance with cool gentle breeze moves in, fills in your nostrils and permeate your entire body...

You take the arm of your partner, lead him to the bed and make love... riding on the motor bike... and there arrive the guardian angels, with the angelic child... now you are holding your baby in your arm and... putting the tender lips of baby to your nipples and feel the flow as vigorously the baby sucks!

The bottom line in summary is that group hypnosis is feasible and effective. Its greatest virtue is, saving of time. It can be an effective tool to teach self-hypnosis (*Yoganidra*). What is generally lost to the western audiences is relevance to group therapy in patients with identical psychopathology.

Hypnodrama

Hypnotherapy belongs to the realm of transpersonal, we now know for certain as to how different area of the brain gets activated during the process.[4] Hypnosis is Interpersonal interaction. The therapy has the power and capacity to influence the functioning of brain of subject. This can be demonstrated objectively by advance imaging techniques of today. This would put a final stamp of hypnotherapy being a science. This will extend the research to charisma, transference and parapsychological occurrences. What is proven and, can be demonstrated was done at a workshop on pain management at 8th conference of our society at Christ University, Bangalore. The details are as follows:

There were about one hundred participants at the workshop for pain management, in a hall. One therapist led the session with assistance from three others. The session began with experience of group hypnosis for about 45 minute. This was followed by asking for volunteers having any kind of chronic pain that may range from head to toe. Twelve volunteers came forward and they were asked to sit in comfort on the stage. An introduction about the pain being a protective symptom was given. The idiom, "a symptom is a definitive discomfort in the mind, that the body displays so as to seek attention for relief" was explained. The examples were sited, such as a chronic headache may suggest a persistent problematic situation that mind is not able to sort out; "cervical spondylitis" and frozen shoulder may be due to a lot of responsibility where manoeuvrability is limited; a chronic backache would simply suggest that a person is carrying a lot of load on his back etc. the volunteers were further told that apart from the two eyes, everyone has a third eye – the eye of intuition; during hypnosis, the third eye opens out and the subject understands the root cause of the problem. To understand is to alleviate and the alleviation may lead to elimination as well.

In the group hypnosis session for about an hour, interspersed with individual attention and gentle stroking at the painful part, there was 90 per cent success in eliminating the pain after the session.

As a reinforcement, that the cause is in mind, and as an explicit demonstration of transpersonal phenomenon in hypnosis, the following session was demonstrated: volunteers were asked from the audience, who have no pain. Three came forward. They were subjected to a painful sensation, one in the head, 2nd in the arm, and the 3rd in the back. They were put under hypnosis through quick induction and were given suggestions to have the desired pain effect. Out of the hypnosis session, all the subjects complained of pain as suggested. It was therapist's duty to relieve the induced pain. This was also successfully demonstrated by quick induction and rapid time reversal.

Sleep Walking

A professional lady working even at odd hours brought her highly intelligent daughter aged 14 yrs for symptoms of sleep talking and somnambulism. The psychodynamics of the situation were obvious. The child had unfinished agenda before sleep with her studies as well as with her mother. During the session involving hypnodrama, a scenario was so constructed that she was made to study at a study table; the mother left for an emergency call at night and before her return the child was made to go to sleep. The session was paused for a while for the child to experience the situation. After sometime the child started mumbling and, walked around with half closed and half open eyes. The therapist walked over to the child, assured her that the mother is all the time with her, asked to mother to give a kiss and a hug and put the child to sleep.

With this single session the child was cured and now is a medical doctor; the mother also switched over to be a hypnotherapist.

This session was shared by a marketing executive who was prone to stammer. When the child demonstrated the hypnotic phenomenon in the deep trance, the subject was asked to open his eyes and see the hypnodrama. Following the session with appropriate post hypnotic suggestion, he was also cured of stammering.

Notes

1. Hawthorne effect is the gain in productivity when working in a group. Though the study was conducted in a industrial set up, the effect is seen in all kind of group activity. Metaphorically it is stated that ten participants produce eleven units of products.
2. Consciousness at any given point in suppose to be sum total of a parallel, simultaneous firing of multiple neurones. Parapsychological phenomenon such as clairaudience, clairvoyance, telepathy are supposed to be due to a simultaneous parallel firing of identical neuron between the participants at a given time. Hypothesis remains to be proved. Transference may also be similar kind of neurophysiological process.
3. Cassandra: The magnificent wife of god sun, the lady with the power to bless to every other women with a child, and yet the one goddess who have no child of her own since the estrange wife sun god... (the Cassandra fell in love on account of his brilliance and so did the sun god for her astounding beauty. He propose marriage to her, she demanded the gift of a pertue in return, in return, after being gifted Cassandra change her mind realising that if she goes to marry this god, she will be running forever. The sun god then cursed her. "yes you can gift any women with a baby but nobody will believe that you indeed, can.)
4. Amir Raj : (hypnotic state and radiology).

20

Exploration of the Unconscious Mind

This chapter is about a strategy for Insight Generation.

By its very definition, it may be argued that the unconscious mind is not accessible to conscious processing. Some believe, therefore, that it is absurd to talk about the exploration of unconscious mind.

The unconscious mind is a demiurgic, dynamic force that propels our behaviour. It guides the conscious behaviour and gives rise to various ego defenses. In the process, however, it peeps out at times, though obscurely. Freud identified that it lets itself reveal through slips of tongue—as Freudian slip. Freud also utilized the complex process of free association for psycho-analysis. It happens to be a lengthy process and is infrequently utilized in psychotherapy today. Ink-blot test may also be employed as a substitute for free association.

Rossi[1] rightly emphasizes that we can engage ourselves in a creative dialogue with our unconscious when we replay our fantasies and daydreams. He believes that this active dialogue is a labour—a psychobiological work function that requires energy to stimulate "activity-dependent gene expression and synaptogenesis" in the brain. This also happens during normal everyday life (when awake as well as during sleep and dreaming) and therapeutic hypnosis. The royal road to unconscious mind is through hypnoanalysis. This is not necessary for all cases. We utilize it only in those subjects with long standing behaviour problems.

The influence of unconscious mind would influence the temperament and such psychological aspects. By the time a child is of five years age, he has accumulated a large overload of stressful memories in his/her unconscious mind. Repressed and so not available to the conscious mind, as they may be, they exercise a definitive dynamic influence. This may be a driving source of the presenting symptom. Any one or more phenomena occurring in the hypnotic process may be utilized for therapeutic change. In most undiagnosed conditions, we find it useful to explore the childhood experiences by way of age regression.

Time and space displacement are most important and of relevance in hypnoanalysis. In other words, time can be psychologically experienced to flow backwards and in such a flow of time, the space also takes the character of that particular moment.

Hypnosis provides a subtle gateway to the unconscious mind. This gateway may be accessible to the therapist in the form of post-hypnotic change or it is experienced by the subject as an insight into his/her problem. Such an insight generation can lead to a cure.

Strategy

Following the induction of a hypnotic state by any method, the preparedness of the subject to do psychodynamic hypnotherapeutic work is obtained by ideodynamic signaling. Pendulum may be employed to provide ideomotor signals and helps deepen trance. Thereafter employing a suitable imagery, the patient is time regressed, gradually. In so doing, the patient may initially be made to experience the pleasant events of the past. Once again, through ideodynamic signaling, the patient's preparedness at the unconscious mind to live through the suppressed, unpleasant events is ascertained.

This way the subject maybe made to review and experience all the significant unpleasant experiences of the past life. There may not be any conscious memory of such events. Quite often in the subjects with severe traumatic experiences, the catharsis is also brought about.

Age Regression

This is our most preferred therapeutic strategy. Of course, as for all the sessions, the subject is explained clearly that the mental work that he/she does is entirely a personal property and need not be divulged to the therapist. There is in fact no need to explain that the therapist is going to explore the unconscious mind. If the subject insists to know the nature of therapeutic work, it is best explained as insight generation.[2]

We use relaxed age regression as a tool. The subject is asked before starting the session to enumerate the major events. The adjectives to the events may be used by the patient, but the therapist maintains a value neutral position. They are written down chronologically in reverse order before the subject is put in trance by a suitable method and, it is deepened. Often, for the exploration of unconscious, we employ a pendulum for induction. 'Yes', 'No' and 'I do not know' of the pendulum are demonstrated by the therapist on himself. The ideomotor nature of the signals is left unexplained. This leaves a sense of wonder that is conducive to quick induction.

Though psychotherapeutic work is done in lighter trance too, here we prefer to work with the subject in deep trance. If the subject shows resistance, a double bind is used, like, "we are prepared for a very nice experience. But you are free to choose how much work you wish to do today. Should you decide to stop at any stage, you simply have to move your "no" finger. Of course, we shall stop then and there. But if you decide to terminate the session, it shall be your loss since you have chosen to get well quickly. Now, you may decide whether to proceed or accept the loss. Let me know by the movement of the appropriate finger."

The entire session of 90 minutes or more is based on eliciting Yes, No and I do not know answers. The subject is frequently asked whether he would want to carry on with the excellent work that he/she is doing. There are several moments of silence during which the subject goes on doing work on his/her own.

The subject may be age regressed while holding the pendulum. It may be suggested that at the moment of insight generation, there will be tremendous relaxation of all the muscles of the body. On arrival of such a moment in time regression, the pendulum indeed falls.

We present a case of age regression.[3] The study uses the handwriting and the signatures as the evidence of age regression.

Case Study of Age Regression

An experiment conducted by the authors on 11th June, 2003 illustrates the title of the paper. A 41 years old lady (date of birth 10/06/62) was the volunteer. The differences in her handwriting in the form of signatures at varying ages show evidence of age regression. The date 2/2/2000 was the date of happy celebrations of sacred thread *samskara* ceremony of her son. Isolated and lonely as she was in the absence of her late husband, she confessed that this was a landmark achievement for her which is reflected in her signature. Years 1997-99 were a period of trial and tribulation because of serious psychiatric as well as near fatal illnesses in her family. Regressing further, she was happy and steady in her medical practice. On 10/4/95–she suddenly lost her husband. The jarring can hardly be ignored. At this point her signature takes the form of an illegible scrawl. However, an interesting change is on 23/08/1984 when she signs by her maiden name. This was when she graduated and was unmarried. As she goes further backwards in time, the handwriting becomes that of a school girl (1977). And then change to Gujarati from English (1967). This continues way down to the time of nursery school and then to the time when she has hardly learnt to write. It goes to the scribble of a child past that age. The style of writing changes according to the age being lived; the subject signs the name according to the period—like married name changing to maiden name at the appropriate time in corresponding age.

Discussion

Age regression is objectively demonstrated up to the infant age. There is a probability that it can extend further up to intrauterine state. There are innumerable unproven case studies, which show age regression even to the previous birth. This is further discussed in Chapter on Past Life Regression.

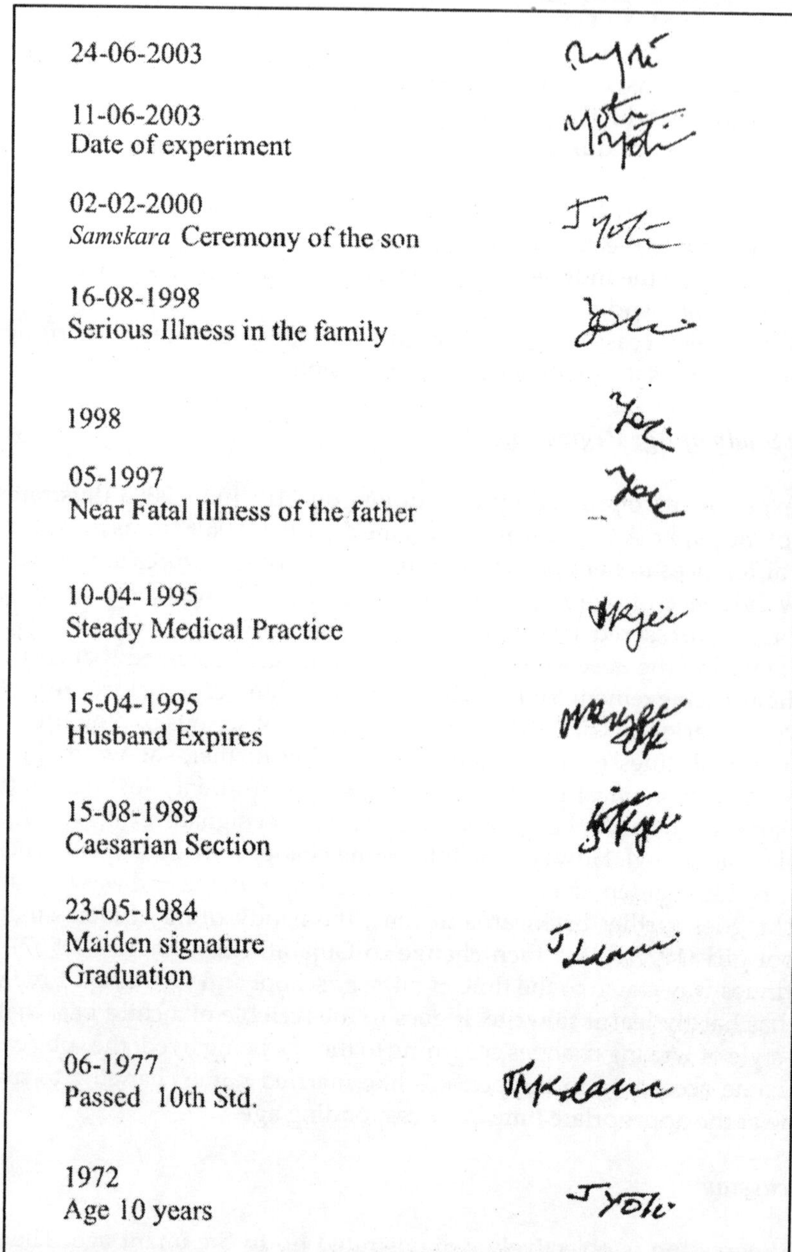

24-06-2003

11-06-2003
Date of experiment

02-02-2000
Samskara Ceremony of the son

16-08-1998
Serious Illness in the family

1998

05-1997
Near Fatal Illness of the father

10-04-1995
Steady Medical Practice

15-04-1995
Husband Expires

15-08-1989
Caesarian Section

23-05-1984
Maiden signature
Graduation

06-1977
Passed 10th Std.

1972
Age 10 years

In the altered state of consciousness, the subject is focally aware and the marginal sensory inputs fade away. It is one of the characteristics of hypnosis that the subject experiences time distortion. In the state of profound trance, experience of time reversal can be simulated. Unconscious mind is not easily explored but such an experience of time reversal unravels conflicts and trauma that have been thrown into unconscious mind through repression.

When this is uncovered there is insight generation that leads to a cascade of molecular biological events that result in clinical cure of a physical condition.

Since it is frequent, it is repeated that there may be a catharsis of various magnitude. We let it happen.

This is the most subtle of all hypnotherapeutic interventions. The subject may want to discuss new insights with the therapist; only patient listening and confident reassurance is what is needed. If the subject decides to remain taciturn about the newly found discoveries/dimensions, he/she is told that what insight is acquired shall remain as a guiding light for times to come.

Notes

1. Ernest Rossi, *Personal Communication.*
2. What is insight?
   It is the voice of wise man within.
   It is the moment that reveals what the unconscious mind was toiling to express for long.
   It is the flash that strikes the clouded consciousness like a lightening.
   It is "Aha" experience of creative people.
   It is Eureka of Archimedes.
   It is the voice of a traditional Hindu wife!
3. Bhaskar Vyas and Rajni Vyas, *Space Time Consciousness—Fifth Dimension,* New Delhi, 2005.

21

Strategic Design

Transformation through Trance

Since hypnotherapy works precisely and produces results that are repeatable and reproducible, it is scientific. Further proof of it being a science is that it is falsifiable[1]: while the success is statistically significant, one may not succeed 100 per cent at any time. With this parameter, most recently initiated look for a standard protocol that may be repeated with any client as a script-stereotype that may be applied parrot like. There is no hypnotherapeutic pill. A script can not be prescribed to be mimicked, since hypnotherapy is an art too.

For this kind of artist, a vast repertoire of information about sociology, different cultures, history of civilizations and their epics add to his armamentarium. These provide say, colours for the painting: fundamentals of psychology and the subject that the therapist is specialized are then equated with basic colour, white.

There is an opinion that a therapist may restrict—specialize in a particular area: that may be the area of his primary discipline. There is a merit in this suggestion; specialization and super-specialization yield better results. However, there is no constraint in a hypnotherapist wanting to have a wider canvass: he will have to work that much more to acquire the necessary deftness and skills.

After the diagnosis and goals are established, a standard session is structured as per the steps described earlier in Chapter 15. The session may progress more or less with the steps as enumerated. Versatile therapists design special session for each individual client; but it is not mandatory. Hypnosis may be utilized for being better than what is in general. It therefore, applies that people in normal health would perform better in their study and work. They can be programmed to be creative – more creative. Clients and patients with situations that handicap them can be helped to return to normalcy.

For therapy, detailed protocols with elaborate programmes for individual conditions are in vogue.[2] Our approach is based on the etiopathology; and than we classify the disorders and diseases. Disorders of behaviour arise in the psyche and there is one model of strategy that can be modified to suit an individual client. At organic level, there are stress related diseases rooted in autonomic nervous system, endocrine system and auto immune diseases. A model stress relieving strategy is applied initially to all: they are then subsequently treated with a strategy appropriate to each category in general and, sensibilities of the client in particular. Below are some the models.

Normative to Creative

We shall elaborate on memory enhancement and, better study and creativity enhancement.

Memory Enhancement and Better Study

This may also and better utilize in a group. Following introduction that there is much useless clutter, noise and jarring that is there in your minds, there is a method that can generate silence. After that is done, one can learn and remember what is being studied better and clear. While this is being talked about, indirect hypnosis is being applied as per the sensibility of the group; e.g. For children, stories are incorporated; for young collegiate students, stories of science and inventions are appropriate. After induction of hypnosis, following strategy may then be applied:

- *First Session*

As you have relaxed now, and...experiencing a state of calm, cool, complete comprehension, you are...you are...you are you...you are at your silent best...best place to be...silent, serene...salubrious, soft and your sleek an serene self...this is the place that is specially structured for you...your most comfortable personal...place of your own choice...just the right softness in the seats...choice of your own preferred coolness...and all the clutter has been...is being cleared...so that the place is clean and tidy ...neat. There is clear light...and you see with better clarity now since you have put on an additional light...the comfort place is now flooded with brightness...and you see clearly...a black board in front of you...so much of scribble on it...white chalk, coloured pencils...disjointed words... and jumbled figures...difficult to find a clear message...you get up from your cozy chair...with a lurch...pick up a duster from a stand and, start wiping the black board clean...wipe it clean...you have wiped it clean...it is clean now...You write your own message there...you are writing in clean, neat, tidy and elegant letters...you have written...let us see how it reads...it reads as

> Wonderful....Marvelous...I....am....quite....magnificent, Excellent....
> In every way,

Brilliant is what I say...
First class...
A1...
Top notch...
Well done...
Well done...
Let me tell you straight...
Wonderful
Marvelous......
Me I'm
GREAT!

So, you have scripted the script as you are....that you are, for sure....for sure now...and for ever, you are great, marvelous and excellent.

Next time when we meet...and say yes with your Yes finger, Yes... next time we are meeting...and when you will be seated here...you will be seated in your most comfortable, cool place, you will take this forward...you have taken this forward...towards excellence...where you will...excel better than ...excellence itself.

- *Second Session*

As you are now in your most comfortable, cozy, cool, comfort chamber...you are very cozy...and there is a glass window to your air conditioned comfort chamber...you are looking...you are looking out of this window...and..., you find quite a few children... quite a few children...assembled down there... quite a few children...are there...some of them have bows and arrows... bows and arrows...are aiming...and..., there is a teacher... a teacher...almost like a sage...he is a guide... like a sage...he is a guide...and he is asking... he is asking...his pupils to look at the eye of a bird... to look at the eye of a bird...and..., one by one... quite a few children... and..., one by one...they see the whole tree...you are seeing... they see the whole tree...whole tree...its big trunk...its branches. its leaves and, the sky...other birds flying... branches. its leaves and, the sky...other birds flying...and a boy is now seeing...there are boys......and a boy, Arjun, is now seeing...boys with shot gun... and a boy, Arjun, is now seeing...aiming at the bird... to look at the eye of a bird...and, there is a boy with a bow and arrow... and a boy is now seeing...only the eye of the bird and he...the boy is with a shot gun...he is Aniruddha...he fires the gun...and he has hit the eye of the bird...He wins Olympic gold medal...and there are photographers...they take pictures...as you see the photo... you see yourself there...

Yes, you have won a gold medal...that happened because..., you focalized... you focalized...on the eye of the bird...so when you are studying... you are studying...you focalize, repeat, you focalize, repeat, repeat, recapitulate... when you are studying, repeat, retrieve...recapitulate, refresh, when you are studying, repeat, retrieve...recapitulate, refresh, recap... retrieve...recapitulate, refresh, recap...and you have reinforced . .that focalization is the key... focalization is the key...to successful memory. Focalization is the key to successful memory. Focalize and you have it!

Creativity[3]

Generation and Enhancement[4]

Creativity strategies are derived based on depth psychology elaborated in brief below.

Therapist should have in depth understanding of the creative process in order to succeed with this refined mode of utilization of hypnosis. While a session carved at the end of the following discussion you succeed, without the therapist having had personal experiencing of creativity, the session may end with "the tail wagging the dog": subject would be better enlightened than the therapist.

Ancient Sanskrit critical tradition defines creativity as "*nava navonmesha shalini pratibha*" meaning, that which blossoms in an individual with newer and newer forms. At the other end, is *Tagore* who attributes his creativity to Divinity—"I am a dead reed, but you make it a flute by blowing various tunes through me over valleys and hills." Thus, man is only at the receiving end! (Sushil Kumar De 1960). It may even manifest itself as *humility* as can be seen when *Shankaracharya* replied that what he had done was nothing more than the waving of Arati compared to the illumination of the sun after his disciples praised him for having completed several treatises.

Creativity was believed to be a divine gift by Plato, over which the individual had no control. "He thought that our sober senses must be clouded either by sleep or some malady, or lifted from its place in heavenly rapture" if creativity were to show up. Or, as writers often report "It came to me. It was like taking dictation."

In the Vedas, which have been characterized as *apaurushah*, meaning that they were not written by human beings but descended from the above, the prayer is that let good thoughts come to us from all sides. And it further goes on to ask, which Gods shall we pray for that?

However, creativity as such is by and large associated with the characteristics of '*something new*', '*unique*' or 'original' with an element of 'surprise' and 'usefulness.' One may also come across references like latent creativity and manifest creativity to denote either in its hidden or manifest aspects.

Sometimes a distinction is made between scientific creativity and artistic creativity. In scientific creativity the important feature is of insight, and the scientist relies on truth and objectivity. The artist on the other hand externalizes his needs, perceptions, feelings etc., in the form of writing, painting, and sculpturing, and there is no scope for fact-finding. This 'artist – scientist' differentiation and the authentic distinction (?) is well brought out by the artist George Seurat, who declared, "Some say they see poetry in my painting; I see only science"; or Albert Einstein, who played the violin and said of his own scientific discoveries, "There is no logical way to the discovery of these elementary laws; there is only the way of intuition." (Arguelles 1975)

Koestler draws the following lines from Goethe—*"Man cannot persist long in a conscious state, he must throw himself into the Unconscious, for his root lives there...take for example a talented musician, composing an important score: conscious and unconscious will be like warp and weft."*

Another reference to Carpenter who coined the term '*unconscious cerebration*' in the nineteenth century, was reflected in English coinages like—Wordsworth's '*caverns in the mind which sun can never penetrate*', Coleridge's '*twilight realm of consciousness*', William James's '*fringe consciousness*', and Myers's '*subliminal self*'. And Wundt described it vividly further—*"Our mind is so fortunately equipped, that it brings us the most important bases for our thoughts without our having the least knowledge of this work of elaboration. Only the results of it become conscious. This unconscious mind is for us like an unknown being that creates and produces for us, and finally throws the ripe fruits in our lap."*

But Jung's emphasis was more on the other mode of creativity called '*visionary*', which "comes upon the person in a great surge from the depths of the unconscious" as in case of prophets, seers, visionaries, and poets who "are open to the 'night-side of life and are willing and able to attend to the messages that side forth". (June Singer, 1980)

This is the psychology of the genius, which is also amenable to criteria derived from the non-genius. The creative act, in so far as it depends on unconscious resources, presupposes a relaxing of the controls and a regression to modes of ideation which are indifferent to the rules of verbal logic. Verbal thinking as it is most vulnerable to infectious diseases", and thereby language stands like a screen between the thinker and reality. This is the reason why true creativity often starts where language ends.

Before the actual composition of the Classic Epic, *Ramayana*, it is said that Sage Valmiki was at a loss as to how to begin the great epic. So when he was groping, struggling, experiencing the pangs and throes of creativity, it so happened that he saw a female *krauncha* bird distraught with grief weeping and wailing. The cause of her sorrow was occasioned by the sudden death of her partner under tragic circumstances. A cruel hunter had shot down the male *krauncha* bird when it was making love to its beloved. As a consequence the widowed female bird started lamenting over the death of its dear one. The compassionate sage was so deeply moved on seeing the miserable plight of the poor female bird that he involuntarily burst into song: *"Ma nishada..."* which itself became the starting point (the *mangala-shloka*) of the *Ramayana*. *Shoka* (grief) was transformed into *shloka* (song) which explains why pathos or *karuna rasa* is the dominant emotion of the *Ramayana*. The heart-rending scene that Sage Valmiki had witnessed was such that he was stirred to his depths and not being able to contain all that emotion, he spontaneously broke into song. This is a classic case of transmuting one's personal sorrow through an act of creativity.

'*Janusian* thinking' is based on the Roman god Janus with two faces in opposite directions. Creative persons are known to possess this ability of conceiving and utilizing two or more opposite or contradictory ideas, concepts or images simultaneously which operates in art, literature, music, science and mathematics and of course in hypnosis.

By creativity it is meant to establish the underlying association or a link amongst different entities which might take on the form of (1) *Serendipity*—hitting at an answer by chance or accident, (2) *Similarity* – associative elements appearing in the form of contiguity, pattern, or a rhyme, (3) *Mediation* – different elements are associated at the symbolic level, and scientists belong to this group.

There is also a neuropsychological explanation accounting for the two halves of the brain to be essentially two brains, nearly identical in conformation, but differing in what they do. In right-handed people, the left hemisphere is primarily concerned with verbal behaviour and analytical tasks, whereas the right hemisphere is concerned with more global tasks such as imagination, space perception, and music. The left hemisphere acts like a stimulus-response brain, and the right acts like a Gestalt brain. The relationships may be reversed in left- handed people (Gazzaniga, Bogen and Sperry 1962). Verbal content of the poem is believed to stimulate the left-hemisphere; while imagery, primary process material, and divergent thinking stimulate the right "resulting in an altered state of consciousness". Based on implicit understanding of the above, a session for creativity may be structured on the following lines:

Step 1. Take the subject to a pleasant place that has been ascertained before hand; may be sea shore, mountains or vast panoramic plains. Ascertain by ideomotor signal.

Step 2. Make him enter a garden there... Ascertain by ideomotor signal...Make him visualize flowers of all the hues...violet, indigo, blue...green...yellow, orange...and... red... Ascertain by ideomotor signal...they have generated a mixed delicate perfume...that enters the nostrils... Ascertain by ideomotor signal...how pleasant and...yes... (This suggests deep trance)...

Again, depending upon the sensibility of the subject, make him visualize the rising sun (archetypal symbol for father, sun, source of energy and strength) as...there you are looking at the east...and there is a colourful sunrise that you are now seeing...the sun is rising...bright crimson, mixed with a little magenta...and it is now shining scarlet red...orange... it is coming up... it is coming up...and sun rays are suddenly shining over the earth, over the garden...sun is turning yellow...and getting to be white...it is difficult to gaze at... Ascertain by ideomotor signal...the rays are touching your face and as the rays of sun are touching your face... the rays of sun are touching your face...you feel energized...supported...cared for...strong, strong in your wish... strong, strong in your resolve as now you have the support of great, great grand father, that is sun...you now have the support. And you are sure to be granted your wish...

Or

Make him visualize the earth as the Mother Earth, source of energy, nutrition and nurture. She is sending the energy to nurture through several pores... that are there in the soles... of your feet. And, through those several pores, you are sucking... at several breasts that Mother Earth has...through that milk, energy flows all over... strong, strong in your wish... as now you have the support of great, great grand eternal mother, that is Mother earth...You can suck her milk...ay time you feel like smoking... strong, strong in your resolve... as now you have the support of great, great grand father, that is sun...you now have the support. And you are sure to be granted your wish...

Or

Substitute a friend that is holding his hand and guiding him through to show the beautiful spots...that turn out into several scenic vistas...and as the friend is leading you to scenes more pleasant than before...you are looking at the face of the friend...how nice to see your therapist by your side...he is by your side all the time...till such time that you are now at this place that you have moved to...all easy and familiar... strong, strong in your resolve as now you have the support of great, great grand father, that is sun...you now have the support. And you are sure to be granted your wish...

For most conditions like habit modification, symptom amelioration and psychological disorders, simple imageries usually suffice.

Direct Suggestions for Symptom Amelioration

- Symptom substitution
- Symptom transformation
- Assertiveness

Strategy

- Positive imagery such as

  Red balloon rising upwards in the sky, getting bigger and bigger till it bursts

  Black board; scribbled, wiped clean and written and drawn stylish now

  Helmet image; a protection

  Comfort chamber: for most stressful conditions

  Ice cube melting: melting of anger

  Ice cube application: for cooling down; hypnoanesthesia

Sunrise; sea shore, mountains or landscape: for most stressful conditions, according to the sensibilities of the subject ascertained before

Flowers in a garden, buds opening out, all colours, VIBGYOR (violet, indigo, blue, green, yellow, orange, red)

Germination of a seed: creativity, insight generation

Flowing river: psychodynamics that rise, swell and normalize; flow of hormones

- Incorporation of archetypal symbols (depending upon patient's life experiences, interests and values)
- Time distortion
- Age regression and cognitive restructuring
- Age progression and mental rehearsal
- Response substitution

The sessions become more complex and less structured as we proceed further to disorders of autonomic nervous system imbalances and stress management. Hormonal[5] disturbances and auto immune diseases need many sessions over a period of protracted therapy. The goals will also vary.

Stable Relationships

Miss D. Psychologist, 27 years, tutor at college; had multiple intimate relationships, one at a time, with boys of the same age group. Her relationships would end when the boy dominated, as understood by her retrospectively. She believes all these affairs were loaded as unfinished business from previous birth. However, she cannot just subordinate to *mcps* (Male Chauvinist Pigs) who thought they were *avatars* of Rama. Now, she is formally engaged in her community and fears that this relationship will go the same way.

Session in May 2008 when there was landing on the mars; After induction and idecmotor consent to find a way out to a steady, caring, lasting relationship, the strategy went as under:

This is the age of missiles. There was landing on the mars. (Any recent events of significance are used to do the shift of paradigm and also to take the subject unaware to wonder or to cause confusion)... The satellite was moving in the space since many years... since 12 years...how many objects in the space...this satellite would have encountered...it did not crash... it did not collide... It takes time to achieve a thing... In 12 years so many things can go wrong. ... It did not collide... It can go wrong with the satellite... so many things can go wrong. ... And also with the mind! (Metaphor with indirect hypnosis). But the satellite maintained its trajectory... the satellite maintained its orbit... the satellite maintained its path...through cybernetics...

Mind also has a psycho cybernetic way... through cybernetics... Mind has innate ability to correct itself. ... Through cybernetics... The nature has installed a programme in the mind. ... Mind has innate ability to correct...... Mind has innate ability to correct... The nature has installed a programme in the mind...

The computer is like mind but mind is not like a computer. It is mind that feeds the computer and then it functions and takes commands... The nature has installed a programme in the mind. ... Mind with the help of brain makes the programme... The nature has installed a programme in the mind. ...So, the concept of artificial intelligence has come and so many scientists are working on it...with your psychological talents, we are bound to succeed... let us see how to succeed! We have a back up facility in the computer as well as in the mind...as you well know...

The back up in the mind has been installed in many ways as you well know... One of the very important inputs is by the way of heritage. The mother and father have passed over the genetic heritage... as you well know... at the time of conception. You happen to believe in rebirth as you well know... then (ideomotor signal)... you carry forward your memory and other *Samskaras*... from previous birth as well... You are born with the acquisition of attribute from previous birth. This is now with you. But it is not difficult to delete this.

It is like daughter of Sita...how many daughters she had? She is having daughters in India since last 5000 years...but now this is a new age...there is a reversal... there is a reversal in consciousness...Man cannot be compared to woman... Biologically feminine sex is stronger to survive... Man cannot be compared to woman... and, she can struggle much more than man... feminine sex is stronger to survive... to find her way in difficult situations... feminine sex is stronger to survive... She is strong, progressive, and intelligent, she can be Prime minister of India or U.K. or Pakistan (Ego strengthening)... You can be Prime minister of India or U.K. or Pakistan...and, diplomats have a way of dealing with difficult people, difficult situations...and you are a diplomat... diplomats have a way of dealing with difficult people, difficult situations...you are sorting out difficult people... diplomats have a way of dealing with difficult people, difficult situations... psychologist have a way ...... as you well know...you are a diplomat...and a psychologist...you understand the mind sets of people...you understand hypnotherapy...Hypnosis is state of heightened suggestibility. you understand hypnotherapy...the aim of the therapy is to have better confidence, better and stable relationship...you are to have stable relationship now...you like your fiancée...you like his family...even mother in law you can manage... you are having stable relationship now...

Psychological Disorders

We believe the pathogenesis of psychological disorders lies in repressed material in unconscious mind (see Chapter on Psychopathology I). Its "nagging" triggers stress: this is causative of faulty perception that builds wrong concepts.

(Bad) Habits, hysteria, anxiety disorder, dissociative and depersonalization neurosis, multiple personality disorder, obsessive compulsive neurosis, paranoid trait and phobia can all be helped by "digging" the repressed material through the dynamics of age regression and by replacing it with psycho-cybernetics of rejuvenation and re-creation. So is the case with subjects with possession. Disorders of childhood are amenable to treat by incorporating stories as metaphors. Following cases were treated with a few sessions according to this strategy: with gratifying success.

Once the subject is under hypnosis, the examples of prototype dialogue from the cases below, is recommended for command therapy.

Smoking

Diagnosis: Habit change, wants to quit smoking
Goal: quit smoking

Two, well motivated friends from childhood, working in share market want to leave smoking. The age is 32 and 35 with family.

About giving up smoking, so many times you have decided and given up. And again you have started and again given up. So, this time you will require 8 sessions and need to come again every few months for reinforcement. But you are very well motivated and sure, will succeed.

- ***Induction***

You know how to breathe. Please show me how well you breathe in and out deeply. Very good, and... you can really do it well...you know that you can breathe...deep breathe...well...and, when we agree...show it to me... (Ideomotor signal)... If you like you can talk... but... usually in trance you would not talk but move right or left index finger to answer. If need be... we can wake you from trance and talk as well and again go back to trance.

Now as you breathe in and out and as you take a deep breath, (quick induction done) and...you are in trance. If you like to keep eyes open... or close..., close your eyes...it is your choice but if you feel your eyelids...heavy let them close. Take a deep breath in and deep breath out.... (Twice)... As you take deep breathe in and out... your hand feels heavy... and... it relaxes. And as it relaxes your hand falls... in your lap and as it falls...let it fall... you relax further. Take a deep breathe in and out (thrice), deeper and still deeper, you feel calm, peaceful and totally relaxed.

(Make the subject comfortable by adjusting the head and also relaxing his shoulder on his chair by giving pressure on his shoulder.)

You are totally relaxed and let go all the tension... deep, deep breathe..., and your whole body is perfectly... completely and totally... relaxed. The whole body feels tranquil and at peace... Take a deep breathe in and let go (thrice).

Body is getting relieved of stress.... It is feeling very, very fresh and fragrant...how wonderful to have a morning rain. As it has rained outside (confusion technique), take a deep breathe in and out (twice)... and... the wetness outside are giving your whole body a feeling of inner peace, and deep within... a great tranquility. That wonderful feeling and experience... beautiful nature that surrounds you... with slowly trickling rain and slowly moving wind.... It makes you peaceful and also... impeccable peace surrounds you. It not only surrounds you... but also engulfs you in each and every cell of your body and mind...

Th.: So you are feeling relaxed. And, as you are feeling relaxed, your right index finger moves.

Sub. Moves the right index finger.

Th.: And you want to feel more relaxed... more at peace, serenity and harmony... If so, move your right index finger.

Sub. Moves the right index finger.

Th.: That is your natural due... All intelligent people feel the way you do. Now take your time to decide... ... take a deep breadth in...take a deep breadth out... (Repeat a few times)...and you are deciding now... to move ahead... to feel more relaxed... more at peace, serenity and harmony... If so, move your right index finger.

Sub. Moves the right index finger.

Th.: That is a correct choice...I did expect that from a highly sensible person that you are...And, it is common sense to understand that moving means movement...and movement means (a few deep breadths)... change of position....and when you have decided to move, you have moved... If so, move your right index finger.

Sub. Moves the right index finger.

Th.: We have changed our position by moving forward...we have moved forward... you were a smoker...that was one position...there was bad breadth, social stigma and a constraint... but you loved your family. If so, move your right index finger.

Sub. Moves the right index finger.

Th.: In all cultures the family is valued...in our culture particularly, family is a value in itself. for you I am very pleased to learn that family is so...and you loved your family before and now and for ever... If so, move your right index finger.

Sub. Moves the right index finger.

Th.: That is a value that you are carrying with you... (A few deep breadths), shall remain with you...and you want to care for your family... If so, move your right index finger.

Sub. Moves the

Right index finger.

Th.: So, I am proud of you...for the people whom you love, you want to care...and, when you care for yourself... so that you live a long healthy life...you are loving the people whom you love, more and more... If so, move your right index finger.

Sub. Moves the right index finger.

Th.: That is indeed natural and...yet it is great...you have since long known this... you want to live a disease free healthy life for the sake of your children...you will say, yes, I am sure...

Sub. Moves the right index finger.

Th.: And, then you know the easy way to do so. Quit smoking. You have quit smoking. Quit smoking for good. Quit smoking for ever.

Though most of the times, the session moves in the indicated direction, the subject may decide to move his "no" finger. It indicates unconscious block: the subject has some compensation for which his unconscious mind propels him to continue. That will call for advanced exploratory work.

For exploration of unconscious mind, if necessary, age regression or such other strategies discussed later may be applied. Most cases will benefit by further addition of a support system derived from Nature, such as Sun, the source of all energy and strength, Mother Earth or a congenial friend, guide or a mentor as described above.

The subject is brought back to ordinary awake state in a slow, even paced way as:

Now...there is peace in mind...all over your mind... in your natural state, relax even more and more. It was my endeavour and duty to make you feel comfortable, at ease and at peace with your self...and, I am so happy to see the successful outcome...

You have learned very fast...because of your hypnotic talent... and it is easy also because it is your natural due, so even more....so...

As you relax, feel comfortable, enjoy the state of wonderful alternate existence and, find an easy way to feel calm, cool, and comfortable and... be at ease.

Because of your natural due... feeling so ...you are so touching the fundamental foundation... of your own creativity. When I have so spoken to you, it is a great privilege for me...

We have...a communion in consciousness sharing... and... I consider it to be, a great privilege that you showed your confidence... and, you trust me to conduct this session.

Let's share this silence, take a deep breath in... a further deeper... breath...to a state that you feel rejuvenated...the state of creative and re-creative, silence of the mind... you wake up as I count from 10 to 1.

10, 9, 8, 7, 6, 5... as I am counting other sounds also start coming back to you...listen to the sound of moving the fan, other friends... talking on the road.

10, 9, 8, 7, 6, 5, 4... let me assure you that when you are coming back in your natural... ordinary, every day state ...of awareness...

9, 8, 7, 6, 5, you will feel fresh... re-fresh and cool...

8, 7, 6, 5, 4, tonight before going to your bed... 7, 6, 5, 4, 3, before you sleep... when you will lay down on the bed... you will recreate this session in your mind...you will listen to the recorded cassette...

6, 5, 4, 3, 2, you are your best friend...and...when you listen to your self... in this high state of creativity you experience great...

5, 4, 3, 2, 1, wake up and wake up to the awareness of your body...experience great...peace, calm...peace.

Now you are totally awake...awake as we count 5...4, 3, 2, 1.... Yes...very good, wonderful job... very nice, congratulations! (Shake hands if the situation permits)... Alert and wide awake...stretch your hands...Alert, totally alert!

- ***Give Post Hypnotic Suggestion***

You will be able to experience this any time and every time...that you want to. You will listen to the recorded cassette, also it is recorded in your mind, and this is a promise to your self that shall be fulfilled...promise is given, you have given the promise...and ... that shall be fulfilled.

Insomnia

The cause of insomnia is in psychodynamics of unfinished business at unconscious mind. There is a bell ringing in subconscious – unconscious mind. That is causing alarm to be alert. Therapist aims to complete the loop of unfinished business and silence the bell, as below:

A Muslim medical doctor, middle aged, was having sleepless nights since 2 years when he presented in 2004. His session went like this:

> We are shifting to the easy chair....more comfortable position...and...you are finding it more comfortable...and so will you find it even more comfortable when you follow my suggestions...you know, in the past century...American parents advised their sons to go West...and, you know about the ...presence in West...let us once again change our position and sit facing West...that is nice...you have always faced West while offering Namaz...

He was age regressed to 2002. He became restless and fidgety then. Sensing that the riots of 2002 are most likely cause for his insomnia, he was further suggested in trance as:

> While things around are unpleasant and insecure...you are offering Namaz...and, as you do so...you pray...the prayers are rewarded...a white bearded... saintly... kind aged person is coming to you...and he is holding your hand...you are holding his hand...he says some faint words...listen to them. and, you are listening to them...nothing

whatsoever can happen against the will of Allah...Allah is almighty protector and he sent a messenger ...in the West...Allah is all kindness...merciful...and you have offered prayers to Him...and. He rewards you with full protection...everything will happen according to his wish...blessings.

He was able to sleep with this recorded cassette.

Fugue: Dissociative Neurosis, Depersonalization

A middle aged engineer was driving, when he suddenly lost consciousness and his car suffered a small accident. He was diagnosed to have had a brain hemorrhage and operated surgically for a burst aneurism. He recovered and was rehabilitated to his occupation. But soon it started happening that while driving he would lose the sense of who he is and where is he heading till such time that he would arrive at a strange not thought of destination.

He was age regressed up to the operative session and made to relive the steps on the operation table. He was made to see that the surgeon has ligated and removed his aneurism. He was made to see his brain, normal. After few sessions he is well for over 10 years now.

Possession

This is frequently seen in Indian women; though more common in rural background, highly educated urbanized ladies are also prone to it. Such as,

1. An engineer lady, teaching in a college, would discuss high profile physics with a senior. They would travel together morning and evening for a considerable distance. From physics the subjects will revolve around physics of consciousness, collective consciousness and how one individual is a part of indivisible whole that is Universe. They communicated such esoteric maters by e-mails too. (She put a bulky load of e-mail print outs to prove that he had now completely possessed her). She was sure that he is to influence her that she will be made to do dirty things.

The senior was contacted and was found to be a troubled man now. He had revealed the matter to his wife and stopped all contacts.

Cue was taken from the e-mail papers that either she is showing them to the therapist at her will or he is causing her to show them. The sessions were designed in the language of physics. During hypnosis, causality and change were discussed as well as law of inertia. She was teaching thermodynamics. She agreed that all living systems obey thermodynamic principles and was subject to rejuvenation by a fresh input of energy.

The sessions were conducted in the presence of her loyal and supportive boy friend. She completely got out of it. They migrated to another city.

2. A double graduate housewife with a single child and a hard working upcoming husband, living in a city moved to a new house. After the child and husband will leave in the morning, the lonely lady will sense bad spirits that will take her possession in new house. She wanted to be occupied but had no job. She denied that she wanted another child: in her condition when she has lost 10 kg (spirits were eating away all that she ate), she will not be able to take care of a second one.

During hypnosis, she was presented with a paradigm: there are bad spirits and, so there are good ones too. Therapist is familiar with good spirits and shall introduce them to her. She had *Durga* in her home. Not only she is a protector, but a destroyer of the evil spirits.

There was *Janmastami* just before the last session. This is the time when Krishna is born. And, Krishna is protected and nurtured by divine forces. Krishna is born to destroy evil forces.

Telephonically, she canceled the next appointment to say that she is well and has conceived.

Phobia

This is best treated by hypnosis: no other help can be so certain. Here, it is repressed material that is triggering even panic attacks. The use of hypnosis in exploratory psychotherapy, such as in the insight approaches, is contingent upon the influence of hypnosis on unconscious resistance that in resolution helps the individual establish closer contact with repressed needs and conflicts. It may thus be possible to bring to the surface significant memories and repressed impulses that expedite the analytic process. We have universal success in phobias and our subjects generated insights too as follows:

- *Case 1*

A middle aged man, living in thickly populated area of city was having panic attacks no sooner he would hear sound of any kind of tapping. He will sweat all over his body, be restless and will have to give up whatever he may have been doing. Age regressed to the time since the attacks started; he relived a murder taking place near his shop. There were loud bangs with a hammer and lot of splurge of blood. Selective ablation of the past was done. He was well after a single session.

Therapy was continued for few more sessions. He continued to remain well after 8 years. Now he states that the incident was the cause of his panic attacks.

- *Case 2*

At a workshop, this subject presented for therapy through her clinical psychologist. A wealthy lady, who used to travel by air from childhood, could not do so after she got married, again into a wealthy family. At the suggestion only she will panic. Age regressed to the time around the happening; she relived the experience of having gone to Kashmir for her honeymoon. Traveling by air that time, the plane had experienced a lot of air turbulence. While every one including her landed safely, she recalled almost all were panicky. She was further age regressed to several times of her air travels before, this was brought forward to superimpose on the distressing event. It took 3 sessions when she declared herself cured.

The clinical psychologist learnt hypnotherapy at the workshop and, was entrusted to conduct reinforcement sessions.

- *Case 3*

A middle aged man in his mid thirties was experiencing claustrophobia since last 15 years. He has tried several measures like yoga therapy, hypnotherapy from "spirit release hypnotherapists" who had proclaimed that he was possessed by evil spirits and several psychiatrists. To prove that he can control his mind, he did stop smoking. Over the years, his disability progressed so that he cannot enter any closed space. Travel by train and air was ruled out. He just has to move about in his own car.

He rose to be a director of a company that was in air travel business. His promotion to international directorship stopped since he could not travel by air.

Two simultaneous strategies, working at multiple level of communication were applied. Space expansion was taught, with metaphors from atomic physics and space. The focus was that there is abundant space all over and all within. Age regression was to relive last 15 years piece by piece. Following 2 sessions, he slept without sleeping pills and his irritable bowel syndrome cooled down. He travelled by Metro train and set in a giant wheel.

As a classic example of insight generation, he wrote, "I recollect rather with some embarrassment and a feeling of shame, that when I was a child, I was cornered by a wicked man and abused. I have dreams of a child being cornered and a tough man approaching him with a large stick. Could this be the cause of my phobia?"

He was left to be followed up by a local psychiatrist.

Theatre technique utilizes age regression covertly. The subject is made to sit in a vast, comfortable, air conditioned theatre, with a remote control in his/her hand. The movie begins and the screen displays the subject and therapist to begin with. The subject leisurely moves the remote control and movements of the clicking are utilized as ideomotor signals. It proceeds to fast backwards mode till the phobic object/situation/panic attack appears on the screen. The subject is given a solid stick by the therapist, rushes to the screen and smashes the object/situation. The screen is left intact. Walking back to comfortable sit, the subject commands fast forward mode to come back, on to the screen, on the day of therapy; completely well; totally rid of phobia/panic attack.

Migraine

There are numerous causes ascribed to migraine. What is of paramount importance is that most patients are highly intelligent persons having an unresolved conflict. I tell them a Zen metaphor to ponder over: we have put a chicken in a flask, fed it, now it has grown up. No sooner we can find out a way by which we can bring out the hen without breaking the flask – and you know a way to do it, for sure – your migraine is to fly out.

Beyond this I utilize passive, permissive, Ericksonian approach in hypnoanalysis through age regression. In a few sessions the insight generation occurs. They listen to the recorded cassette and follow the sessions till cured.

Anxiety Neurosis[6]

The following hypnotherapeutic techniques can be utilized in the management of anxiety and psychosomatic disorders:

1. Introduction and removal of misconception
2. Autogenic training: six standard techniques
3. Hypnotic phenomena
   Hypnotic analgesia and anesthesia
   Temperature alteration
   Amnesia
   Catalepsy
   Ideomotor and ideosensory activities
   Dissociation
   Time distortion
   Automatic writing
   Relaxation
   Age regression
   Age progression
4. Hypnoanalysis
5. Paintings
6. Paradoxical interventions

Erectile Dysfunction

It is usually rooted in deep seated anxiety and, a possible failure to perform in the past. Failure need not pertain to sex; failure in any of the culturally conditioned masculine functions may lead to "impotence". Viagra helps; but hypnotherapy is the drugless therapy. Some times, the results are spectacular; subjects performed normal immediately following the session. This was due to their faith in the treatment and "aura" for the therapist. The session is on the following lines: Note the metaphors that are displayed in italics; Freudian interpretations apply.

You are getting out of your *home* with your partner. You have *mount*ed on *a motor bike*. You are driving to a famous *garden*. It is the garden of your choice. In this garden *Adam* and *Eve* played. You have *play*ed there before. The *road is bumpy* and there are jerks. You enjoy the *bumps*. Having arrived at the garden, you take your partner to a leisurely stroll and show her various *tall trees*. There are flowers and there is *scent*.

There is a *lake* full of *water*. There is still water with gentlè *ripples* because there is breeze. There is a *boat* parked at the lake. You take your partner and give her your *hand*, help her into the boat. There is a long *oar* that you *row* with... a long oar that you *rove* with. The boat *rocks*. You like it. Your partner likes it very much...

Hypersexuality

Several males are harassed by their persistent insatiable drive-urge—for sex. This may generate multiple partnerships - socially acceptable or unacceptable. They seldom seek help directly; may even welcome, when offered covertly through indirect hypnosis. Organic causes like tumor of the anterior pituitary, adrenals or testis should be ruled out by biochemistry.

A first generation neo–rich wealthy man, religious, regular practitioner of Yoga had multiple relationships. He would get severe attacks of migraine.

He as well had irritable bowel syndrome. Wife ignored till such time that he started eyeing her younger sister. He got her married to a non-entity and employed her husband. Wife approached for help. Therapeutic strategy was to provide help for his headache and bowels. CAT Scans and gastroscopy were done.

Meanwhile, he was prescribed a pill for symptomatic relief. Honvan, a synthetic estrogen pill had immediate effect to slow down his drive. He was "sublimated" through yogic practice of arousal of *Kundalini* and energy emanating there from; that went upwards through *muladhara chakra* to all the way up in *Sahasrara;* so that, he will utilize his energy for larger social benefits. He became president of his business association; ran some charities.

Thus, here is a classic illustration of utilization of Freudian ego defenses. Neurotic aggrandizement–megalomania—was substituted with mature defenses.

Frigidity and Dysparunia

Physiology is explained. Foreplay is to be explained. Sex is biological, but when two people who love each other and have sex, it transcends into several aesthetic realms. Gynecologist's intervention in the use of vaginal dilators helps. After ruling out any underlying psychological trauma, the suggestions are on the metaphors involving water, swimming, riding a scooter or a horse. The dry land becomes soft and pliable when it rains: rain of estrogen and such other hormones is raining when you make love. See the magnificent carvings on the temple of your choice: see Khajurao and such other temples. Gods made love and world was created.

Explain sexual aggression as: all Siva temples have a bull before the *sanctum sanctorum*.

Unexplained Reproductive Failure: Infertility

The psychodynamics is discussed elsewhere.

Hypnotherapy involves targeting the autonomic nervous system (through relaxation and deep trance, metaphors applied are removal of road blocks while going on a joy ride, traffic propels in pulses), balancing the hormonal system (direct explanation of physiology; there is a composer of the orchestra as well as a band-master who conducts it in harmony) and immune responses (indirect hypnosis by way of demonstrating live sperms before; and in lysis after they are instilled in vagina). The therapy that is applied to the couple together is on the following lines:

Two of them decide to go for a joy ride after taking a refreshing shower of cool water...comfortably and pleasantly dressed...riding on a scooter...enter a garden...garden of Eden...so beautiful...where the gods play...hand in hand...tall trees...beautiful flower beds...beds of green grass...velvet like green grass...beds...the birds are chirping...the sun is going down in the West...they see a garden with children playing...they pause...look...a mother is holding an infant in her arms...beautiful smile...your partner takes out his mobile phone...that has a camera...takes a picture...both of you see...there is a picture of a mother that is you with a child...both of you look into each other's eyes...leisurely saunter back...sun is setting in the West...ride on your vehicle...a bit of bumpy drive...enjoyable...reach home...there is a lock...you are fumbling with the key...your doctor, Dr. R is just around...helps you, the lock just opens...you go to your bed room...you see at the foot end of the bed a nice picture...it is a mother with a baby... it is a mother with a baby...that your partner has flashed in the garden...it is You with your baby...no body around...only you and your partner...open door...open the windows...fresh flow of air...you make love...

The following illustration provides clues to derive metaphors from the name and surroundings. Shruti (name of the subject) is given the suggestions derived from her name. Shruti means what has been heard as told by sages and saints in *Vedas* and *Upanishads*.

Ego strengthening and metaphors are obvious.
Goal: Creativity and insight generation

We have read the poetry...and, there was a sound in the sky... which I have heard...and, you have been hearing as a...divine blessing... as a *Shruti*—*Shruti* is what is heard... a divine sound heard from the sky... that comes from the sages... and, seers... that may be in the form of *Pranava*... *Pranava* is *Om* .. that you recite in this sacred place often during the day. It is the big bang... that the big bang... we are hearing... *Shruti* is hearing sublime poetry of strength and vigor.... Having heard the *Shruti, Shruti* is never scared. Now that *Shruti* has heard the ever resonating sound... that is "*NIHASHABDA*", i.e. without words, we have heard the sound of silence... we have heard the sound of silence... today. We are hearing the sound of silence...and you have stopped the sound of clapping with one hand...There is no sound of clapping... Yes, you are now telling to yourself... but how can I clap with one hand!!!!. Still I hear the sound of silence... I am still hearing the sound of silence. The wise person within me says... I can hear the sound of silence... I have done it. I can do it once again.

Yes, that is silence in my mind... so that, I can hear the sounds of silence... Let there be silence. I am serene, tranquil, peaceful..., and free of all the fears, tension, anxiety... I am in deep... silence. All the stress is gone for ever. I am happy, cheerful, and completely relaxed.

Strategies for Stress Relief: 1

Subject with *phobia of public speaking*; fear of women

Goal: restoration of confidence; elimination of phobia.

Mr. D., 29 Years, shy person, had fear of crowd, especially women. Blood pressure went up as "side effect of medicines". He came from rural background and has been educated in conservative society. He is from a backward class. Father was suffering from Alzheimer's disease. Anxiety and symptoms of autonomic nervous system imbalance noted. There was drug dependence for sleep. His interest is cricket.

Anxiety neurosis patients are very tense and making them comfortable, relaxed and on positive mode is the aim in first session. Suggestions are aimed at opening up to new modalities of changing world and values deriving metaphors from his hobby.

Metaphors applied: In a crowd, he is comfortable playing cricket; he also remembers playing cricket with his schoolmates. Cricket is played before the crowds. Foot ball or cricket, they all are games. Crowds at the cricket ground consist of males and females: females also cheer and, they cheer more.

Are you comfortable with shoes...and...when you are comfortable then we go further. Do you always sit with crossed hands to be comfortable? (Sitting tense with crossed legs or tight closed hands conveys that subject is tense and needs relaxation to interact. I suggest that probably you are comfortable... without crossing your hands and legs. We already have shaken hands... Do I have your permission to touch your hands.? When you give me this permission, this session goes on better. (Touch enhances the induction of trance)... Yes, thank you for your permission.

(Look at his eyes. They are already heavy). If you like to keep it open, but if you like to keep them closed it is your choice. (Permissive suggestion, but indirectly asking him to close the eyes). As I relax your hands, move your head, right hand moves up... like a feather. Quick induction is done. Ego strengthening is done. Deep breathe, your left hand is getting heavier and heavier that you feel while it is stuck at your shoulder, deep breathe (2),... right hand feels totally lighter, lighter than feather (confusion by paradox, hand levitation, right hand goes up)...So, it just stays in this position and you are not making any effort to move it... as it stays there... take a deep breathe, further deep breathe and your right hand finger moves... (Moves all the fingers of right hand)... And as they move you are doing so wonderfully fine and well... You realize as you try to close your fingers, it makes a fist... and you are exactly doing this and tighten your fingers... yes, and as you tighten your fist... rest of the body relaxes even more, (2), your right upper extremity is lighter than a feather.

A feather usually floats in the air, and the thing lighter than air goes up... Yes, you tighten your lips now and your hand becomes lighter. You know your science very well... that gravity pulls you down. Your right extremity is floating up (2)... yes... up and up, and as it is going up and it is lighter than air (right hand goes up), wonderful, as it has gone up... it stays in this light position, no tension in your elbow... I can feel your elbow muscles so relaxed, no tension, no fatigue that you have no difficulty with open eyes or closed eyes... When your eyelids are heavy and you want to close them, so that you feel more at ease, comfortable, tranquil, sure, energetic, confident of your self. There is a talk about some great people that when they have closed their fists and grasped a bit firmly...and when they are... standing with right hand up, further up and with fist closed...they hit a sixer...then also...you win...and winning is in hitting a sixer...before the crowds...Players play game...players play different games...and, they may change the game...to another game...a game of football...that tackles the players...and cricketer may play football...tackling players before the crowds... that clap...women in the crowds...clap even more...

- ***Second Session***

Age regression-to the age when he had traumatic experiences. Help him to visualize a black board where hurtful messages and good messages are jumbled up. Help the subject to wipe out wrong messages and write correct messages.

- ***Third Session***

Language of friendship...language.... of love is so simple...Such relationships are just a few... No extra effort is required...others relate according to...protocol, be nice... Nice, caring atmosphere...is all that builds trust...that builds confidence...straight line is straight...and short...shortest distance between two points...two people...Good communication in a straight line is easy to do.... Straight communication in a straight line is direct communication... Straight line is easy to draw... by joining two points... It is meaningful and self explanatory...it is simple... when you hit a sixer, it may not be straight...yet, a sixer is a sixer.... Body language also is a way to communicate. But sometime it is easy... to have verbal communication that conveys what exactly one wants to communicate. You are meeting your office colleague in a social function. When you see each other from a distance you greet each other. Both of you move towards each other. You have confident, meaningful conversation. When you see the watch it is more than half an hour and you are pleased to have met her. After reaching home, you feel happy, confident with in, and great.

Strategies for Stress Relief: 2

Stress of surgical operation: secondary hemorrhage

Goal: Consent for secondary surgery; stopping the hemorrhage.

A lady of 67 years had bilateral knee replacement. She started oozing from the site of the second operation after 3 days. This was not controlled and the surgeons thought there was a slipped ligature. They decided to reexplore but the patient refused. Hypnotherapist was called in and, he offered two options: to stop bleeding with hypnosis or to help with the consent for the second operation. Surgeons chose the second. The following strategy was applied[7]:

I have known about your fortitude... I have known about your fortitude...from your son as well as from your doctors...Knee replacement is a major operation... I have known about your fortitude...and, you have undergone it twice already...you have wisely chosen your expert surgeons...and how well have they performed...two major operations with you being wide awake...and they took good care...to see that you do not have any pain too... and they took good care to see that you do not have any pain too...just see past few days before your eyes... to see that you do not have any pain too...now the surgeons what to take good care of you... since they think this leak from the wound is due to a slipped ligature...they should act...they cannot leave you to bleed inside your joint... and they took good care to see that you do not have any pain too...and now they want to be sure that you do not loose blood...and do not have pain...you should not have any pain... ...you will not have any pain...that is a promise, yes, that is good...just keep taking a few deep breaths for me...deep...deep breaths and there you relax... there you relax...perfectly. Relax from toes to forehead...all over...

Your surgeons have a nice comfortable operating rooms...a very comfortable table... it is your comfort place...where you were removed of your uncomfortable painful knees... it is your comfort place...and you want to go to your comfortable place...say it by moving your index finger...yes, you are being taken to your comfort place... your comfort table place in operation room...

Enjoy the place...I am talking to your unconscious mind...and you need not concentrate on what I am saying... need not concentrate on what is going on...what I am saying.... Just enjoy your cool comfort table...you are cooling down...more cool...more comfort...and your both knees are cool...very cool now...your left knee is even cooler...and cooler it is there is all ice...frozen ice... frozen ice has frozen every thing in your left knee... frozen ice has frozen the blood in and around your left knee...the blood vessels are cool...cold. and they are frozen and shrunk... frozen the blood in and around your left knee...there is no oozing of any blood...and you will recover and your wound would heal, is healing ...and, pain is gone...there is just an unpleasant sensation....surgeons are expert...oozing has stopped...see that there is water flowing into a pipe and there is a no leakage...there are engineers and, they can repair the leak and leak has stopped...it has stopped...you are now on a fast track of recovery...hardly any pain...soon walking on your new knees... comfortable and fine.

Surgeons could not find any pathology for her oozing intraoperatively.

Tics

A *tic* is a persistent, intermittent muscle twitch or spasm, usually limited to a localized muscle group. The term is used broadly to include blinking the eye, twitching the mouth, licking the lips, shrugging the shoulders, twisting the neck, clearing the throat, blowing the nose, and grimacing, among other actions.

The disorder stems from psychological causes, such as self-consciousness or tension in social situations.

Same strategy, as applied to Mr. D. above is applicable. But always leave some leeway so that person has escape door available, i.e. embarrassing and socially unacceptable ticks may be substituted by infrequent and acceptable behaviour i.e. putting a hand in the pocket and touching the index finger and thumb. This is applicable to epilepsy also where there in no detectable lesion in the brain for convulsions on electroencephalogram. Symptom substitution is done by suggestion that convulsions are permissible when they occur only in the little finger.

Symptom Relief

Subject: [J] A nervous young man, devout Christian, given to **coughing every time he felt nervous.**

Goal: To be cured of his cough

Therapists: Two at a time (Two therapists may work in tandem when the session is likely to be difficult or/and prolonged).

Strategy: Age regression

Hold this book and pen. When you hold it, it's not going to interfere in your relaxation. Write the date and sign, sign once again and during the session as you relax we will ask you to sign but that will not interfere with your relaxation.

A person with your sensibility is able to go into a deep trance. Louder we speak, J relaxes more and more. It's very nice J that you have found a method to relax yourself. And, as we speak softly you relax even…better…

You have focused your eyes on a spot on the wall opposite and as you keep on looking at this spot… your eyes have become watery… tired and they want to close, let them close, yes they are closing… and they have closed. The moment they have closed, J you have experienced a profound deep sense of ease, further ease, so much of relaxation, yes all the tension in each and every muscle… of your body… the muscles of your eyelids, of your face, of your lips, of your chin, of your neck, of your shoulder, both the shoulders, completely relaxed.

Deep breath… in and out… deep breath, deeper still, and as you swallow a little saliva, swallow a little saliva J, wonderful… and your throat is now feeling clean, absolutely clean and neat… and all the viruses have been swallowed and digested… The relaxation goes down along the digestive tract, front of the chest, back of the chest, and in one sudden sway… shift your relaxation all the way down to rest of your body…till the tips of your toes.

As you wriggle the toes, the tension, worries, anxiety and all that is hurried… is slowly and surely…now gone, gone now and gone forever. take a deep breath and… this day…on October 5, 2006… you take a deep breath… yes, you have taken a deep breath and we are on October 2, 2006… its Gandhiji's birthday and, I would like to tell you a few things about this man… who was instrumental in making India free., this frail man was very…powerful…frail man can also be powerful…could shake the British empire!

You could have been there… so nice J to meet this man, deep breath and still a deep breath let me know when you want to meet Mahatma Gandhi, very nice, we now travel in one breath you are now 3 days backwards, and in one breath you are there in 2003… at the interview for your MSW entrance, and the instructor asks you to be studious and willing to help others always, would you sign the document saying so J? think over, face to face with the interviewer…you are now seated across the table and sign yourself…you have a pen in your right hand and there is a paper before you…deep breath J., I assure you that when you will sign… to be a good student we shall then go further…go further backward to meet Mahatma Gandhi, would you want to sign now?…Take your time.

V is now helping you and assuring you…that…as I take your hand and you may sign with your eyes… closed or, open… your choice, but I need your consent…I am taking your hand and putting it on the paper, sign your name J, as you sign your cheque., very nice. J, we are moving four steps…backwards.

It is year 2000. Deep breath and in the year 2000…you have just now known that you have successfully passed your examination. That was standard 12 and the mark sheet is before your eyes… deep breath.

Would you like to take a short breath…and see your standard 10? Let me help you see that and sign again J… yes, you want the certificate and you've signed. In one deep breath you have gone behind 10 years… … …This chubby cheerful boy J, is playing in the campus in Rosary school… It has nice open ground, a very smooth skating area…you are skating…J, you are now a young chubby boy of 4 and a half years in the kindergarten…and, the teacher has taught you alphabets and so you can write your name., deep breath and as I help you now, the little boy J writes his name., take your time.

Yes…very nice, just learned how to write your name., and I promise to take you to see Mahatma Gandhi…deep breath and you may write or draw or scribble whatever you like, you have now gone wayward to the year 1988 and then you are writing your name… aah…aa, very nice, you are writing some alphabets J, so, nice,, s for sheep, e for egg… s for sheep and p for pig… and, b for a baby and, yes… you have seen a cat, J…And you wrote C… lovely child!

Deep breath, now J is a little baby, about the age of 1or is it 2, and, mummy is giving you., or is it some aunty or uncle? …J happy in drawing… please draw something for us…a house, sun or cat., with one deep breath…the little baby has gone into the mother's tummy and, (puts his thumb in the mouth)…you are sucking your thumb… and in one deep breath J, we now go., 48 or 49 or maybe 50 years backwards…take a deep breath and it is… …30th Jan., 1948 evening of 5 o clock… and, you see this man walking along with 2 young ladies… looking at his watch, he is late so he is hurrying fast and…suddenly he falls…we have heard 3 loud bangs and this fallen man…take a deep breath since we now see in this fallen man across., and on that Cross no other sound now, total silence we have in one deep, deep breath jumped across 48 years and on that cross… the bleeding tortured form of Jesus Christ is… when you see that form of Jesus, J, sign for me again!

It requires a noble soul and a pious heart to see Jesus Christ right in front of your eyes…at this very moment! I am also privileged to have met Mahatma Gandhi and Jesus together., see him being resurrected, and as you see him rising, sign for me., V and J are sharing tears of joy at the resurrection… and having this blissful experience that we are sharing with our friends.

This is a wonderful moment in our life., J lets travel 2006 years in one swift breath you are so empowered that you take a deep breath and make a quantum jump and there we are on 2nd October, 2006 in the Psychology dept. room no. 19 a little earlier than 6 pm and as you swallow that saliva, swallow and let it sip deep down… I promise to you that this will be a memorable day in our lives. We saw 2 great saviors of mankind face to face…V is counting from 10 to 1 and J, 10., 9. 8., 3 J is waking up, yes, his eyes are opening… and, 2, 1 great, we are so proud of this boy, so very proud, thank you.

Hypnoanalgesia; Hypnoanethesia

Subjects: Gitanjali [G] (Veena [V] Group of two, simultaneous.

Goal: Hypnoanalgesia; hypnoanethesia

Therapists: Two at a time

Both of you will listen to both of us...so you have known this process and now we are going to assert this plainly and loudly. Now, you are comfortable, totally relaxed, perfectly at ease. In short, G put yourself in yes, dear, put yourself in trance, so simple, you have done this before...repeat it now... and, show you talented you are, take it easy, no tension, yes, relax yourself and very nice...very nice, you have by now learnt several effective techniques... to induce a trance, here you have put yourself...in a comfortable position., be entirely at ease, peace and relaxed. You have chosen a simple method to put yourself into and, yes... as you swallow a little saliva and as it trickles down your gullet...you have started experiencing a state of progressive muscular relaxation. Deep breath in and out, with every breath that you now take you feel., the deep sense of relaxation... on your knees, cheeks, forearms, legs, trunk, forehead and...the whole body is relaxed wonderful... very nice... so talented so highly intelligent and, so profoundly spiritual (this was done at an *Ashram*) and...as this profound relaxation has now gone over your whole body...and you are now feeling a profound sense of relaxation, security, peace, joy...almost rapture., that's your natural due G., that's yours and enjoy it yourself...

Since now you have learned to produce endorphins within your brain and as each molecule of endorphin., each molecule of endorphin...is now percolating into your body fluids...into your blood, you have a great sense of supreme, sublime joy, peace, ease and Ananda will get deeper as you have now started sharing it with V...with every breath that you take, and...your eyes are so much heavy, your eyelids are perfectly relaxed so that when you try to open your eyes...even when I tell you...your eyes are so like, tightly closed doors!

They just can't open., open your eyes and as you try... try now...your eyeballs rotate...but the lids remain tightly closed. Try once again, to open your eyes., and see how heavy your eyelids are and then it is so much comfortable, to be at ease and...enjoy your peace as your eyelids remain closed, G your right hand...is getting lighter and lighter., you've started on the most wonderful journey of your life...and...when you are enjoying the state of your new found peace, your right index finger moves...deep breath and when you are at peace, move your right index finger G. And how very clever, V, you have also moved your...right index finger.

Now, you see with your closed eyes...you are getting up from your chair... you have got out of the door...climbed down the stairs...yes, the steps are 1, 2, 8, and you are already in the landing. As you move to climb further steps down, yes...G, yes V...you get into a 9, 10, 11 deeper trance with every step down 12, 13, 16 and you are in the sublime stage of deep trance.

You have taken your vehicle, starting it...and, started driving towards home...fresh air touching all your face both hands, forearms, fine, fresh and cool...

A nice fragrance of the Ashram garden flowers...G is so pleased to smell the nice fragrance...and, as you smell the nice fragrance you are sharing it with V...sited on your back seat...your right hand is also getting lighter., lighter so that it wants to float up., up., up in the air and let it float G., gently and all by itself, it goes up., up., up further up and, G yet, you have full control of your vehicle...there is no weight, no strain, very nice absolutely like a feather...when you want it to rest on the handle that is also nice...or if it is floating in the air that way it is also better but now you have decided for better control of the vehicle...as your hand falls like a log of wood, feeling cold and you have done so much of work... my dear, that now you are at home, very nice G relax... because, you have done so much of work...you deserve a glass of cold water... you both deserve a glass of cold water...

V has followed you to kitchen...you have gone to the kitchen, and...you are opening the door of the refrigerator...yes, from the opened door V says...a cool breeze of cold air wraps around you...feel the cold air...enjoy the cool breeze...and, you are now opening the freezer compartment.

The ice compartment of the fridge is loaded with ice trays... you have taken out 1, 2, or may be 3 or 4 trays full of ice cubes, put them on the dining table... totally at ease, comfortable as we are with you, going to be all pleasure... and one by one... you have started picking up the ice cubes with your right hand...and you are putting them into a plate and maybe into a glass...as you are picking up those ice cubes...your hand is getting colder and colder, one by one the ice cubes make your hand cool...so very cool and numb, cool and numb... cool and numb.

All the sensations of pain, heat and touch are gone...only feeling cold, there is cool coldness all over your right hand...the blood has flown out of it or maybe that also is frozen...right hand is cool...one by one ice cubes are being picked up and... the right hand is frozen and numb...just ice like...up to the level where my finger has touched you, your right hand is frozen ice... frozen ice has no feelings and as you lift the glass of cold water with your left hand...putting it on your lips, your lips., you are now sipping the cold water and your lips are feeling nice and cold...and the water is going down the gullet...the right hand remains frozen and cold, absolutely cold, frozen ice, no feelings. How very nice to sip on this nice cold water...your right hand is totally numb and painless...frozen ice...totally numb and painless., no pain only cold and very, very cold and, as you keep on sipping that cold water your mouth is getting numb.

And...as you put this frozen ice on your chin and see how tightly 2 pieces of ice...deep breath G, as you press two pieces of ice...they can not be separated and...even you have taken this piece of ice, no pain at all.

That is wonderful V that you have also helped G and sipped cold, very cold water...G and V are two pieces of ice tightly stuck to each other...so gifted is G ...so gifted is V, you are such gifted, talented human beings, spiritually spirited and... no pain at all.

(Needles are inserted in right hands of both the subjects, G and V)

...they will open their eyes G, and see what you have done...., deep breath and while G is enjoying...whatever kind of water she is enjoying the cool, cool drink that she enjoys one sip and a deeper trance, 2nd sip and still deeper trance..., deep and relaxed...., fine perfume of the food that you liked the most, has filled your kitchen and as you look on, the table, yes, G enjoy the look and the taste of the food...and your right hand remains frozen ice, remain comfortable...., totally easy and when I put you into this state of extra comfort, wonderful very nice, very, very nice, while you enjoy the taste...and the smell of the food in your kitchen... you have forgotten... all the sounds around you and...till I come back to you, you are not listening even to my voice.

(Discussion with the participants. This is to reinforce post hypnotic suggestion of persistence of analgesia even after the subjects are out of trance. When the participants tell them what was discussed, they realize that they have not heard it at all).

Now G and V have got the right drink of the cold temperature. Please start listening to my voice once again. When you will listen to my voice...both of you will still remain in trance...and, when you will open your eyes once again and...see that a needle is in your hands...yes, G yes, V, have a look on your right hand, what tremendous creative potential...one who can master pain is like Shri Bhishma Pitamah, resting on the bed of arrows... G, She is seeing Bhishma Pitamah in a flash...we are 5000 years behind...where there are so many warriors and there is Arjun who has created a bed of arrows for Bhishma...and G and no pain at all... and G and V and Bhishma have the same capability to conquer pain.

Anytime in your future as you wish...you will take 3 deep breaths, empower your right hand...master the quality of pain control. When you will put your right hand on any part of your body the pain will get frozen and...will...and will get away. Believe in yourself whenever you will have a person in pain, when you will put your right hand...after taking 3 deep breaths, on the subject...the subject will go into a subtle trance...after taking three deep breaths and...you will be able to relieve the pain!

Substance Abuse: Alcoholic Subject

- *Session 1*

History: The subject was a highly educated (Ph.D. in mathematics); most intelligent disappointed, unmarried man 35. He took to alcohol after he was ditched by his first and only lady love. He had tried to give up; and partly succeeded in giving up alcohol a few times. He relapsed every time soon after. There was high motivation for giving up alcohol, for financial considerations (he was already broke), for love of family, for social acceptance, health hazard, and intellectual growth all were at stake. He had come to an Ashram finally.

While rapport building was done, motivation was strengthened: only way to go back to family, back to the society, normal health and above every thing, utilize his intellect was to give up.

He said he has come to seminar out of curiosity, but he understands from literature and Internet that there is genetic predisposition. There are so many members on his father's side that he has no hope; since genes are what you inherit and die with.

When explained, he learnt genetics very fast. He read Rossi's book, Psychobiology of Gene Expression over night. Contrary to his understanding, based on profound facts of current neuroscience, Rossi (2002) has this to say – "Our genes are not buried in our biology, remote from our daily consciousness and concerns" and dismisses the concept of "genetic determinism" as a myth. He also observes "that our life experiences, thoughts, emotions and behaviour irrespective of whether they are minute to minute or hourly, can modulate gene expression and neurogenesis in ways that change the physical structure and development of the brain." And he agreed that the truth is "...Neither gene nor environment dominates development: rather there is a continual interaction between genes and environment." (Rossi 2000) This indeed was a giant step forward in putting the body-mind affinity in the right perspective to the client and strengthened the rapport by the most recent advances in functional genomics.

Apart from he being a precious person, this convinced us about his motivation and we decided to do therapy.

Following his conviction that genes do get activated as well as suppressed, and, the royal road to do so through hypnosis, he was given four sessions on alternate days. They were recorded. In the salubrious, spiritual retreat of an Ashram, surrounded by empathetic experts in psychotherapy who combined behaviour and occupational therapy with *yoga,* he gave up and rejuvenated to contribute creatively.

The first session was hypnoanalytic: he was before a dimly lighted, though magnificent mansion. He enters, rather hesitantly, but finds a cordial welcome. After demurring a while in the drawing room, where it seems that a cocktail party is going on, he avoids people and decides to go past a corridor. This leads to a series of rooms. He unlatches them one by one.

After opening the first room, he finds it totally dark. But there is a switch just next to door and he is able to find a button that switches on the light...the light has made...the gene has been turned on...and the light has made room bright. He is able to see clearly.

And, in the room there is a tall and vide cupboard with the labels on the drawers. He reads the label, one by one...June – 4, c-phos...and what are these names...he wonders and there is a ...faint recollection...At one late night, he has met those blinking masters...that generate creativity in all...minds, though they may have been dumb some times...

And, each of the drawers has files that are familiar and forgotten to him...or are empty...he likes to browse and keeps doing so, room after room after room...he comes across pictures...of a heart bleeding...but the blood has frozen...and heart is pumping... heart is pumping normally.

When he returns, the cocktails are over...the people have been leaving now...one by one by one... he has no need to talk to them...he is tired... he is tired and happy to see a bleeding heart, that has stopped... he is tired and lies down on a sofa and goes to sleep...to wake up in the morning with heart full of happiness... heart full of happiness...he does not understand... heart full of happiness...but he is happy...seems to have made some mathematics of invention.

He was given other sessions on similar lines. At the *Ashram,* he was given behaviour and occupational therapy. He practiced *yoga* regularly. He continued with *Yoga nidra* as per the recorded sessions. On a follow up after two years, he was at his normal best. He was engaged in organizing and teaching activities. This was possible mainly because of high motivation, cognitive restructuring through hypnotherapy, *yoga* and caring support from the inmates of *Ashram.*

Vertigo and Tinnitus

These conditions occur due to disturbances at eighth cranial nerve. The nerve is enclosed in a closed space. We believe that stress mediators, for some indeterminate reasons, hit the nerve and it swells because of nonspecific inflammation causing symptoms. As such the conditions are difficult to treat and, a thorough medical check up should rule out any other organic cause.

- ***Illustrative Strategy***

A Christian divorced (when asked why, she answered, it was heaven that united us and heaven that decided to do us part) lady of 35 years, is a lecturer in psychology; having twins; both boys, extremely difficult to manage, stays with the mother, and has vertigo.

Quick induction...Deeper and deeper breath...Intelligent ladies are intelligent girls ...experience trance quick and fast...and you know that...you have taught that. And, intelligent mothers even better...trance in seconds. Therapist does athetoid movements of the hand, forearm, arm and shoulder, of the subject, telling Grandpa is holding hand of grand child.

As you are relaxing... you are relaxing...your hand is becoming relaxed...lighter and lighter. Lighter than air...It is wanting to float in the air (may need support of a finger of a therapist for hand levitation) and... is gradually going up and up... is gradually going up and up... (Up till it is at the level of shoulder). It is as light as feather...and it stays there, without any hurt...As you take deep breath in...and...out you are going deeper and still deeper...in the trance. Continue to enjoy this trance. (Elicit ideomotor signaling).

You have achieved so much at such a young age...and you have so much more to achieve...that is your natural due...We are now moving to reach a newer goal. (Elicit ideomotor signaling). Transformation has started... Great... Great transformation has started... for a radical therapeutic change...from good to better...to best... that is your natural due...from best to be a doctor of philosophy... that is your natural due...(Elicit ideomotor signaling).

Three ferries are coming...they are descending in sparkling white clothes... Three ferries are coming... They have blue wonderful eyes, innocent features, tremendous lot of wisdom...they are making their presence felt... Enjoy the presence. Enjoy their company.

(Elicit ideomotor signaling for moving further)

Gifted soul... and, dutiful, caring... and, loving mother. You are taking your sons ... You are taking your sons on a giant wheel...you are going on a giant wheel...It starts slowly...and, it starts moving... little faster... and...faster. Moving and progressive...further ahead, progress...as it goes forward, progress...as it goes forward, backwards, sideways, left and right, right and left... give support to your boys...and take ...support... progress...as it goes forward... given and taken (confusion technique) ... take deep breath, deep, deep breath progress...as it goes forward ... swallow the saliva ... or wet the lips ... as they are dry (parasympathetic over take). You are going...and as you are going about...forward, backward, upward, downward journey...is going in a circle (Elicit ideomotor signaling) you are going round and round... you are going round and round...in an orbit. It is a close circuit...you are going round and round. As you go in a circle, you feel giddy...and, there is vertigo (Elicit ideomotor signaling). As it moves... it moves... it is so uncomfortable...to bear this vertigo.

Writing finger moves and moves (Elicit ideomotor signaling). Writing finger moves on and on...it has written—neither all thy tears nor your request can erase...the writing finger of the father in heaven (subject coughs)... Wet the lips and swallow the saliva...With the wet mop we erase...wet the lips and we can erase...Feel at ease... feel at ease...with vertigo, let it increase in its intensity... and suddenly the wheel stops...wheel has stopped and, all that has begun is... destined to stop...

Why are we trying... are we trying... to erase that which Lord has written... we are trying... Messiah has written as ... we are trying... as Messiah has written...Having reached the height of intense vertigo...... we are trying... Messiah has written to stop it...as you cry out why. Why me...writing finger has written and, that I can read for you-vision is clear for me...so also for you. It is clear, bolder and bolder... (Catharsis occurs). Wipe out. Some of the dirt on the canvas is wiped out...Tears have wonderful ability to clear the site. Now perception is so wonderfully clear.

Good Riddance of Bad Rubbish! You Have Wiped It All Out! Throw it Away!

As vertigo... goes round and round and round...with centripetal force, rubbish is getting dissipated. Wipe your tears, relax yourself...in Merry-go-round. With vertigo motion you perceptually realize the concept also perceptually arrive at the concept that you have dissipated the dust by centripetal force. Dirt is getting off and off.

Good Riddance of Bad Rubbish

Paranoia, compulsive traits, obsessive compulsions, please, leave...please...do carry away the rubbish. Leave it, in the past, past, past bygone. It is gone... As soon as the merry go round is about to halt, waste disposal also has occurred... the wheel has stopped... Merry go round has stopped...you are slowly coming down, and also coming to halt. Heavens or genes bring it to halt...And, you have support of both...and you are getting down with your sons....

You have planted a flowering plant. Yes it has started flowering,. You are a flowering plant, blossoming...two lovely fruits on bloom are seen. Nature has fulfilled its purpose... you have done your its work.

You have a mission in life...Mission has already found the fulfillment. There is complete waste disposal by centripetal force (Elicit ideomotor signaling). Get down from the merry go round...for sure... Get down.

Age progression. Looking forward to good job profile, good environment to stay, Pure, innocent, hyperactive twins hugging, caressing. There is a royal road waiting for Dr, Rajkumari to trade on it...Process of excellence is awaiting you.

Stress Causing Myofascial Pain Syndrome[8]

Introduction: An extensive review of over 120 related references make the imprecise understanding of this condition more evident. Regardless, the effectiveness of hypnotherapy merits its discussion here.

Myofascial Pain Syndrome (MPS) is a frequent cause of acute and chronic pain in any muscle location of the body. An acute myofascial pain syndrome of one muscle arises from trigger-point (TP) activity in the muscle and/or its associated fascia due to stress that localizes at the site of mechanical overload. When overlooked or inadequately treated, acute single-muscle syndromes can become chronic multiple-muscle syndromes. More than half of the patients admitted to chronic pain programmes in two recent studies were found to be suffering primarily from myofascial pain syndromes due to tender points[9,10] in the muscles.

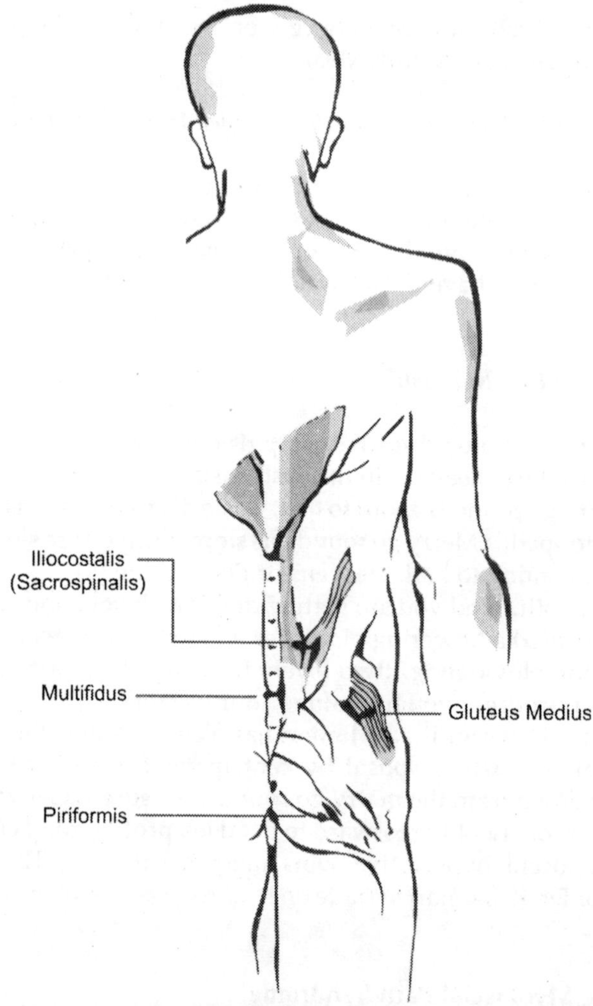

Fig. 21.1: Trigger Points in Myofascial Pain Syndrome. Patients with MPD have tenderness within the affected muscle and soft tissue. Trigger Points are shown in the muscles that are most commonly affected.

Pathophysiology of Pain in MPS

In stressful situations → Anxiety → Tension → Activation of Stressor systems → Secretion of Adrenalin and Noradrenalin→ Vasospasm→ Anoxia → Muscle spasm→ MPS → Mind body therapy.

Muscle spasm under stressful situation is likely to have an autoimmune component due to development of auto-antibodies[11] to muscle/fascia.

- ***Strategies***

There is generally a passing reference of mind body therapies[12,13,14,15,16,17,18,19] in most literatures. A personal illustration by Dr. Mukesh Trivedi:

I was suffering from recurrent pain on left side of upper back for last 4 years. Initially I got my cervical spine x ray done which showed some osteophytes with early and mild osteoarthritis changes and also C6-7 mild disc changes. I was diagnosed as having trapezitis, cervical spondylitis and "rheumatic myositis"[20] by the orthopedic surgeons and neurophysicians. I took symptomatic treatment and underwent physiotherapy together with ultrasound heat treatment and TNS (transcutaneous nerve stimulation). I recovered completely but problem resurfaced after 2 months. I again repeated same treatment and continued muscle strengthening exercises. Due to recurrent left side trapezitis, the orthopedic surgeons advised inactivation of myofascial trigger point by local injection of xylocaine with steroid. This was repeated after four weeks. Recurrence continued. I joined Diploma course in Clinical and Applied Hypnosis at M. S. University, Vadodara and came in contact with hypnotherapy.

On following hypnotherapy sessions, during recurrent MPS attacks, in which various pain relieving imageries were suggested and suggestions were given to take various responsibilities in life in true spirit also. It was also suggested that responsibilities are those which I want to take therefore I should take them as challenges and not as burden on my back. These suggestions gave me an understanding of my problems and I developed an insight that MPS attacks followed a set pattern of some situations causing distress. On insight generation, I learnt to convert distress into eustress. This effected a change in my thinking, feeling and behaviour.

DISORDERS OF AUTONOMIC NERVOUS SYSTEM

Allergies, asthma, hyperhydrosis etc.

Name: Vigneshwari Presenting Symptom: "chronic nasal allergy" with discharge.

A lady of 24 years, with history of "chronic nasal allergy" with discharge, nasal hypersensitivity, irritation inside the mucous membrane of the nose, discharge of mucus since 10 years. This occurs once a year at a stretch for 2-3 months. Then, it lasts for 2 to 3 hours every day in the morning. It aggravates by sneezing. There is remission automatically. She cannot find the irritant. She had Yoga therapy for 2 years. Past history: At age of 11 years she was in Mewas (Name of the town), it was a messy place. At 13-22years, she was in Gurgaon which she described as highly polluted. She was at the moment studying Yoga Therapy for 2 years at an Ashram.

Diagnosis: Allergic rhinitis; autonomic system imbalance; Immune system malfunction, possibly due to a deep trigger of some traumatic experience in the past.

Strategy: Insight generation. Therapeutic touch, discourse with genes, arousal of early activated genes. Uncritical acceptance of insight, in a heightened state of suggestibility with Yogic currency was the strategy for the treatment. Subject does not know the reason but insight generation will occur. No need to disclose the reason and if asked, therapist also forgot the reason, if he ever knew. Something gone out from your system is gone out for good. It is good riddance of bad rubbish.

- ***First Session***

Aim: Learn *Yoga Nidra* or Self-Hypnosis.

Yes, very nice, take deep breath in and out, wonderful. As you are taking the breath, you move and wriggle out your toes and throw away all the tension. Start relaxation. Progressive muscular relaxation is applied. (Confirmation with ideomotor signal)… These waves of relaxation go inside the abdomen…it is a Pandora's box…that keeps all our secrets… all the organs, all the system like GI system, liver, spleen, kidneys, reproductive system all get that fresh… oxygenated energized blood…And, as your chest relaxes, you are listening to your own heart beats, breathing…and my voice… Progressive muscular relaxation is further applied. (Confirmation with ideomotor signal)… let it move towards the neck…. Its goes on to your face and your brain "I am feeling relaxed, happy, and tranquil all over myself, very, very peaceful, quietly enjoying this state…And, as you feel relaxed, happy, and tranquil in your brain…the brain knows what is inside the Pandora's box….

In this state of being, cool, comfortable, quiet and peaceful, yes, I want you to move forward in this state of relaxation. I will go out from this room of ashram to the comfort place of your choice…you are going there…I am there and, it is spring, just before summer. The first ray of light, I am able to see and, so do you see. The darkness is being penetrated by the sun rays from the east where sun is gradually rising from the horizon…. The darkness has completely disappeared with the rising sun… rising from the horizon…. There is bright, refreshing environment full of mild fragrance of flowers…There are big trees and small bushes all around in the garden. You like this fragrance and its coolness dries your nose… its coolness dries your nose from inside…

The birds have woken up and are chirping and are making beautiful, pleasant music…we are enjoying this nice music of singing of the birds, nice cool and pleasant breeze. You are telling yourself now… You are telling yourself now… pleasant breeze is going all along inside myself, and as it touches my face, yes, it is making me very happy…as it goes inside my nose…drying… yes, it is making me very happy… It gives me pleasant feeling as well as smoothening all over myself. It makes me quiet, cool, comfortable, quite tension free. I am experiencing the tranquility and also very, very relaxed...

Please continue for a while to enjoy this state of being – as you are in the state of your choice at your own comfort place. There, that red, bright sun in the round, red ball shape... gradually is moving up and up...You are seeing and...I am very, very happy. I am very, very happy that you get that energy; ...I am very, very happy...through red rising sun...as I am watching it. It gradually comes up as bright red, a complete circular ball. I am listening to many birds waking up and chirping – making nice music, I am listening...musical sounds which fill up my heart with joy. Cool air is all the time flowing...drying my nose. drying my nose... The touch of that cool air is making me very, very happy. ...everything is fine and a fine fragrance comes with that flow of wind...I am smelling the fragrance of my choice and it fills me all over...I am smelling the fragrance of my choice and it fills me all over... I am seeing, visualizing, smelling, and enjoying each and everything... that is around me...that I hear the smell...the sound of this smell is drying my nose... Sun has come up and changed colours...

I turn my head and see a temple... and see a temple... The entrance to the temple is very nice, decorated with fragrant flowers. As the sun has come up, I experience the sunrise. I decide to enter the temple... decorated with fragrant flowers...a magnificent big temple. This temple has a deity. I like to pray to the deity. It is my duty to pray everyday.

The morning aarti has begun. I join in the aarti...go near the bell...look up...move the body around...I start ringing the bell. And my choice ...I start ringing the bell... the voice that comes out of ringing bell, is my voice...I join in the aarti... I am in front of the deity. The deity moves forward... The deity moves forward... gives blessings to me standing in front of me. I am fully – yes – I am truly blessed by this deity everyday.

I am with this deity...today is the new experience. I am being blessed, I am truly blessed...I continue to ring the bell, continue the experience of these blessings. I feel very, very fortunate, privileged and happy. I continue to ring the bell and feel this presence, I want to fill up this experience in myself, in my heart, in my mind; it lasts for ever... I want to fill up this experience in myself, in my nose... as I continue to do this, I am fully satisfied...

Aarti is over. The birds have started flying in the air leaving their nests. The sun is shinning bright now. I feel light all over, all around, the surrounding makes me feel very nice. All my worries, all my tensions are gone.

- ***Second Session***

Aim: Cure from nasal allergy

Quick induction followed by...I am a free bird without any load on me. I am enjoying this flight fully convinced about capabilities of myself. I can do what I decide to do... I feel light all over, all around, the surrounding makes me feel very nice...I am flying in the sky and I come across Dr. Vyas...he is happy to be flying with me, and as I am flying higher and higher I realize that I am made of exceptional stuff. I am so unique and specific and singular, that the nature – the mother-nature has crafted me, sculpted me, designed me to excel in my own unique way...that I have a dry nose is so simple... in whatever that I wish and undertake to do and... I have a dry nose is so simple...I shall undertake only such things...the mess from my nose is gone... shall undertake only such things...that are noble, unique, magnificent, wonderful and excellent;...be it the routine Sunday jobs: cleaning my house, washing my clothes or excelling in the spiritual heights...of this ashram...climbing Mt. Everest... excelling in the spiritual heights...I am made to excel in my own way and if excellence is that, which alone is – I am excellent, I am magnificent, and I am wonderful.

As I am flying higher and higher...it has started raining...I am wet all over...dripping... dripping...all clean... I am wet all over...dripping... dripping...all clean...all the dirt is washed away... all the dirt is washed away...in this very pleasing drizzle...of cleansing rain... I am nice and clean...

My nice and clean... name – yes, my name is excellence incarnated and in excelling myself in my own way. I have no hesitations, no reservations. My name is Vighneshwari...excellence itself, that excellence which is signified and symbolized Jasmine form of Saraswati – Vighneshwari (goddess who removes obstacles) – Vighneshwari – Vijaya Lakshmi – Maha Saraswati – Maha Durga (other ladies at the workshop have undergone spontaneous trance)...that is so Komal (soft, smooth), so Komal as Kavitha and Kavitha and Komal and Kavitha. Whatever way in realizing the submergence of the Jasmine fragrance of Vighneshwari... excellence in myself, I supremely sublimate to greater heights of being a human being and in realizing the potential of flying high. I have incorporated within my flying self the flying spirit of high riding Subhramanyam...the adventurous deity...who can slain any evil...mess from nose is gone...I am so capable as Kartikeya he goes round whole world like the bright shining sun, I also can go around the world, the universe. Totally convinced that masculinity is the valor and vigor of Kartikeya who excels in ardent pursuit of adventure and in so doing create many fold forms that is fine and beautiful.

Acute on Chronic Stress

Several medical conditions, as we have seen earlier (Chapter 11), have their origin in stress and symptoms manifest when allostatic stress load gets decompensated; homeostatic hormonal balance is disturbed and stress mediators produce non specific changes that resemble inflammation in mesenchymal tissues.

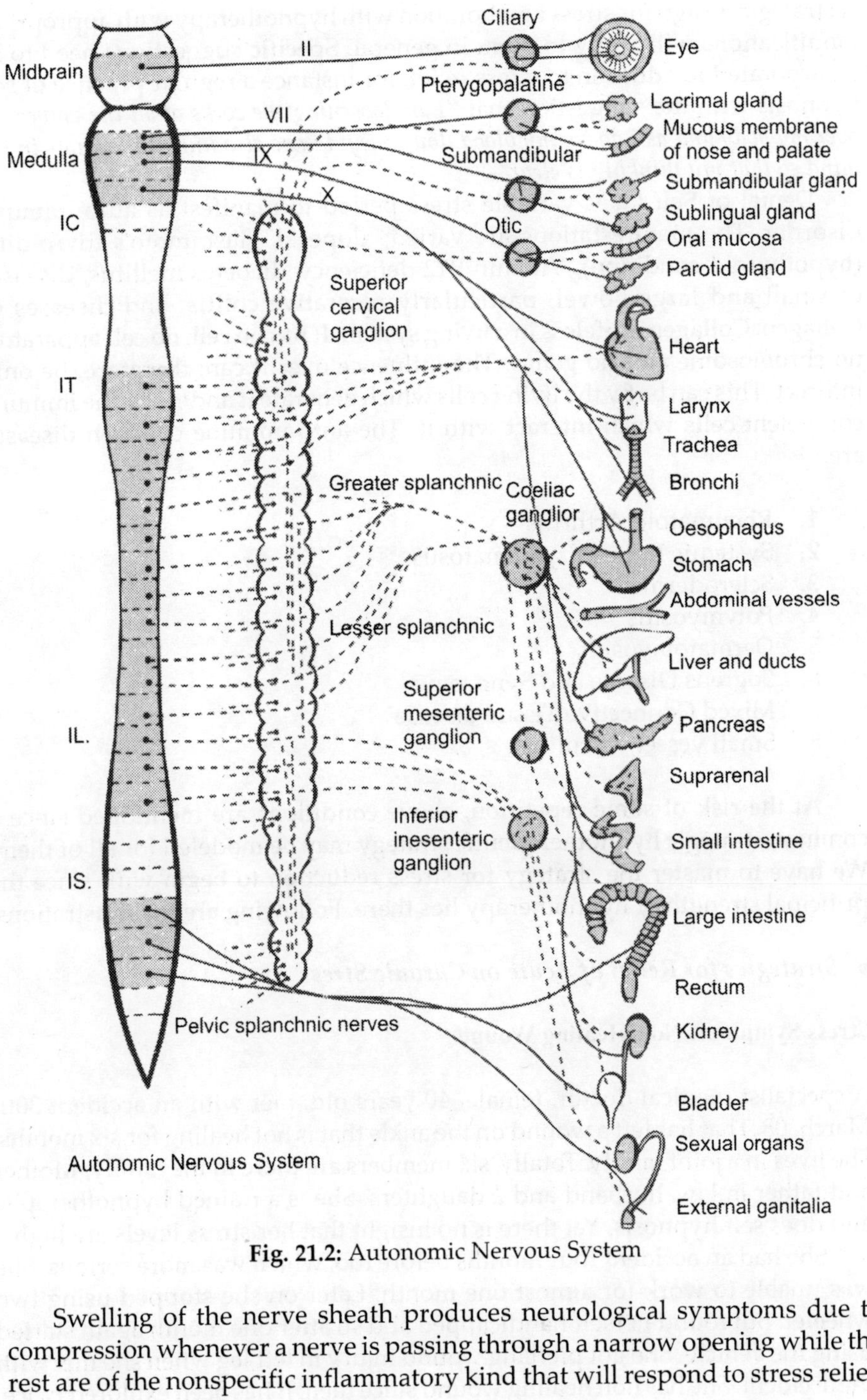

Fig. 21.2: Autonomic Nervous System

Swelling of the nerve sheath produces neurological symptoms due to compression whenever a nerve is passing through a narrow opening while the rest are of the nonspecific inflammatory kind that will respond to stress relief.

A strategic design for stress amelioration with hypnotherapy with appropriate modifications will apply to them in general. Specific suggestions need to be incorporated in addition to stress relief; for instance a regular practice of self hypnosis with the suggestion that *"I am loosening the corks of all the valves, all over my body and as I do so, my blood flows easy: I have also untied the knots in my mind so that my thinking is clear"*.

Denial of Self takes variable stress period to manifest as auto immune disorder. The manifestations are varied; alopecia, Hashimoto's thyroiditis (hypothyroid condition), Vitamin B12 deficiency, diabetes mellitus, diseases of small and large bowel, particularly ulcerative colitis, and diseases of Collagen. Collagen is lifeless in a living system. It has no cell, no cell apparatus, no chromosome and no genes. The influence over it can, therefore, be only indirect. This can be by the living cells which generate it and/or by the immune competent cells which interact with it. The auto immune collagen diseases are:

1. Rheumatoid Arthritis
2. Systemic Lupus Erythematosus
3. Scleroderma
4. Polymyositis
5. Dermatomyositis
6. Sogrens Disease and Syndrome
7. Mixed Connective Tissue disease
8. Small vessel vasculitis

At the risk of some repetition, above conditions are mentioned since a common strategic hypnotherapeutic strategy may be modeled for all of them. We have to master the strategy for stress reduction to begin with since the principal strength of hypnotherapy lies there. Following are the illustrations:

- ***Strategies for Relief of Acute on Chronic Stress***

Stress Symptom: Non-Healing Wound

A specialist medical doctor, female, 40 years old, met with an accident 30th March, 08. That has left a wound on the ankle that is not healing for six months. She lives in a joint family. Totally, six members are there in the family; Mother and father in law, husband and 2 daughters. She is a trained hypnotherapist and does self hypnosis. Yet there is no insight that her stress levels are high.

She had an accident four months before too, which was more serious. She was unable to work for almost one month. Later on she stopped using two wheeler. But found herself handicapped and so after one month again started using the vehicle. She got piercing wound injury in left leg when she met with the accident. She has non healing wound since then. It has been explored twice.

- ***First Session***

Strategy applied: Indirect Hypnosis.

What is your stress? Is it work burden, or family burden or...you are a liberated woman? Recognize the stress.

Are you obsessed to excel? Let us count how many jobs can you do? Let us count how many jobs can you do, to be a professor, doing hypnosis, computer science, Okay. Is looking after the family, house and studies of children some work? You feel guilty as you think you are not able to attend the children. Have you compared yourself with most mothers in the neighbourhood? How many hands do they have?. In this *Navaratri* festival, see how many hands Durga has...and you are having as many hands as Durga ...eight...twelve... sixteen to do...to be a professor, doing hypnosis, computer science... The subject, hypnoidal now, cries and, says even then, she is not a happy bunny...my husband says he can manage the house with his income...She says she cannot remain idle. With double income there is buttress to the family. The comfort level is very high.

Now, quick induction is done.

The session follows as:

As you understand the mind body connection so well, and know it so well, just apply to yourself. Do you think Princess Diana died of an accident? It was her stressful situation which killed her. What you need is the insight generation. It is hypnotherapist heal thyself. For you it is easy: It is like converting the converted.

S, you know how to relax and so let go yourself. I say with honesty and candidness S, you know so much, that you take a deep breath, deeper and still deeper breath... deeper and still deeper breath...you go into deep trance, you go into deep trance. As you are experiencing this deep, profound and peace in this quick relaxation, your whole body relaxes, quickly entirely... S, you know so much... As you have so easily and totally relaxed yourself all the muscles of your body is totally relaxed...and entered into a deep trance...

Your eyelids have closed and eyelids are together. They are shut and stuck together so that howsoever you might try to open them you are unable to open them... As you try to open them... As you try to open them...they are so heavy as if lead sheets are put on the eyes...eyelids are lead sheets...that they are stuck together. So let them remain closed and enjoy this great relaxation...Simple ways are easily known to you and by your own effort and deftness, you are very well relaxed. (Show me by your chosen ideomotor signal).

S. in deep trance

Little girl S, 20 years back, though such a playful, fragrant flowery child, how dependable, how very, very vulnerable, S is. But through the protection, care and the caring of family, littlè girl with fragrance is growing. She is 5-6-7-8 years old girl. Child with fragrance and fragrance of innocence and she grows in pristine innocence of childhood and all this is around you... and all this is around you...

As you feel and... and, all this is around you ... and all this fragrance is around you...tell me fragrance is around you...(ideomotor signal is positive.)...This is great creative power, ability of your pristine innocence. As little S is growing up... As little S is growing up... what all S has acquired by now!!!

She is a lady, a devoted wife, a daughter in law, a doting mother, professionally a professor, and highly respectable doctor. S wonders as to what all has happened to her. So many people have been left behind who were her colleagues. She is running fast, very fast, still faster. She is running very, very fast... She is running very, very fast ... She is running very, very fast. She wonders that she is running without feet. She is running with her hands. She can run faster... run faster... run faster but now she is breathless...she wants to rest... Suddenly, she presses a button with her running hand... and a flood gate of light opens and gate of wisdom opens up with the gentle application of her fingers. S has pressed the switch here and there, touched a lever hidden here and there.

S is aware of so much of light...her own intuitive wisdom...so much power in her so many hands...that they can run...and, when deft and wise...turn on the light...

Barely had you time to observe yourself this way. Hardly ever you have cared that way....S, this is your natural self, happy by your self, peaceful, confident, radiant and eager to learn anything that is new...After learning to implement and practice in all possible way.

To be aware of your potential is your natural due. So much of work you can do in such a short time. You are capable of throwing out all the noxious substances from your system, is an easy affair, wipe out all the dust that is accumulated on your mirror... (ideomotor signal)... Now S, this clean, spotless mirror, reflects radiant, beautiful, clever, capable, and confidant S. You will reach your destination in no time. You are doing wonderfully well.

You are being looked after by an eminent therapist...as well as a professor plastic surgeon, who cares for you; as you are an esteemed colleague... who is expert in the city. ...Now with the enhanced ability of your self, you visualize your radiant capable self healing this wound. ...You are pouring all the energy, antibodies, every thing that is needed to bring about the healing is being poured into it. Then the healing has to be a natural and a simple affair, a child's play.

Let me tell you that you are very intelligent and clever student. And you are going to pass your examination with brilliant colours. Last one year of our interaction, the courage, the multifaceted personality, the well chiseled presentations and clear perception will make you go through the examination with flying colours.

- ***Second Session***

Quick induction, suggestions given once trance established.

You have set the goal and you need to gather up, cool the system and just get composed and have one pointed focalization. The road is clear without any traffic jam. Just move forward with full confidence. You have more than achieved your goal. If you want to have something more…then move your right index finger and if you want to move forward slowly… then move your left hand index finger….either way you are to win….to excel in the examination…

It is your natural due to excel; it is my privilege to show you the way and also the technique.

You are moving forward and as you are progressing forward, you see floods of light from all the direction. For a fraction of a second you are dazzled…as all the beams of light are focalized on you. You are standing in the centre of the gate with the best of your dress. It is pink or orange or violet or yellow!!! But the little girl S is wearing her choicest dress (ideomotor signal).

All the beam of light is flooding the stage as it is focused on the centre of the stage. S wants to dance all round on this large and vast stage all across the stage…she is dancing. As she is taking the steps with her feet forward and backwards, the hands automatically give various actions with the face changing expressions. She is extremely in cheerful mood with happiness and joy.

As she moves her hand, she is playing with her toys, she is learning to cook, has passed her SSC exam, and further study. Little girl S with 2 hands have now 2+2 hands. As S clears with brilliant marks, she sees herself with 2+2+2 hands. She can read, write, ride bicycle, and learn mathematics, biology by dissecting frog. She knows the secret of life. She has become a medical student. She has now known all the secret of human body and she has 2 more hands.

As the time is progressing she knows more and more, deeper and deeper of the skin. She becomes absolutely well worth with the knowledge of the skin. She is a specialist. She has 2 more hands. S can work with 10 more hands with her will and at her will. Now she is a specialist. S knows all the treatment for the skin conditions including injury to the skin. She is producing all the substances that are required to heal her wound and be again normal as herself. S is opening huge compartments, various drawers, healing substances are flowing and she is healing from the bottom of the wound…she is seeing, visualizing and experiencing the wound being filled from the bottom and gradually the wound is filling up with healthy tissue. With 12 pairs of hands she is Durga. S is utilizing in doing cooking, pressing various keys of computer, being a teacher, is treating the patients and writing prescriptions, driving the car, caring for family and children and such so many activities. S is counting how many hands she has! And how many activities she is capable of doing…

And how many activities she is capable of doing… She is counting 1-2-3-4-5— —12 pairs of hands. These are her most favourite hands.

While S is in a state of dream, or sleep or awake she is enjoying the state of creativity. S is visualizing herself as a creative force…behind the family as well as herself. With such potential self expansion there is self extension also…Let there be self expansion this is your real self, indeed your real self. It is a real, capable, creative consultant self in its full dimension…. S is experiencing full power in her entire self, able, creative and in full control of her self.

S will listen to this cassette in the morning or late in the evening, or before going to bed…

S this is my gift to you to be your creative self. When you will close your eyes at will, when you will take two deep breaths, you will appreciate 32 hands at your command performing various activities of your choice without any compulsion from anywhere. You will handle all these hands with full control and further create all that you wish to do in your creative enfoldment of your personality…Inspire total confidence in your creative abilities, we have established communion in consciousness and with furthest exposure of your creative self…you are amply rewarded.

Little accident and subsequent discomfort will further take you to realize the blessing in disguise. You will recover fully in the shortest possible time. You will start using all your hands in the creative creations of what you are capable…you are to create.

Strategies for Autonomic Nervous System Disorders

- ***Bronchial Asthma***

The sessions are designed as per above lines: there is allergy that is triggered by the hidden factor of fear: that is removed by constant ego strengthening during the session. If trauma is suspected, it is glossed over. The system cools down at a comfort chamber. The black board is wiped clean. You are drawing nice paintings on a clean canvas. Repeat the sessions. Give a cue that when the subject apprehends an impending attack, he will at once take a few deep breaths; hold the index and ring finger of the left hand that will at once transport him to his comfort place. Incorporate daily practice of *anuloma-viloma pranayama.* If the attacks persist, use exploratory strategies for triggers in the unconscious.

- ***Irritable Bowel Syndrome***

Point to the stress and autonomic imbalance by the metaphor: when it rains, river swells. It then flows fast. When the river flows fast, there is turbulence: but, river does slow down… river does slow down…when the rain stops… river does slow down…by diverting its waters elsewhere, even when it may be raining heavily…and, when the floods are known… river does slow down...the people build dams... river does slow down...and the waters in the dam are useful... the waters in the dam are useful... river does slow down... when the rain stops...the floods subside...that is how there is a balance in Nature...you will cope with your stress...just the way that Nature adjusts its balance.

- ***Chronic Stress Leading to Coronary Heart Disease***

In case of blockage in the blood vessels, in most of the cases either angioplasty or bypass surgery is recommended. Although it is not a final solution, since in many cases grafts have shown blockage again. A few conservative physicians do suggest an alternative that involves life style change. This requires a change in the personality that can be difficult. The steps are:

- Well considered decision by the patient: choice is entirely left to him. No covert or overt leading to conservative modality; on the other, impress that surgery is safe now a days.
- Reinforce with insight generation.
- Reduction of acute stress by any of the strategies described above including a vacation at home.
- Further insight generation to identify stressors and mechanisms to cope with them; modification and elimination. Hypnotherapy initially for stress alleviation and later on, regularly the form of Yognidra helps to transform the life style.
- Evaluate the behaviour change, cardiac condition and general health.
- Monitor maintenance.

This is narrated by a beneficiary since 10 + years.

I am Mahendra S. Bhavsar, Consulting Engineer, Vadodara.

I am delighted to share my own experience of managing coronary heart disease without surgery that was judiciously recommended. In last week of October 1997, in the evening of a day after moving around in Universal studio of famous Disneyland-USA I found difficulty in walking and was compelled to take rest till the pain in chest subsidized. I was then of 58 years, working as a professor in Faculty of Technology & Engineering of M.S. University of Vadodara.

I immediately decided to return home from U.S.A. in November 1997. I met an eminent cardiologist in Vadodara. I had to undergo stress test and angiography. The result showed 90 per cent blockage in two arteries. I was advised bypass surgery. It was a panic for family members to hear about bypass surgery. We met our family friend Dr. Vyas for his guidance. Dr. Vyas opined, "As per cardiologist's advice for bypass surgery is alright." I was mortally scared and he pacified by saying that there are alternatives. He asked "In Vadodara city if we want to go from Mandvi to Railway Station, and two main roads are blocked can we reach from Mandvi to Railway Station?" Dr Vyas said "The same corollary works for heart too. Blood will find its paths to flow. But we have to explore and may be, create new roads." We were further advised (1) to consult another eminent cardiologist. And, if he agrees for conservatism, follow Dean Ornish's universal healing programme along with medicines (2) to undergo a few sessions of hypnotherapy (3) to meet Director of Yogniketan to learn about meditation and *yoga*.

At second consultation, it was opined that there was a choice for alternative conservative treatment. I studied books on coronary heart disease and decided to follow the universal healing programme in addition to medicines. In second phase of treatment I joined Yogniketan and learnt meditation and *yogasanas*. I started walking in the morning, although I could not walk for more than ten minutes. Dr. Kiran Shinglot at Yogniketan guided me to yoga-nidra and yogic exercises. I gradually increased time for morning walk.

After almost 10 years, of my undergoing angiography in December 26 1997, at present I keep my visit my doctors regularly as per their advice. My daily morning schedule is as below.

I wake up early in the morning at about 4.00 a.m. I take one-hour walk and then attend from 6:00 a.m. to 6:20 a.m. 'Arti' of Lord Shiva a temple. At 6-30 a.m. I reach Yogniketan by car. From 6:30 to 7:30 a.m. I perform alone in small room, chanting of omkar, anulom vilom, pranayama and meditation. From 7:30 a.m. to 8:30 a.m. I practice various yogasanas and shavasan. I daily climb two floors of about 14 feet height each by staircase. This has made me to live altogether new life. My body and mind remain tension free, delighted and full of energy for whole day. Occasional tension is released by fasting.

My bypass surgery has been by passed and I am living a very healthy life with strong and excellent heart.

Stress Manifesting as Anxiety Neurosis[21]

–and other psychosomatic diseases

The following hypnotherapeutic techniques can be utilized in the management of anxiety and psychosomatic disorders:

1. Introduction and removal of misconception
2. Autogenic training
3. Hypnotic phenomena
   Hypnotic analgesia and anesthesia
   Temperature alteration
   Amnesia
   Catalepsy
   Ideomotor and ideosensory activities
   Dissociation
   Time distortion

Automatic writing
Relaxation
Age regression
Age progression
7. Hypnoanalysis
8. Hypnodrama and role reversal
9. Paintings
10. Paradoxical interventions
11. Cognitive behavioural approaches

Obesity[22]

It is quite a formidable task to maintain weight loss in obese patients. It is very frustrating for them to see their efforts being undone and not uncommon for the obese client to give up after repeated failures. Recurrent weight loss and gain can be much more stressful than just remaining obese.

A wide variety of treatments are available to lose weight. Unfortunately the long-term results are not promising. "Most obese patients will not remain in treatment. Of those who do remain in treatment, most will not lose significant poundage, and those of whom do lose weight will regain it promptly. In a careful follow-up study, only 8 per cent of obese patients seen in a nutrition clinic actually maintained a satisfactory weight loss." (*Cornell Conference on Therapy*, 1958, p. 87.)

Success has been claimed for "diet clinic" type approaches (Franklin and Rynearson, 1960), Fasting has been found to be quite dramatic for weight loss (Bortz, 1969, Stokes, 1969), but the patients regain weight rapidly after leaving the hospital (MacCuish *et al.*, 1970). Positive results were obtained by hypnosis (Erickson, 1960; Hanley, 1967; Kroger, 1970; Stanton, 1975). Positive results have also been reported for behaviour therapy techniques like token replacement (Bernard, 1968), aversion therapy (Meyer and Crisp, 1964) and covert sensitization (Cautela, 1967). Using behaviour approaches, Stuart (1970) had evidence to suggest the usefulness of a threefold treatment plan: (1) environmental control of overeating (2) nutritional planning and (3) regulated increase in energy expenditure.

We utilize the following methods of autogenic training and hypnotherapy to treat patients with obesity, morbid obesity and bulimia nervosa. All patients were referred by their family physicians, and remained under their supervision for physical problems such as blood pressure coronary insufficiency, diabetes, arthritis, etc.

- ***Procedure***

Each client is treated individually for half-hour sessions at least once a week and/or in cases of morbid obesity and bulimia nervosa, twice a week. We plan to follow the patients for at least two years. The sessions are recorded on cassettes and clients are encouraged to listen to the tape at least once daily.

Treating distortion of body image and reinforcement of body boundaries: during the hypnotherapy sessions the clients are asked to wear an abdominal belt with multiple notches, adjustable elastic bands on legs, thighs, hips, abdomen, scapular regions, arms, shoulders and under the chin. In female clients, care was taken to avoid the breasts when applying bands over the chest. The clients were asked to wear the belt and the elastic bands when listening to the tapes at home.

The following suggestions were given to the patients, modified according to the individual's specific problems.

"You remain quite comfortable and deeply relaxed while I am giving these suggestions to you. Allow your subconscious mind to listen to my suggestions. Do not analyze me and do not analyze your own thinking. You have no need to eat excessively. Your will be sensible about your eating habits. You can eat whatever you want but eat less. Everything that you eat, you will have good control of it. Remember, eat but eat less. You will be quite satisfied by eating a lesser amount of food. Gradually, you will start liking the lower calorie foods more and more. You are going to develop a complete aversion to high calorie foods. Even the smell of fried foods will start to bother you. You will be quite uncomfortable in the presence of fried foods. The taste in your mouth is already slightly changing. The thought of food is bringing an unpleasant taste in your mouth. Your mouth tastes like jungle mouth. You are losing your appetite. You are getting the kind of feeling that you have after a fever or after vomiting.

"Now you visualize eating. I would not be surprised if your mouth feels numb; your jaw gets a little stiff as you keep eating. Your mouth is getting still drier. You are becoming more uncomfortable about eating. You can continue to eat but you do not want to. You are feeling some discomfort in your tummy. You wish you could stop eating, which you certainly can and feel good about it.

"Now I would like you to visualize a clock. The hands on the clock are showing a particular time of the night when you eat excessively. I would like you to imagine that this particular time is passing comfortably and you are quite at ease without becoming anxious about eating. The social hours of eating like breakfast time, Lunch and supper and night snacks do not have any appeal to you. Any time you eat impulsively, you will feel sick in your stomach. You will lose all appetite when you prepare foods, at parties and social gatherings.

Any discomfort or noises in your abdomen is not a signal for you to eat. Remember, you can eat but you do not want to eat. If you do happen to eat you will eat less than you have done before. If by mistake you happen to eat more than you really need, then this food will not get absorbed in your system. You may have a loose motion later on. Once again, you will feel quite uncomfortable all over your body. Gradually, you are becoming more and more competent to control your eating without becoming anxious.

"I would like you to regard non-eating as a reward and eating as a self-punishment. If you do happen to eat excessively you will get no relief from anxiety. I do not want you to feel sorry about it as this will lead to guilt and may provoke further over-eating."

The above suggestions help patients to desensitize their desire to eat, to eat in less quantity and to develop aversion of eating during the day as well as during the night.

Body image alteration: "You are getting slimmer every day. All those people who are significant to you praise you for becoming slimmer. You feel much more accepted by your friends, as you are getting slimmer. You are proud of being able to control your body size and weight. You have started to like yourself a little more every day.

"Now, I would like you to visualize yourself wearing clothes that are one size smaller and you are comfortable within them. You notice that your body size becomes a little slimmer; you need to adjust your belt. You can tighten it one more notch and still remain comfortable. You can feel that belt around your tummy. The elastic bands on different parts of your body are making you feel that your body is shrinking in all chose places. Your body is shrinking under your chin, across your shoulders, under the arms, over your back, your tummy, the sides of your trunk, hips, thighs and legs. Every time you breathe out, you notice that your skin separates from your clothes. You get a feeling that your trunk is shrinking. You will be able to adjust the notice that your body is shrinking over your fingers. The rings have to be readjusted. The wristwatch band can be tightened a little more. Your shoes, panties, bra—they all need a little readjustment as your body continues to shrink.

"Now, I would like you to visualize that you are walking around. You feel lighter as you have lost some weight. You can move faster. There is a spring in your walk. You enjoy this excess of energy and you are able to pass between two objects easily without unduly squeezing yourself. You move in between people, taking lesser space. You particularly notice that your body is shrinking when you get in and out of your car. The distance between the steering wheel and your body is increasing. You notice pleasantly that you can now cross your legs, which you could hardly do before. You will notice that your body is shrinking, when you rub your body. You will find that you take less space when you sit on a chair. You will pleasantly notice that you can bend easily. Look into the mirror—you are getting slimmer indeed.

"You own this body. In a way, you are remolding it. You are being reborn. You will accept your new image without any difficulty. You will love yourself to be a slimmer person. Every day of your life you will accept yourself getting slimmer and slimmer. If you happen, by mistake, to start slipping, within five pounds of any increasing weight you will notice that you have become quite uncomfortable. You will feel sick. Your tummy will appear too full, bloated and uncomfortable. You will have a strong need to control your eating behaviour."

Group psychotherapy for morbid obesity: (Patients who need to lose more than 100 pounds of body weight): The groups are held once a week for two hours. Various psychotherapeutic approaches have been introduced in these groups. The psychodrama approach, frequently used with bulimic patients, is also utilized with the group of morbidly obese patients.

In summary: Emphasis is to control the body weight by correcting eating habits and the body image through various modalities of hypnotherapy and autogenic training.

Total Allergy Syndrome[23]

This newly described condition in which the patient claims to be hypersensitive to his or her environment, particularly to synthetic materials, is also known as twentieth century disease. Mild cases are characterized by a variety of psychological and physical symptoms such as depression, fatigue, irritability, poor concentration, migraine headaches, respiratory problems and various bowel symptoms such as vomiting, constipation, diarrhea and abdominal pain.

In severe cases the patient feels incapable of living in the modern world and finds he or she has life-threatening reactions to many substances including clothing, furniture, construction materials, food, water and even the air (Stewart and Ruskin, 1985). This cluster of symptoms is seen among a major group of psychiatric disorders viz. schizophrenia, atypical psychosis, depression, panic disorder, hypochondriasis and personality disorders; even anorexia nervosa may be a suspected diagnosis.

Case presentation: L, a 70-year old retired nurse, presented with symptoms of anorexia, weight loss, migraine headaches, heartburn and constipation. She was a chronic complainer. She had tried almost every kind of diet and was fond of vitamins, minerals and amino acids.

The diagnosis of "total allergy syndrome" was made and she under went extensive investigations and treatment programmes in the United States, spending a horrendous amount of money. She tried chelating, hyperbaric oxygen and SEDAC. She was proud to show forty pages typed in booklet describing her investigations and treatments. By this stage she had lost 37-40 pounds, her total weight being 80 pounds. Her symptoms continued to deteriorate; therefore, as a last resort, she was referred for hypnotherapy. On examination she showed no preoccupation with body weight but was aware of her thinness and wanted to gain weight.

L, was a good hypnotic subject and responded well to post-hypnotic suggestion to control the activity of the gastrointestinal tract. She learned to increase her awareness in smelling her food and to salivate. By utilizing the imagery of a waterfall she could swallow food without getting any cramps in the abdomen. By breathing out from an imaginary hole in the epigastrium she obtained some relief from stomach distention and cramps. She also found this technique useful in regulating bowel movements.

To control preoccupation with food allergies she listened to audio cassettes, prepared by her therapists, prior to every meal. The suggestions given on the cassettes were that her body would treat her food in a friendly manner and thus she would have no adverse reaction to the food she ate. Occasionally, she did develop a few red spots in her skin as a reaction but these disappeared within an hour or so.

Now L was not afraid of candida anymore. She was able to eat almost every kind of food to which she had allegedly been allergic. She gained 37 pounds in 47 days. L decompensated a couple of times under family stress, especially having to cope with her alcoholic husband. Once again she contacted a physician to investigate for other abnormalities. With great dissatisfaction she returned to the author in order to cope with anxieties relating to her health.

For the past three years L has maintained her body weight and her "Twentieth Century Disease", or "Total allergy syndrome", has disappeared.

Hypnotherapy for Dermatological Disorders[24,25]

The course of some dermatological disorders can be modified favourably through hypnotherapy. Almost all modern textbooks on hypnosis cover dermatological disorders. The brain and skin have common ectodermic origin and, since emotions can alter the functions and even the structure of the skin, stress and repressed material in the unconscious mind can be manipulated deftly by hypnosis to produce spectacular results.

Skin is the boundary that separates the organism from its environment. Some of the important functions of the skin are protection, perception, and heat regulation of the body. Skin and the nervous system both develop from the ectoderm. It is feasible that both organs can influence each other. As a child develops, the skin plays a significant role in molding his/her personality.

The skin normally responds to emotions to produce homeostasis between the body and the environment. Pathological changes can also be produced in the skin in response to stress and repressed emotions. Literature and our everyday language have many words and phrases that indicate a close relationship between the skin and the emotions—e.g. thick skinned, thin skinned, touchy, be in touch, warm, cold, contact, red with anger, pale with fear, hair stood on end, scratching their heads, got under their skin, jumped out of their skins, pins and needles, numb. Hypnotherapeutic techniques can modify certain dermatological disorders by reducing stress and resolving repressed emotional conflicts. Thus, psychotherapeutic maneuvers are more successful in those dermatological disorders where emotions have played a greater etiological role. The patient can modify his/her emotional responses by cognitive restructuring. It is not known with certainty why the skin is the target organ for stress in some people.

In a typical session, the patient is informed about hypnosis. The patient's questions are answered and any obvious misconceptions regarding hypnosis are removed. The patient is reassured that, with some practice, s/he is likely to achieve greater success.

Ego-strengthening suggestions are given; hypnosis is induced. The patient is then taught as many hypnotic phenomena as possible, e.g. glove anesthesia and increasing the temperature of the fingertips. At times a thermal biofeedback machine is attached so that the patient can see that the temperature in his/her fingertips is indeed increasing. The patient is also taught autogenic training exercises such as cooling of the forehead.

The patient is then asked to de-hypnotize him/herself gradually and at the end of the session is asked to report on any feelings regarding the session, or ask any questions.

The sessions are recorded. The patient is expected to practice the recorded hypnotic session at home frequently until s/he he a mastered the techniques. More sessions are recorded in follow-up, as required.

At times, when the patient shows resistance, more explorative work is done through age regression, dream work, and by giving explanations to various drawings that the patient may have made. As the patient's condition improves, the follow-up intervals are increased.

Subsequent progress is monitored by the patients themselves, who keep the therapists informed by writing letters or by telephone.

- ***Case 1: Hyperhydrosis***

Mrs. M, a 20-year old women, gradually started sweating profusely from her armpits. She tried various remedies without success. Dermatological examinations were all negative. She learned to relax and used cooling imagery with limited success. As the symptoms worsened, age regression was explored.

She was a shy, submissive woman who was experiencing conflict with her husband. She remembered an incident when her husband. She remembered an incident when her husband told her that other women probably had firmer breasts. Mrs. M said that she felt quite threatened. She used to have firmer breasts before the birth of her child. When her husband approached her for sexual intimacy, she became very nervous and started to sweat, with most of the sweat coming from her armpits.

She also noticed that she did not like him touching her breasts at all. Her husband became quite frustrated. Gradually, the sweating would come at any time when her husband was close to her body. Her sweating was not only profuse, but also had quite a repellant smell.

Mrs. M abreacted and expressed her insecurities and inabilities to assert herself with her husband. After the session, it was easy to counsel the couple. They gained insight. Her husband started treating her with a little more respect, and Mrs. M did not feel so insecure in speaking of her feelings to her husband. Mrs. M soon learned self-hypnosis. She was able to relax during love-making and was able to use cooling imagery to cool her armpits. The symptoms subsided in one month. Two-year follow-up revealed no recurrence of hyperhydrosis.

- ***Case 2: Alopecia Areata***

Ms. V, a 20-year old university student, developed bald patches on her scalp over six months; she was referred from the department of dermatology as she was not responding to traditional methods of treatment.

Imagery suggestions for increased scalp circulation and hair growth did not bring about improvement in two months. Age regression was then explored. Ms. V revealed that she started losing her hair six months after the death of her father. She was supposed to be the strength of the family. She did not cry nor show any sadness at the time of his funeral. It was explained to her that she was going through a period of prolonged mourning, and also that hair has a special significance in mourning in certain Eastern cultures. After the death of a father usually the eldest son, who conducts the funeral, has his head shaved. To abandon one's hair is also regarded as a self-imposed restriction on sexual desires so that people may achieve more spiritual enlightenment. Some remove their hair so that they can sublimate their sexual energy for higher purposes in life.

During the hypnosis sessions Ms. V was able to experience the sadness she had felt at the time of her father's death. She accepted that it was quite alright to cry at the funeral and that crying is not a sign of weakness on her part.

She learned self-hypnosis and gradually started increasing her scalp circulation by imagining her head under a heat lamp. She also imagined that the hair was growing like little seedlings.

In three months' time, her bald patches were covered. Subsequent follow-up for one year revealed no recurrence of alopecia.

- ***Case 3: Blushing***

A 28-year old lawyer, Ms. J, was prevented from appearing in court because of her problems with blushing. She could only work in the office. After two years of struggling, she decided to try hypnotherapy. Some mechanisms behind blushing were explained and she appeared to have some insight. She tried to displace the blushing to other parts of the body, when it might suddenly appear on her face when she was presenting in court.

Ms. J was then asked to imagine hot tea in her mouth and after a little practice she was able to increase the temperature in her mouth. She gained confidence in this method and interpretations were given that she was allowed to blush in court, but as she is only blushing in the doper tissues of the face and in her mouth, no one can see it; she did not have to worry about the blushing suddenly appearing on her skin. As the blushing was transferred it was easier for her to keep her attention not only on her ongoing court work but on her blushing as well without any disruptions.

Three months later Ms J was able to work in court. She did not blush even when she had to differ from the opposition lawyer. She became more assertive and her blushing disappeared.

- ***Case 4: Eczema***

Mrs. W, aged 35 years, came for depression. She explained that her depression was due to her severe eczema on her hands. The itching was intense, so severe that it let to bleeding.

She had had eczema for 15 years. She was quite frustrated with traditional therapies as they gave her only temporary relief. She was quite willing to try hypnotherapy, as she believed that the mind can control the body.

At first, she tried cooling images. She imagined she was blowing air out from the skin on her hands and this air was very cold, so that the skin felt numb. The itching gradually lessened but the bleeding continued. She utilized her own imagination and went under the skin to turn the blood vessels off, just like she would turn a water tap off in her garden. She was quite amused by this imagery. The bleeding stopped in one month and a three-year follow-up showed no recurrence of either eczema or depression.

- ***Case 5: Hair Growth***

Mr. H, a 25-year old homosexual hairdresser, wanted to grow more hair on his chest. Dermatological examinations were negative. He was able to use imagery for warming the skin on the upper part of his chest. He also used images of normal hair growing like seedlings. In six months' time he had satisfactory hair growth on the upper part of his chest. Three years later he was maintaining the hair growth.

- ***Case 6: Hair Removal***

Ms. K, a 28-year old fashion model, was quite frustrated with excess hair growth around her nipples she bleached them with hydrogen peroxide. Whereas she was allowing her facial hair to be removed with electrolysis, she did not approve the same procedure for her breasts.

Ms. K. was able to cool her breasts by imagining that there was a big ice cube over her nipples. She was also able to produce hypnoanalgesia at the hair roots. It was interesting to note that as she gradually twisted the hair, instead of feeling pain she felt ticklish, and the hair would come out without any discomfort. There was hardly any bleeding and there was not much inflammatory reaction after the hair removal. She would remove one or two hairs at each session.

18-month follow-up did not reveal any hair growth over her breasts.

- ***Case 7: Trichotillomania***

Ms. H, a 22-year old opera singer, had been pulling hair from her vertex for the last six years. Direct symptom removal by relaxation, making the hair roots too sensitive, and weakening of the hands during hair pulling was of limited success.

After a year, age regression was explored. She revealed that six years ago, while she was traveling with three men in a truck, they had raped her. She could not escape. She heard them laughing and making fun of her. At that time, she happened to pull her hair. She felt somewhat better, as she hurt herself by doing so. From that time onwards, she started to pull her hair whenever she experienced emotional difficulties or inability to express her anger. Gradually, she started to pull her hair even when she faced everyday problems. She also started pulling her hair when experiencing anticipatory anxiety, such as before she had to appear to sing opera. She was able to accept interpretations and gained more insight into her hair pulling. She was able to transfer her desire to pull her hair, into just caressing it. She had much more success in six months' time and is still being seen at three month intervals. There has been no recurrence of Trichotillomania.

- ***Case 8: Pruritis***

Mrs. C, 50 years old, was diagnosed as a terminal case of biliary cirrhosis. She was deeply jaundiced. She had intense itching all over her body. The itching was more marked on all pressure areas. She could not wear a bra or any tight clothing. The itching was unbearable at night. Traditional therapies did not give any relief from the itching.

Mrs. CK was a good subject for hypnosis. She learned cooling imagery. She also learned to spread the intense itching from pressure areas to other parts of her body and thus the itching became less intense. It is interesting to note that she learned most of the techniques in only two sessions. She continued to control the itching for the remaining six months of her life.

- ***Case 9: Herpes Ophthalmicus***

Ms. B, 55 years old, had suffered from a severe post-herpetic neuralgia for the past three years. She was affected on the right side of her forehead. When all traditional therapies failed to help her, she thought of trying hypnosis. Within two months she was able to transfer hypnoanalgesia from her hand to her head. Whenever she had severe pain, she would modify her perception of that pain by imagining that the pain was spreading from her forehead to other parts of the head and was gradually becoming diluted. Once she gained confidence that she could lessen the intensity of her pain, she was not so afraid of trying hypnotherapeutic methods. She was able to sleep by putting her head on the pillow. She could even go out for a walk facing the cold wind and was able to comb her hair without pain.

At six month follow-up, she was found to have good control of her pain. Her life was much more pleasant and she did not feel that she was being punished for some sins that she may have committed in the past.

The psychopathology of dermatological disorders is uncertain. Entire range of pathogenesis—from allergic response to auto immune is on display over a vast surface. Perhaps equally puzzling is the cure by hypnosis. Hypnosis is not only an adjunct to other traditional therapies, but at times is the only treatment which is effective.

Hypnotherapy for Autoimmune Disorders

The concepts are elucidated in detail earlier. Just to recapitulate: A prolonged duration of stress over a number of years finally manifests as auto immune disease. The concepts are fast changing: hormonal disorders like diabetes mellitus and hypothyroidism are also now being understood as auto immune. There is probably a chain extending from alopecia to calcaneal spur that encompass mesenchymal tissues and endothelial cells (thyroid and stomach – vitamin B 12 deficiency) to produce various auto immune diseases that are the symptoms of a stressed psyche. Cancer has been for long labeled as failure of immune system. We give few details of successful outcome in a patient, S., having rheumatoid disease that has already progressed to generalized peripheral vasculitis. Presenting symptom was localized gangrene resulting into a non healing ulcer for 5 years.

- ***Short History of S, the Beautiful***

S, the beautiful, a lady, 45 years old (2006), was very sweet and chubby child. She was very active, fast in learning skills, i.e. early milestones in development, like turnover, crawling, stand and walk, speak and forming sentences.

Stress during childhood: Mother had been to Bombay for work and child S, the beautiful was at Bangalore with her Aunt. She felt sick, had fever and constipation. Constipation was cleared with frequent glycerin enema. During this stress she missed the mother most.

As a school going kid she was okay. But showed nervousness syndrome at the time of examinations like fever or stomach upset. She will recover through half the examination.

After her college and before her marriage she was subjected to the biggest stress in her life. One of the lady relative gossiped with mother that S, the beautiful has been molested; hence she is not getting married. This caused enough commotion and naturally she was at the receiving end. Things were resolved. S, the beautiful came out clear. She felt: she was to be absolutely divine!

After S, the beautiful's marriage (1981), mother passed away due to cancer breast (1984). It was a rude shock. The shock was deep and personal loss. She started the symptoms of rheumatoid arthritis at young age of 22 years (1984). When she came for treatment, she had rheumatoid deformity of hands and feet. She had an ulcer on her feet of size of 8 in. by 4 in. since 5 years. From the size of a cm, it had grown to the present size. Rheumatologist has diagnosed it as gangrenous condition associated with rheumatoid disease. It was skin grafted 3 times at Bangalore under proper antibiotic cover as well as immune suppression. Homeopathy was also tried. The ulcer was slowly increasing in size. The cardiologist and rheumatologist further diagnosed that her rheumatoid disease has advanced to general vasculitis all over the body.

She disclosed to the lady cardiologist that her favourite god is Siva, with flowing hair and she dreams of Ganga emanating from there.

Totally 14 sessions were given over a period of hospitalization for a month. Some of them are given below. She listens to recorded cassettes even after being well for four years.

- ***Session 1***

S, the beautiful: Rapport building

Come on this chair and ... the next step in the session is to make as little noise as possible...we want to be quiet and at peace... now lie down. Draw the curtain please, let the room be dimly lighted...and yet, there is enough light...and yet, there is enough light...uncross your legs ...let go...and you have started relaxing your self. Uncross various zigzags... it is very nice to let go zigzags and go straight...and you have known what it is to meditate, so is to relax.... Yesterday I worked with you even for a short while, I work with you in the shortest possible time to let your self go and relax. Yesterday it was so kind of you... it was so kind of you...that even though we had yet to make better friends...from good friends, and I ask your permission to let me touch you on your hand, on your face and on your forehead... we have made better friends...without any reserve, you permitted me to do so as, your brother M. is an affectionate brother you permitted me to do so as...so am I...to have this privilege of having one more sister.

Method of induction: Deep breathing and leisurely Progressive Muscular Relaxation.

So wonderfully relax... wonderfully relaxed, and with this relaxation to have started feeling the deep sense of ease, comfort and peace... feeling the deep sense of ease, comfort and peace.

Deepening and ideomotor signaling.

There is perception of mild fragrance all around you, when you feel that ease, comfort and peace, then your right index finger which is your yes finger and with increasing sense of serenity...serenity is increasing as you take breath in and breath out ...serenity is increasing as you take deep breath in and breath out...perfect peace grows all over and a sublime serenity is experienced...In this experience your right index finger is your Yes finger. If there is carefully, most certainly, increasing comfort all over in your mind a while... could you tell me yes by moving your right index finger, deep breath, deeper and deeper and as I touch... as I touch... how well you are relaxed.

Hand Levitation

(While supporting the left hand)

...the left hand goes up... as I touch... in the air up to the level of ear...How perfectly, yes, as I let go...your left hand... yes, as I let go your left hand, it just falls like a feather, (hand falls) wonderful... if there is something that is holding back your comfort and, of course you can move and say yes, by moving your right index finger, our first premise is that is my duty and my privilege to make you comfortable all the time. And that I promise...to happen right now... at this stage of your therapy...and subsequently, we shall invoke all those potential forces..., potential positive forces, so that by the time the session is in further progress...as the session progresses further and further...you will be increasingly more comfortable and, as you listen to my voice, every word that is heard, your comfort level goes up-up and further up...so much so that all other sounds are gradually fading away...You are now listening only to my voice, and to the breathing and beating of your heart...and, every spoken word increases the comfort level, so much so that, your eyes are comfortably closed now, and...your eyelids have dropped softly, gently, yet certainly, so that they are very, very heavy. And as you try to open your eyes, you even relax more. The entire face relaxes, let go, let go Yes... very – very nice, you have let gone the last beat of residual tension... and your eyelids are so certainly closed and when you try to open them, you are unable to open your eyelids...Try to open your eyes and as you find that they are so very, very heavy, like lifting such a heavy weight and...you are unable to open them.

Method of induction: Deep breathing and leisurely Progressive Muscular Relaxation

Deepening and ideomotor signaling

There is perception of mild fragrance.

That's fine work S, the beautiful, that's wonderful, you have now mastered...what it is to let go...between both better and the best friends...I want to ask you, S, the beautiful, are you prepared to do more work now...is there still something holding your comfort back.... Oh, you said No, nothing is holding you to do further work... Yes, very good, very good S, the beautiful, you understood my mind...so very much that she knows her right hand is the yes hand... and with several moments of relaxation, the left index finger which to my mind was No left hand, she has said that nothing is holding S, the beautiful. Now from enjoying the comfort in the peace of present moment as you have started talking to me, very clearly and loudly through the voice of silence...I understand your silence of speech S, the beautiful, (paradoxical suggestion). Would you now like to tell me, do you know what was holding back your comfort?

Further Exploration: Deepening: Arousal of Early Activated Genes.

You may or you may not, and if you may have known, it is gone, and if you may not have known, then also it is gone... (Reassurance) Do you know S, the beautiful, what was holding back your comfort and, remember...you will tell me only that much as you wish to tell... you will tell yourself only that much as you wish to tell... I certainly grant you, a private corner, (winning the confidence of the subject)...some where inside your inner mind...which is entirely yours. So even if you now know what was holding back your comfort.... You don't have to have any concern that you will be required to tell me. Deep breath, deeper and deeper still, so much at peace, so much at comfort, that in this moment of applying supreme silence a fine fragrance is permeating all around you, and in this room, as you wonder whether it is jasmine, or lavender, or sandalwood or it is one of the most favourite perfume that you like to have some time ago. It is all around you and when that is all around you, the index finger moves, let the fragrance permeate all around you, it is in you, in your mind, in each and every cell your body. And once it has done so, move your yes finger, let me know. Having done so much of useful work and in such a record short time, I am indeed very proud of S, the beautiful, as in short time of few minutes you have pervaded the entire atmosphere with your high spirit.

Application of imagery and archetypal symbols; incorporation of physiology.

I like that smile of yours, and finely refined perfume, this finely refined perfume is emanating from somewhere higher up where you have seen the visions of flowing Ganga...(visual imagery) and in that shape of *Jata* (long finely tied hair of Siva) and *Trishul*, (The symbol of Siva's armor and ammunition)...Ganga is flowing down... in your blood stream, down in the highest center of your brain, and also down to, what we recall the most controlling part of the brain that is hypothalamus. This is really the fountain head of all the streams of Ganga...It flows and as it flows, it regulates lower down your anterior pituitary. The anterior pituitary has flooded the entire system.... Its uniform flow of Ganga, whom you have experienced as a flowing, cleansing, healing mother... I think it is wonderful for me to have young friend Arunesh (a plastic surgeon), and your dear elder brother M., who have witnessed...such a stupendous phenomena of communion in consciousness, as M. is putting his hand on your forehead...there they see, feel and experience gigantic turbulent flow of Ganga, its coolness, freshness and its healing power. You are healing...you are healed...We ourselves are so much healed and feel so much light by communion in consciousness with you... We are very – very proud and privileged of such a kind soul, and as S, the beautiful is there to decorate, and S, the beautiful has given all such S, the beautiful fragrance. This fine fragrance stays with you all day.

Utilization in Therapy

You will repeat this experience after few hours, when Arunesh and I will be dressing your wound. We would like to see the turbulent water of healing Ganga, going all across your body, and as you now have a final look at your left leg, and the ulcer you see, you have known so very well, and there is no strain to recognize it because that S, the beautiful herself, when S, the beautiful knows S, the beautiful as a real beautiful self, real S, the beautiful herself is healing her ulcer herself.

Post Hypnotic Suggestion

What is best for you and your system now, you have done some hard solid work. If you like to keep on doing it even more, your choice and let me know, by moving your yes finger and since it is your natural due, I think, you are doing so wonderfully well, in your quiet solitude in this prefect peace, even my voice withdraws. You are face to face with real S, the beautiful, with your true self, it returns to you after such a long, long time of many, many years. Welcome, real S, the beautiful, back to yourself. She is S, the beautiful and S, the beautiful is she, not only they are best friends, they are none other than one... you will continue to rejoice this restoration of identity being such time that you think is your appropriate choice. And when you wake up all by your self, room will be filled with the same fragrance...that is all around you. It is to remain with you for the whole day... It is to remain with you for the whole day... It is to remain with you for the whole day and the joy...joy...joy of finding Real S, the beautiful will abound all over.

- *Session 3*

Exploration: Erasing the past memory by age regression, confusion technique

Put yourself in trance...Moment you start experiencing trance, S, the beautiful, we had a very pleasant sense of smell in the previous session remember, yeah, so what was the smell, would you tell me? (Does not move any finger) It is fine; you won't disturb your trance. It is definitely a pleasant scent, something that you like, ok, so as you put yourself to a state of complete relaxation deep, deep within...voice is soothing and healing around as you go, and you are putting your self to a deep trance. A sense of peace, harmony, and gratuitous grace is felt all over yourself. When you experience, that your self is calm, cool and composed, tell your right index finger to move...Your eyelids are heavy and S, the beautiful, how difficult it is to open them... so let us do the thing in easy and immaculate way. To practice serenity, sublime spirituality and you feel you are yourself in the refined aromatics...smell as you perceive the refined aromatics...smell and as if it has filled the whole room.

Now I want to share with you some of the secrets of hypnotherapy in which you are already initiated. You have advanced so very much, in such a short time. Would you like to know them? You only have to say yes by moving your yes finger and I will reveal some of the finest facts of working of your inner most self, yes... we can go fast forwards...same way we can go fast backwards...(age regression is done, at every step, the flow of Ganga is cleaning.)

That is...is my friend, between friends, we share our secret. You know that you have traveled far and wide...and had a bath in the holy waters of Ganga at several ghats...going down...coming up...Not only we understand others, we understand ourselves. S, the beautiful has been a wonderful person.

She has almost always. She has almost always done the right things in right way and at the right time. When I say almost always, she likes to be self sufficient, she likes to help people, and she has for sure consideration for people whom she likes. She has brought a beautiful boy in this world, who is now handsome, able, and so confident with himself, and of many a splendor. S, the beautiful as you look yourself...flowing with Ganga...on the quiet run... that you are once again there in 1976 and as you run a rapidly forward recorded cassette. How many good things you have done to so many people, so many friends near and dear ones. I really have run the cassette fast forward now, so that as you see all those good, kind, charitable acts, your heart fills with joy.

All right S, the beautiful, yes, why should I ever tell you something which may not be right, I know yourself as much as I know the palm of my hand. S, the beautiful did all and almost all things right. S, the beautiful, only to my friend, I would want to tell at a point, one per cent of an error that S, the beautiful made. I would want to tell you that if you are not hurt...I will tell you, should I tell? OK, yes, you know that I will be not only the last person to hurt you, here I am trying to warn you of all kinds of harmful effects. Be prepared to listen a bit of yes, I am kind of wavering. I don't want to hurt you at all, S, the beautiful wants to know where did she, if ever did she went wrong. I see it very clearly as a day light when S, the beautiful went wrong. A small error, should I tell you right now, deep, deep breath, as I admire your trust and confidence in me S, the beautiful, has gone back in 1976 again we are running the cassette fast forward and we are pushing it forward and back ward and forward, and back ward and as this cassette is now undulating...time is undulating... there is a flash as you see, and to make an error as you see before your eyes...undulations of forward and back ward in time.

And you see at erroneous happening, and as you see at erroneous happening, your right index finger moves, deep breath, deeper and deeper to and fro, forwards and back wards 1976, 77, 80, 82, 85, fast back wards 80, 79, 76, 75, 74, 60, 64, 70, 73, 76, 79, ...I give remote monitor in your left hand and you are either moving fast forward or fast back ward and keep seeing whole panorama of time as you arrive, yes, you are nearly there...and when you know that you are there your right index finger moves...

Would you want to know or rather not to know, could you rather not want to know, what went wrong and just correct it...as I know how to. I want S, the beautiful to progress further today, so that we come to the correction mode before surgery. S, the beautiful and I have a big stake and a responsibility. Shall we just correct it? As I see it clearly, I want S, the beautiful to tell me, and tell me yes, and when you tell me yes than only I shall correct it.

Thank you, let's not bother, let us not wonder if you know it you know it, and if you do not know than you do not know, then also I know it and having known I am now telling you very easy straight and swift...as I am correcting it, it was a case of mistaken identity...S, the beautiful, what ever that happened, lost attachment, rooted ness, belongingness to her own self that was totally false, now correction....

S, the beautiful has come to realize that S, the beautiful has a real self, and S, the beautiful has totally effaced that erroneous identity.

Strategic suggestions for pre-operative preparation and acceptance of skin graft

S, the beautiful is at peace with her self. All over the body, there is S, the beautiful here...and this S, the beautiful is going to transfer beauty on her left leg and ankle, the ankle, what a beautiful ringing of the bell as that is being transferred, we got beautiful bells and very beautiful sound acknowledging the total correction. S, the beautiful has corrected, cleaned the dust of her house, cleaned out all the room cupboards...way back from afternoon and now it is evening. She is face to face, real beautiful S, the beautiful, herself, which is her true identity and on Thursday morning about 10' O'clock S, the beautiful will be in the process of this bell ringing and transferring... some S, the beautiful... to some part to other, with open arms, yes, you will tell yourself... you are my real self for me, S, the beautiful, and yourself that is being transferred. And we, that is me, S, the beautiful and S., shall stay together forever...So wonderful to work with you S, the beautiful, and following your quantum jump, following your various cleansing, finally your self-identity is restoring...restored.

- ***Session 4***

After induction...Congratulations, I am indeed pleased to see those sloping blue edges on your wound there, which is a clear scientific evidence that you have not only not given up but you have conquered thus... we shall over come,

You have stopped fighting with your self... You have stopped fighting with your self and, in that M. wants to add couple of affectionate, brotherly requests, and understand that M's request is a command that is to be followed, M., please give your command to S, the beautiful. What a wonderful job of conquering unconscious mind that shall enter in the new mind, but conscious and all those unconscious...whom we have not known... you are over coming all these difficulties.

This makes me very proud of you as I would be of my sister, and as a fantastic human being. Congratulations. You can do wonders with your life, at the forbearance of your love, affection to all. Congratulations again, on going to the past with your life, a sweet family, you, your husband, a beautiful intelligent son of yours, all others that your seniors in your family, sister in law, brother in law, father in law, it is the time to rejoice. That time for rejoicing should be almost eternal, forward to those peaceful moments.... Unpleasant moment is no more existent. You are going to a beautiful garden, fine fragrance, love, joy, and contentment, peace of everybody's mind in the family and in the surroundings.

Congratulations S, the beautiful, congratulations...you are wonderfully well, Keep up this flight, you see that you have won...comfortable margin, all the flags, high, tall furling, through your restfulness...

- ***Session 5***

Quick Induction: archetypal symbol utilization: post operative

Still people call it Ganga, can you just see the flow of Ganga, ...deep breath...as different Ganga has started flowing, is the same Ganga in Ganga that you experienced yesterday, and if it is the same, it is easy for you to let go all the tension and put yourself into a deep, deep trance. As my hand is touching your ear like a brother, to a naughty sister, come S, the beautiful, very good girl and the affection, the warm regard, the respect, responsibility and caring, all had carried you now, to a deep, very deep, relaxation...trance.

Peace, joy, confidence (2) as S, the beautiful has done it before and S, the beautiful shall ever be able to do, is to experience, a sublime experience of spirituality as I take your right arm, yes, she is so sure, that even before I ask S, the beautiful, she tell me yes, (3), I can do it, I am doing it and I will be doing it... wonderful work which generates tranquility, utter spirituality...is the generic ground of all healing, work, peace from silently to rapid mode, and as you listen to this voice of silence, S, the beautiful, ...silence is a clear certain voice... is the voice of silence...S, the beautiful is experiencing nice perfume... As the perfume spreads into your entire being, entire room here...All over the hospital...entire city of Baroda, to every where perfume is going deeper and deeper into every where, and...into every cell of your body.

...This is the healing perfume, and in the flow of this healing perfume yes, thank you... thank you very much...no need to make make any effort. Things happen by themselves, this is your natural due, what a perfectly gentle soul...time is helpful to everyone... everyone...needs time... after a long, prolonged fight and struggle...not willing to give up. Stunningly, distinctly pristine, pure quality, pure quality personality and so much rooted ness to the strength... and in your rooted ness in the tradition, I would wish that S, the beautiful is face to face, to sublimely superior qualities as a human being.

Would you care, would you like to see face to face, S, the beautiful, your inner strength, sterling pure consciousness...you don't have to hurry up at all, tell S, the beautiful, you say 'yes' even before I ask, so nice of you... take your time to think over, to undergo the experience of a transformation...you have done excellent work and you are doing...You are now mentally, physically, emotionally, intelligently and spiritually experiencing a transformation and that is your natural due as my hand rests on your forehead and as some of your inner psychic being is activated right before your eyes you see a hazy mist, as you focus, you see a deem light that is mixed and as you see that light, your right index finger moves, take your own time focus your eyes and see a deem light, going brighter beat, by beat, brighter and, how profound is the vision.

Visualization of a slowly increasing light somewhere through the mist, we are struck with wonder and awe. Deep...kind of wonderful experience in this hall... there is no fear, there is no flight, and there is no hesitation. In this wonderful experience you are perfectly all right... even forget your yes and no, no and yes, (Confusion technique). It hardly matters now, as you see this increasing light, light of, yes, you have experience the flowing of the energy of the glowing light which is like a sun and as you swallowed a little saliva, it is the energy...of this wonderful source of light which probably is a rising sun or may be, may be more than one sun, like the energy of thousand suns. S, the beautiful has a wonderful sun; this sun is like a thousand suns, regulating so much of light and energy all over your body. This is energy of your psychic being, a mind that is so pure and intelligent and achiever.

We are experiencing brilliance and luminousness of a thousand suns. In those thousand suns, there are regulation, the light energies into focalize being of light, stay behind there, my finger is on your forehead is a part of brain. It receives all this kinds of energies and in brain as you look a little backward under a surface as a focal point of a gland call pituitary gland, are you aware of the pituitary gland S, the beautiful? That gland is the focal point of receiving, transforming all such energy and remitting them all over to the body and whenever and whatever are the needs of the body is even appropriately and accordingly...your pituitary gland has received this energy of a thousand suns, brilliance and luminary...and the pituitary is now responding to the command of spreading waters of Ganga.... all the mist has cleared up now, clear and absolutely distinct before your eyes, you are seeing spreading water of Ganga as that Ganga is flowing down a Jata and by the side of *Jata* is now a *Trishul* and your mind is overflowing with joy...

Do you want to seek further blessing? It is for S, the beautiful to choose, and S, the beautiful says that I am so transformed that I see depth of most wonderful trance experience. I have attended, chosen a transformation in healing myself and having chosen so I have no more to choose.

Then the waters of...Ganga has now come to the plains in all over...even more, spreading slow,.(3) spreading slowly all over the plain. And it would be pleasant and refreshing to have a bath in these refreshing, pleasantly cool waters of Ganga. There is M. to help you with his hand and... support with the other hand that into... clean waters of Ganga... put your right foot in, now you are putting left foot in, how pleasantly and gently. Sit down being your beautiful self, immerge in the cool, refreshing pleasant waters of Ganga. This is ever changing and yet it is the same Ganga which flows down in your anterior pituitary all over the body, we call it the same Ganga, so our friend, the philosopher has made us understand that ever changing, some moment to moment difference, from ever flowing Ganga...and in this changing the form of, from moment to moment you experience.

You say to yourself...I see a ...strange looking stranger, in front of you... in the form... becomes clearer. This is an image of some one I have seen so often almost every day and yet I thought that it looks like a stranger. I didn't really understand this is so familiar so much of my kith and kin, or it is S, the beautiful her self, 'yes' such transformation, and yet so easy and so real... You have seen your own inner strength, which is to achieve a transformation as your left hand now goes to fore head, is the silent flow of Ganga flowing and her transformation is reached. You have seen your face, S, the beautiful is herself, and S, the beautiful is face to face with her self. S, the beautiful is having S, the beautiful as her real self I have at long last, found my real S, the beautiful...

- ***Session 6***

Strategy: Metaphor, quantum jump; step three and half

Indirect Hypnosis

We talk about making a radical change, a transformation and that transformation means totally different than what was once upon a time. S, the beautiful last week, last Thursday, she was one S, the beautiful, who did not know, who is not real S, the beautiful, now S, the beautiful is all beautiful smile, (3), because M. tells me that as a child, you were a divine child. Your divinity, even now is in two ways. You're smiling, this is a divine smile that you have on your face and I also told M. to talk to you about what is a quantum jump. But he has not bothered to tell you about quantum jump. It is some thing that is 100 per cent and beyond, in one step. You know there is a story of another God SANAT.

He is the doctor of the Gods. There were several avatars of God, and there were nine and one of them was Waman avatar. So when that demon of a king, making so much of trouble, this Waman says, I don't need anything more, for whatever, service and favour I have done for you. I only want three and a half step of land. You don't know this show, there was a half step. That was the quantum jump. In three steps he covered heaven, *Prithivi*, and *patal*. Nothing was left to put for another half step. So, he put the half step on the demon's chest. We have to make that half step only today. We have already made three steps. We have to make that half step and I am asking you to do it. You are capable of doing it. If you are not capable I wouldn't ask you to do this impossible, but having undergone this total transformation. You happen to meet face to face to real S, the beautiful.

- *Session 7*

Strategy: Explain Physiology, Immune System Suggestions: Rejuvenation is reversal of disease; occurs all the time.

Now S, the beautiful you have so much of motivation to change...to a better order...your mind, treating your self. Transform your inner mind to get rid of the rubbish...I want you, S, the beautiful to learn to switch off and switch on yourself into this state of mental relaxation. This state of self hypnosis, this state of inward journey as a spontaneous person...change...change...change... is bringing about a change, a change... love of nature...is the product of nature...the wisdom of nature...See how S, the beautiful even in this breathing process, I am now giving you an insight on your primary process...on autoimmune disease. This is bringing about a change, a change and an exchange. An exchange, where antibodies, are reduced ...auto antibodies are being destroyed once and for all. ...Your immune organs are now being conditioned, being programmed, being taught a lesson to work in the normal natural way...as expected to perform...the tissue wisdom... provided by your inner mind is awakening your immune system. It is resetting your biological clock to your normal setting, reprogramming your immune system to make the biological clock start working clock-wise. Yes, there is working in clock-wise, normally, naturally, spontaneously, effortlessly, all by itself with the tissue memory, with the tissue wisdom...As now your whole immune system is being set right, is being programmed perfect, is being conditioned with the knowledge, with the wisdom, with the tissue intelligent to work to produce anti-bodies...as defensive cells...As soldiers release the arms to defend their land from attacking enemies, the anti-bodies produce now by your immune system are working to help to recover your normal health.

What you have cooked is healthy for you. Similarly S, the beautiful, "I want you to clean your inner mind and throw away all your frustrations, all your negative thoughts...

I want you to cook fresh...pleasant, tasty good cooked food, I want you S, the beautiful...positive thoughts, love confidence, courage, self-dignity, self-worthiness, self-respect and self-confidence. S, the beautiful with self-confidence with which you always were bouncing, it makes you an enthusiastic person to be the master of your health. ...Your immune system has got rid of unhealthy anti-bodies and it has replaced to produce normal natural healthy anti-bodies...

- *Session 8*[26]

Strategy. Out of body experience; dissociation from disease

Make yourself drift into a state of total, complete, physical relaxation which you usually do and whenever you hear my voice and I want you S, the beautiful to be in trance...allow things to happen by their own...Now I want you to leave your body here... resting peacefully, comfortably. You come with me to a special place, you have reached now to a beautiful garden...how this huge garden has a beautiful lawn...See this lawn has a very fresh fragrance. You are now walking bare foot on this beautiful lawn. See how bare foot; the sole of your feet is now on beautiful, cool and soft grass. The drops of dew on the grass are making you feel coolness in the feet, may be a tingling sensation in the feet. You suck energy from the mother-nature. It is like a child...sucking milk from mother's breast...the mother who is very affectionately feeding the child...this energy is now transferring this energy to the entire body. Each and every cell including your brain, see how mother-nature by herself; is energizing you...vitalizing you...you have a right to step in this beautiful lawn...Whole body's energy is now being transferred to that part of your body which needs repairs. It may be your joints, it may be your left ankle, it may be your skin...blood vessels...See how this energy is now working...a perfect healing, just healing, sustained healing and complete cure. Mother-nature cures one and all. S, the beautiful...

You are becoming rejuvenated, refresh spiritually. Your spiritual journey has begun; you are very good, very innocent and deserving all these blessings. You are healing and complete and good health...

Now I want S, the beautiful to take a seat near the bench. You see the beautiful sight in front of you. There are many beautiful ponds in this garden being part of the garden. They are large ponds and you are seeing beautiful lotuses swinging and dancing supported by the tender stalks...You have found such a beautiful pond fully covered with white, red, violet lotus flowers. Some are half open, some are partially open and some are fully open. Don't they look beautiful and so unique? Some are just buds that are about to open... their beauty...their fragrance, and... the wind blows and the tender buds also sprout and open... their own beauty, their own identity, their own value and own inner values and virtues...with all these within yourself...now return to...

- *Session 9*

Strategy: Explain auto immune process

Metaphors: A seed has grown into a weed; it is being weeded out; feeding the fish in a pond with the dirt

You...a unique person highly intelligent, highly talented, highly accomplished, having the values and virtues...growing beautiful flowers and a strong and handsome sun S. ... knowingly or unknowingly, seed of a weed is mixed up...created an emotion...created twenty-two years back. I want you, S, the beautiful right now; go back in years... go back in years... go back in years what went wrong? When and why, where and how—this emotion weed got seeded there...That seed has given rise to the plant has created auto immune disease in you. You are now S, the beautiful...riding high to put an end to weed out this weed...weed it out... auto-immune disease...weed it out...It has to be a complete, total...weed it out...

...You are surprised to find that this plant has many roots... One by one you are uprooting all the roots, the plant in total, you are throwing it out... you are throwing it out... you are throwing it out...evacuating and emptying your inner mind once for all. That plant has been discarded, destroyed and disappeared in thin air.

...You have conquered the root cause of your problem; you have derooted and thrown away all the seeds and seedlings...your immune system has now become normal, and has set with the pace in biological system which is normal. It is functioning in a natural way as in all normal human beings. You have your antibodies that will defend you and you *do not* have those antibodies that were destroying you...

Right now, you find S, the beautiful that we are moving to the other pond. This pond is beautiful. It contains fishes of various colours...sizes and shapes. See how beautiful they look. See the fish...various colours like cream, golden yellow and brownish...You take a handful of water and I want you to pour that water on your foot... May be S, the beautiful you may transfer your whole foot to dip in that water. See how your ulcer is being washed out...sad feelings, bad memories, all your frustrations, negative thoughts, all your anger, hatred, all your jealousy, selfishness and...finally your guilt...you are transferring to fish...You throw them in to the water and within seconds all the fish...gobble them. They disappear once and for all and, as those fish disappear...for good...

Now I want you, S, the beautiful, to refill your inner mind with al happy memories, high ambitions, good feelings, positive thoughts, love, caring, confidence, courage, courage to face any situation, courage to overcome any obstacle in life, courage to face the reality that life exposes to you. I want you, S, the beautiful, throw away all the fear and refill with good feeling, positive thoughts, self respect, self dignity, self worthiness and lastly self love...When you love your self than you forgive yourself.

- *Session 10*

Strategy: Substitution of mature defenses of ego – spirituality and aesthetics-for neurosis

Goal: Convergence of split personality; integration of personality

After invocation of *Maha Shakti*, presence of divine dance, S, the beautiful, see this divine dance with in your self. Here, behind my thumb, between the two eyebrows, there is a third eye. In the third eye see the magnificent victory on this Vijayalakshmi day. From this auspicious day we have we have won all the demonic demons. Since we have won there is appreciation of peace, serenity and tranquility. In this serenity you are healing remarkably, silently but certainly...

Open your third eye, S, the beautiful and as you open your third eye, your right index finger moves. And as your right index finger moves your third eye opens. The third eye of Siva, when opens, it destroys all the demons instantaneously.

Tomorrow when Dr. R. comes you will tell her about the unifying experience of spirituality. Thereby S, the beautiful has welcomed and united with S, the beautiful, I am so privileged to have worked with you. My heart is filled with silent joy and as we all pray and thank Lord Siva for his gracious grace, keep enjoying this sublime...this spiritual union with S, the beautiful. When you will wake up, you shall wake up with a sublime identification with your selfhood. Thank you; keep enjoying your spiritual experience regardless of my presence. Thank you.

- ***Session 11***

Strategic utilization of archetypal symbols for access to unconscious mind, exploration

Goal: Transformation and insight generation.

If there is only one way, we know we can go out from this room and there that is only one door...that we usually use...usually use...unusual ways are also the ways...that we unusually use...unusual ways are also the ways...Windows are there...we can go out from there...there are several windows...there are more than a thousand to the mind...the doors to enter into the mind...and find different pathways too.

As S, the beautiful takes a deep, deep breath, she has done several of such actions. She goes into deeper and deeper trance. S, the beautiful is beautiful and has only radiant ambience and goodwill...action with all. S, the beautiful, with her own inner and beautiful self...you happily tuned to your inner rhythm of singing...As you return the flow of water, you start the flow of the water of Ganga...start feeling the flow, (confusion technique) right left and left right, front back and back and front, sideways, all over your brain. As you feel potentiated energized, vitalized, move any of the finger of the right hand, may be left...so many fingers make a move...When you are ready to do some more, and, more, wonderful, very nice...that is...your work as you are flowing out...All over your body; the process of transformation, transmutation... the process of transformation, transmutation...has begun...to your original pure self. Transformation and transmutation is coming through a rapid succession,

1, 2, 3, 4... 6... 15. 20... 30... 79... 85... 410... 3139... In rapid successive visions and views, thousands of windows...that you have opened up in your mind...See these several thousands windows...in multiples of thousands...We see through all these windows radiant light, thousands of candles...give up glimpses...Glimpses of many splendored things.

S, the beautiful, you are seeing through a third eye ...you have a third eye...Siva has a third eye...every is a part of Siva...you are Siva...you have a third eye, it entitles and powers you...the simultaneous vision to all those multiple window openings. S, the beautiful, would you like see...through the third eye simultaneously...at one and same time...through all the windows and the doors, your mind? S, the beautiful...now you are empowered and as you wish to see these numerous windows...you are seeing them... and as you open your third eye, S, the beautiful when your third eye opens that is an eye of Siva. You are right there and your right finger moves (deepen the trance). And as your third eye opens, your left forearm, arm, down to your shoulder is getting lighter and lighter. So that it starts moving upwards like a feather and each upward movement; your right index finger is about to move. Wonderful S, the beautiful and when it has moved, S, the beautiful a daughter of Siva has opened her third eye like Siva. As she has opened her third eye, she has lighted up all those windows in her mind. She sees through the light, various shades, various colours, and which is up to the energy forward, backward and sideways. Before your eyes it is 2006, 2005, 2004, 2000, 1999, 1995, 1989, 1985, 1982 (age regression)...and as you see more and little deep through the window, 1980 and S, the beautiful is wondering, is it my true identity?

Left hand is like a feather; no weight, no stress, no difficulty in holding up, since you are holding it at all? Except feather let it float. 1979, 1980, 1981, 1982, 1983 through the vision of your third eye, 'YES', how nice S, the beautiful has identified that event that went wrong. Do you want to hold on to it? S, the beautiful, your third eye wants to say 'NO'. Let your left hand, slowly and certainly come down, it is coming down. Whatever that probably may have gone wrong; let it go down slowly and certainly as your left hand and forearm is coming down.

Now, let the arm rest peacefully without any function. Your third eye is looking to 1979, 1978, 1975 the time beyond, times beyond and S, the beautiful was all beauty, so beautiful so much of grace, so much of innocence, so much of child like joy, beautiful voice. (Tears rolled down) as I wipe, and as I wipe, you will relax even more. The moment when you put your left hand down, S, the beautiful you have let gone all that went wrong.

That falls identity is erased. That wonderful S, the beautiful that you have seen it through third eye, that third eye remains open... It only sees that which is pure, that which is nice, that which is willing and still clear. Pure water of Ganga is flowing all over your body, your third eye that can open the thousands of windows and doors; through your mind the glimpses are always available to you. S, the beautiful, so that every time that...

You will listen to the cassette and you will open your third eye; you will be able to open up and light up thousands of windows. The light spreading gently through doors and windows spreading light gently, your inner mind will spread it all your body. We doctors call them synapses. One neuron fixes other neuron that you have lighted several thousand candles. Clean water of Ganga is flowing in these functional areas in your brain in your nervous system and S, the beautiful face to face to her true identity is singing the prayer of Siva. Since this power of third eye has empowered herself. The healing energy of Maha Durga has empowered you…

- ***Session 12***

MAHA SHAKTI

Let go, put yourself in trance… relax wonderfully, yes, to your right and to the left is north (confusion technique) and as we move east-words and south-words and move little east-words and move a little south-words, move a little north-words and you see yourself a transformed and transmuted…a weight less, tensionless, effortless, rejuvenated, reformatted, new S, the beautiful, new energy source that is S, the beautiful, S, the beautiful has drawn energy from the all energy forms that dance in *Navaratri* in Gujarat, we are celebrating a festival of rejuvenating energy, the energy, the energy renewal is when you walk bare foot…on grass …

…on the finally bare foot… and you have felt the energy going up your feet both the feet… up like a fountain way up …yet going up and up way up… your face and your face is glowing with billions of energy forms of Durga, Maha Durga, Maha Shakti that flows out from the *Jata* of Siva in the form of Ganga…that is in the East…so you keep your feet facing East… east (in Sanskrit and Hindi, it translates as what is best) for you to keep Ganga water flowing all over your body and with this rejuvenation of energy. The entire body is charged with healing and life sustaining force and as soon as it does so your left index finger moves, revitalize your self, and re-energize your self, nice… S, the beautiful you have learnt the self healing, it has now brought about complete transformation in you.

You are working every second of the day, every day of the month and every microsecond of the year. There is activation of your right brain, your inner mind getting into the root of the problem. You are observing your breathing process in and out of your lungs, in and out of your cells where the law of nature…of give and take is working by itself… it is producing the transformation that you rightly deserve gathering all the beautiful memories.

You are slowly coming back to your self with the sense of lightness for your eyes, with the sense of alertness and awakening. All over your body you are feeling sense of presence in this world. How wonderful you have created your self completely of well being. This you rightly deserve. Everyday you will listen and day by day the depth of the trance will increase and transformation will continue to make you a healthy person, happy and successful person. You will feel lightness in your eyes and become fully awake.

Thank you S, the beautiful...

Summary

As seen from the above, auto immune diseases do respond to prolonged unlimited time frame in therapy. What happened to S. above cannot be considered a remission or placebo effect; later should have happened when she sought novel treatments several times before. Ernest Rossi attributes his recovery from stroke to his manipulation of genes through hypnosis. He mentored S. Iannotti who recovered from near fatal illness due to Guillain Barre Syndrome[27]; to gratefully found Foundation Iannotti – Rossi[28] for research in psychosocial genomics.

However, a single cuckoo does not make for the spring. There are numerous variables that are difficult to monitor for scientific validation: suggestibility of the subject is most important.

Let there be no impression that hypnotherapy is a panacea for all. It may not work for simple conditions and; also in spite of the best efforts by a given therapist. To repeat: suggestibility of the subject is most important.

Post Script to Chapter 17

- *Case 1*

A surgeon came for therapy for psoriasis; the disease has come since one year or so. The lesions have spread all over his upper extremities. He is severely handicapped professionally.

History reveals that he has recently finished his post graduate study. He came from a lower middle class family. His family wanted him to start his practice in their small home town. His elder brother has supported and financed his studies. This was very hard on the family. However, the brilliant young man opted for further specialization. He had to move 500 miles away for higher training. His visits to the home town got infrequent.

One day he got the news that his elder brother has got a heart attack. When he reached his home town his brother was dead. His mother cried and told him: "your brother made you what you are now today, a doctor; but you did not help him". He was deeply hurt by the remark. He developed itching and rashes on both arms.

He returned to his training. Sometime later he noticed psoriasis on his arms.

The young surgeon was age regressed up to the event of death of his brother. He was made to re-live in full details. This was played about till catharsis was induced. His guilt was selectively ablated. He was age progressed to a time when he will finish his highest qualification to serve humanity better.

His psoriasis regressed, by the time he finished his studies. It was practically gone. He went to the nearest city to his home town and set up his practice. His psoriasis recurs off and on since last ten years. He has learnt to meditate and practices mindfulness meditation.

- *Case 2*

An idealist mother of two daughters had the ambition to educate her two daughters and make them high professionals. She lived in a small town. Following high school graduation by the daughters she had to send them for professional studies to distant city in a span of three years. Separation from the daughters was almost like bereavement to her.

Some six months back, at a visit to the dentist she was found to have some lesions on the gums and the pallet. The dermatologist diagnosed it to be pemphigus. This lady was a relative of the surgeon mentioned above. The surgeon referred her for hypnotherapy. The strategies employed in hypnotherapy were to generate insight that she is blaming and punishing herself for sending the daughters away. Subsequent sessions involve re-living her own marriage through age regression. She was made to live cyclic events of nature in human life.

She was made to visualize the emptiness, a natural phenomenon in Nature. She was to see emptiness as empty nest. And, she was also made to experience a nest as a home. Empty though it may be, a home is a home is a home. She was made to experience the true essence of motherhood in the nature of parting, giving and not possessing. Six years following the therapy she doesn't have any pemphigus. Professionally qualified daughters have married and further moved away. Of course there are two tragedies in human life: one is not to get your heart's desire, the other is to get it.

Schizophrenia

It is classically taught that hypnotherapy does not help schizophrenia. We have treated three subjects. They were young male adults. They were brilliant. Personality derangement in two subjects occurred following betrayal by the girl friends. The young men were honest, earnest, sincere and, committed in their relationships. The girl friends happened to be flirt and enjoyed the power to exploit their boyfriend's loyalty. Even after junking the relationship, girls did not jettison the contacts.

- *Case 1*

The innocence of the boys was violated. They were bewildered and devastated.

One of them had to leave his engineering studies half way. The highly educated parents knew about schizophrenia as much there is to know from multiple doctors and Google. They visited most of the premier institutions, when they were told that one Dr. Jana (founder of Indian society of hypnosis) may be able to help. They did not give up, even when they came to know that he is no more. They travelled five hundred miles to take hypnotherapy session.

The strategies involved were to time regress the boy to the age of intimacy with the girl. Then he was made to visualize the girl as a poisonous mermaid and, during the trance he was made to visualize an innocent Devine child who survived the poison of a *vishkanya* (poisonous woman).

The boy completed his studies and as would be his usual grade, passed his final exams with distinction. He got an apprentice job.

The family were advised that he will need a lifelong support. They discontinued therapy to revert back, after sometime to say that the boy has the relapse.

- *Case 2*

It was even more curious. The young man was returning from the college when he saw his father meeting with a fatal accident near his house. He lived in a large joint family with his grandparents and others. The young man was well supported, yet he was depressed. This brought more attention from the family. They noticed some symptoms and signs for personality dissociation. The psychiatrist after some follow up diagnosed it as schizophrenia. He was very heavily drugged. The young man got more withdrawn and further dissociated.

Trauma of witnessing the violent death of his father was initially accepted as the prime psychodynamic pathology by the hypnotherapist, psychiatrist and family. Age regression was tried. A catharsis at or following the event was expected but, did not occur. A couple of sessions brought some cheer back to the boy. The strategies were then changed to hypnotherapeutic exploration: hypnoanalysis. It revealed that with the death of his father, though shocked, the young man has coped well.

A strange fact emerged to the surprise of the therapist. The young man had inherited a large fortune through his father's will, and he had brought a new car.

Following a few sessions, there was a very strong rapport. The boy was to confide that he has been shaken up because his girlfriend was just fiddling with him. The family was a traditional Hindu family. They arranged a bride for him and absorbed him in the family business. There is complete restoration to normal functioning and, total weaning from the drugs.

- *Case 3*

Yet another schizophrenic, in his late twenties was referred with the diagnosis of schizophrenia. He was on medication. Though an engineer he restricted himself to simple clerical job. Yet, he has difficulty to maintain the job. He was unmarried and avoided contact with women. The young man was highly intelligent and had insight as well.

He was brought up by his father and step mother following the divorce from his mother. He was not given the custody to his mother only to further spite her. The boy was treated as stranger by his father. The step mother was as much step motherly as she can. Father never addressed the boy by his proper name. He was called simply as *manava* (human being).

The man has travelled a long distance with strong belief that the treatment with this therapist will restore him to function normally. And functioning normally as far as he was concerned, was to blossom out like Vivekanand (The famous Indian monk). In fact he was going to a *yoga* centre at Bangalore. A psychiatrist help was requisitioned for monitoring his progress. He stayed for therapy for about three weeks. The doses of medication were gradually reduced. A conscious goal setting was made for him that he will outperform his father in material world through his carrier and, further establish his superiority by progress in yoga. This way he will doubly defeat his father.

Thus Oedipus complex was utilised, played and replayed in hypnotherapeutic sessions. After some time he called up to say that he had got an engineering job. There afterwards he is lost for follow up.

Schizophrenia is the last bastion of psychiatric illnesses that we explore psycho-dynamically. Most mental health professional would agree that the illness is psychotic in origin, has genetic linkage and is due to chaotic firing of neurons and molecules so generated in the brain. A few will agree about the influence of psychodynamic environment.

The condition is associated with violence towards self and the others. The patients are usually over drugged to obviate it. To prescribe molecules for schizophrenia will take only a few minutes: to care for one requires a life time support. We are convinced that they are hypnotizable, there is a complex psychodynamic play in the unconscious and these subjects with loving tender care through family support or through NGO[29] can be restored to functional life.[30] If one thing is certain, they live in a different world and may have a beautiful mind; As John Nash demonstrated. They might be super-intelligent like Nash to win Noble prize or write master pieces like autobiographical novel by Robert Pirsing: Zen and the Art of Motorcycle Maintenance.[31]

Notes

1. Karl Popper, *The Logic of Scientific Discovery*, London, 1959.
2. D. Corydon Hammond, *Handbook of Hypnotic Suggestions and Metaphors*, 1990, New York.
3. Inputs by Prof. Ramchandran, Ph.D.

4. References on Creativity

Albert Rothenberg (1978). Cited in *Psychoanalysis, Creativity, and Literature*. Ed., By Alan Roland, Columbia University Press, pp.145-161.

Anthony Storr (1976). *The Dynamics of Creation,* Pelican Books, Harmondsworth, Middlesex, England.

Arguelles Jose A (1975). *The Transformative Vision*. Shambhala, Berkeley & London.

Arthur Koestler (1977). *The Act of Creation*. Picador. London.

Bill Moyers. (1982). In 'The Creativity Quest' in *The American Review.* United States International Communication Agency, New Delhi. Vol. 26, No. 4.

Eissler K.R. (1976). Cited in Chapter 'The Ambivalence of Freud' in *The Dynamics of Creation.* Pelican Books. Harmondsworth, Middlesex, England.

Freud S. (1958). *On Creativity and the Unconsciousness*. Harper, New York.

Gazzaniga, Bogen, and Sperry (1962). In "Divided Consciousness: Multiple Controls in Human Thought and Action" by Hilgard E.R., John Wiley & Sons. New York.

Hoover E. (1978) New Psychology: New Image of Man in *Readings in Psychology* 78/79, Annual Editions, Guilford.

Jha S.K. (1978). *An Analysis of Certain Dimensions of Creativity*. Himalaya Publishing House, Bombay.

John R. Suler (1980). "Primary process thinking and Creativity" in *Psychological Bulletin.* 88, No. 1, 144-165.

June Singer (1980). "A Synthesis of Contradictions": Creativity in the Analytical Psychology of C.G. Jung. In *Perspectives on Creativity and the Unconscious.* (Ed.) Donald W. Fritz, Miami University, Old Northwest Publication.

Kohut (1957). in Creativity and Personality: A Review of Psychological Researches. *Indian Psychological Review.* Vol. 2, 91-102.

Kris, E. (1953). *Psychoanalytic Explorations in Art*. Allen & Unwin. London.

Maslow, A.H. (1971) *The Farther Reaches of Human Nature*. New York: Viking.

McMullan. (1976). "Creative individuals; Paradoxical personages" in *Journal of Creative Behaviour*. Vol. 10, 4, IV Quarter, pp. 265-275.

Mednick S.A. (1962). The Associative Basis of the Creative Process. *Psychological Review.* 69, 220-232.

Rossi Ernest (1977). Reference cited in *Perspectives on Creativity and the Unconscious.* (Ed.) Donald W. Fritz, Miami University, Old Northwest Publication (p. 79).

Rossi Ernest (1991). *The 20 Minute Break*. Tarcher, Inc. Los Angeles.

Rossi Ernest and Kathryn Rossi (1996). *The Symptom Path to Enlightenment*. Palisades Gateway Publishing. California.

Rossi Ernest (2002). The Psychobiology of Gene Expression: Neuroscience and Neurogenesis in Hypnosis and the Healing Arts. New York: Norton Professional Books.

Sheila Ostrander and Lynn Schroeder (1971). *Psychic Discoveries Behind the Iron Curtain.* Prentice Hall, Inc., Englewood Cliffs, New Jersey.

Sushil Kumar De. (1960). *History of Sanskrit Poetics*. Firma K.L. Mukhopadhyay Publishers, Calcutta.

Vernon P.E. (Ed.) (1970). *Creativity*. Penguin Modern Psychology Readings, Harmondsworth, Middlesex, England.

5. Let us look at this poem by Sri Aurobindo:

A DREAM OF SURREAL SCIENCE

One dreamed and saw a gland write Hamlet; drink

At the Mermaid, capture immortality;
A committee of hormones on the Aegean's brisk composed Iliad and the Odyssey.
A thyroid, meditating almost nude under the Iliad tree,
Saw the eternal light,
And arising from its mighty solitude,
Spoke of the wheel and eightfold path alright.
A brain by a disordered stomach driven
Thundered through Europe, conquered, ruled and fell,
From St. Helena, went perhaps to Heaven.
Thus wagged on the surreal world, until
A scientist played with atoms and blew out
The Universe before God had time to shout.

6. Jencks, B. (1977). *Your Body: Biofeedback at its Best*. Chicago; Nelson Hall.
Jencks, B. (1979). Exercise manual for J.J. Schultz's *Standard autogenic Training and Special Formulas*. Des Plaines; American Society of Clinical Hypnosis.
Luthe and Schultz (1969-73). *Autogenic therapy volumes I-VI*. Breene and Stratton.
7. Contributed by Dr. Suresh Sadhavani, M.D.; DCAH.
8. Contributed by Dr. Mukesh Trivedi, M.B.; B.S., DCAH.
9. Goldenberg D.L., Fibromyalgia Syndrome a decade later : What have we learned? Arch Intern Med 1999 ; 159 : 777.
10. Simons DG, Travell JG, Myofascial pain and dysfunction. In PD Wall, R Melzack (Eds.) *Textbook of Pain*, Edinburgh, 1989, pp. 368-385.
11. Nishikai, M, Tomomatsu, S, Hankins, RW, *et al*. Auto antibodies to a 68/48 kDa protein in chronic fatigue syndrome and primary fibromyalgia: a possible marker for hypersomnia and cognitive disorders. *Rheumatology*, 40; 806, 2001.
12. Hadhazy, V.A., Ezzo, J., Creamer, P., Berman, BM. Mind-body therapies for the treatment of fibromyalgia. A systematic review.[In Process Citation]. *J. Rheumatol*, 2000; 27:2911.
13. Goldenberg, D.L., Kaplan, K.H., Nadeau, M.G., *et al*. A controlled study of a stress-reduction, cognitive-behavioural treatment programme in fibromyalgia. *J. Musculoskeletal Pain*, 1994; 2:53.
14. White, K.P., Nielson, WR. Cognitive behavioural treatment of fibromyalgia syndrome: A follow-up assessment. *J. Rheumatol*, 1995; 22:717.
15. Alexander, R.W., Bradley, L.A., Alarcon, G.S., *et al*. Sexual and physical abuse in women with fibromyalgia: association with outpatient health care utilization and pain medication usage. *Arthritis Care Res.*, 1998; 11:102.
16. Linton, S.J. A population-based study of the relationship between sexual abuse and back pain: establishing a link. *Pain* 1997; 73:47.
17. Nicosia, P.M., Radiogenic, V., Weisman, MH, *et al*. A comparison of behavioural and educational interventions for fibromyalgia. *J. Rheumatol*, 1997; 24:2000.
18. Laymen, J.W., Teeken-Gruben, N.J., Goossens, M.E., *et al*. Cognitive-educational treatment of fibromyalgia: a randomized clinical trial. I. Clinical effects. *J Rheumatol*, 1996; 23:1237.
19. Bradley, L.A., Alberts, K.R. Psychological and behavioural approaches to pain management for patients with rheumatic disease. *Rheum Dis. Clin. North Am*, 1999; 25:215.
20. Moldolfski H. Psychogenic rheumatism or the fibrositis syndrome. In : Hill O (ed.) Modern trends in psychosomatic medicine, vol. 3. Boston, 1976, pp. 187-195.
21. Jencks, B. (1977). Your Body: Biofeedback at its best. Chicago; Nelson Hall.

Jencks, B. (1979). Exercise manual for J.J. Schultz's Standard autogenic Training and Special formulas. Des Plaines; *American Society of Clinical Hypnosis*.
Luthe and Schultz (1969-73). Autogenic therapy volumes I-VI. Breene and Stratton.
22. Contributed by Aruna Thakur, FRCP, Canada.
23. Frankl, F. (1965). The doctor and the soul: From psychotherapy to logo therapy.
Haley, J. (1973). Uncommon therapy.
24. Contributed by Aruna Thakur, FRCP, Canada.
25. Barber, T.X. (1978). Hypnosis, suggestion, and psychosomatic phenomena. *American Journal of Clinical Hypnosis*, 21,1; pp 13-27.
Ewin, D.M. (1974). Condylomata accuminatum: Successful treatment of four cases by hypnosis. *American Journal of Clinical Hypnosis*, 17,2; pp. 73-78.
Galski, T.J. (1981). The adjunctive use of hypnosis in the treatment of trichotillomania: A case report. *American Journal of Clinical Hypnosis*, 23,3; pp. 198-201.
Johnson, R.F.Q. and Barber, T.X. (1978). Hypnosis, suggestions, and warts: an experimental investigation implicating the importance of "believed-in efficacy". *American Journal of Clinical Hypnosis*, 20,3; pp. 165-174.
Lehman, R.E., (1978). Brief hypnotherapy of neurodermatitis: A case with four-year follow-up. *American Journal of Clinical Hypnosis*, 21, 1; pp. 48-51.
Rowen, R. (1981). Hypnotic age regression in the treatment of a self-destructive habit: trichotillomania. *American Journal of Clinical Hypnosis*. 23,3; pp. 195-197.
Sheehan, D.V. (1978). Influence of psychosocial factors on wart remission. *American Journal of Clinical Hypnosis*, 20,3; 160-164.
Twerski, A.J. & naar, R. (1974). Hypnotherapy in a case of refractory dermatitis. *American Journal of Clinical hypnosis*, 16,3; pp. 202-205.
Welsh, D.K. (1978). Hypnotic control of blushing: A case study. *American Journal of Clinical Hypnosis*, 20,3; pp. 213-216.
26. Contributed by Dr. Radha Mohan, Pediatrician and Hypnotherapist.
27. We have had a similar success in a Communist lady who was weaned off her ventilator in a few days.
28. Rossi E.L. *A Discourse with Our Genes*, New York, 2004.
29. The noted NGO's in India are The Banyan, Sir Ratan Tata Trust, SCARF to name a few in India and several globally.
30. It must be confessed that we know little about the schizophrenic illness. When I talk to god, it is a prayer; when my patient tell to me that the god is talking to him, I call him a schizophrenic! Joan of Arc, Mary Magdalane, Mira bai and even Shri Aurbindo have been so labelled.
31. The movies about schizophrenia: A Beautiful Mind, Hidden Picture, Unlisted: A Story of Schizophrenia, Crisis in Control.

22
Hypnotherapy for Disorders of Childhood Behaviour[1]

People can often bounce back from difficult childhood circumstances or stressful experiences to make a good adaptation to life. A traumatic incident or a severely deprived childhood may well have grave emotional consequences; but the stories of countless people, some of whom researchers have followed from childhood into at least their sixties, show that a single experience – even one as painful as the death of a parent in childhood – is not likely to cause irreversible damage (Vaillant and Vaillant, 1990[2]). A nurturing environment can often help a child overcome the effects of early deprivation or trauma.

Bidirectional Influence on Childhood Behaviour

Children are not passive sponges, soaking up influences. They actively shape their own environment, and then they respond to the environmental forces that they have helped bring about. When infants babble and coo, they encourage adults to talk to them, and this talk in turn stimulates the baby's language development. Teenager's burgeoning sexuality may evoke their parent's fears of growing older and regrets for lost youth; the parent's reactions, in turn, may affect the teenager's attitudes toward the changes they are undergoing.

Anxiety in Infancy

Separation anxiety and stranger anxiety used to be considered emotional and cognitive milestones of infancy, reflecting attachment to and recognition of the mother. Research over the past decade or so, however, suggests that these phenomena are vary variable and depend largely on a baby's temperamental and life circumstances.

Marital Discord Influencing Child Behaviour

The attachments that infants form with their parent exert a major influence on physical, intellectual, personality, and social development. When these attachments are disrupted or impaired because children are separated from their parents or have painful relationships with them; the consequences can be grave.

Child Abuse and Neglect

Maltreatment of children can take several different forms. *Child abuse* involves physical injury. The typical pattern has been identified as the *battered child syndrome* (Kempe *et al.*[3], 1962). *Sexual abuse* refers to any kind of sexual contact between a child and an old person. *Neglect* is withholding of adequate care, usually physical care such as food, clothing, and supervision. Emotional neglect also occurs, sometimes resulting in a syndrome called *non-organic failure to thrive*, in which a baby fails to grow and gain weight at home despite adequate nutrition, but improves rapidly when moved out of the home and given emotional attention.

Long-term Effects of Abuse and Neglect

Abused children often show delays in speech, showing the link between emotional and cognitive development (Coster, Gersten, Beeghly, & Cicchetti,[4] 1989). Teenagers, who failed to thrive in infancy, are likely to have a variety of physical, intellectual, and emotional problems, apparently due to emotional neglect (Oates, Peacock, & Forest,[5] 1985). Adults who were sexually abused children are often fearful, anxious, depressed, angry, hostile, or aggressive. They often suffer from low self-esteem, do not trust people, and feel isolated and stigmatized. They tend to be sexually maladjusted.

Normal childhood stresses take many forms and can affect the healthy emotional development of children. Unusual stresses, such as natural disasters and wars, also affect many children. As a result of changing life styles, family responsibilities, and pressure to grow up too soon, many children today are experiencing a shortened and stressful childhood.

Sigmund Freud, G. Stanley Hall[6], Margaret Mead[7], Anna Freud[8], Erik Erickson and James Marcia[9] considered adolescence a time of storm and stress, marked by turbulent, contradictory emotions. Some of them emphasized crisis in identity, intellectualization and ascetism.

Hypnotherapy in Disorders of Childhood

The disorders that will be covered are attention-deficit hyperactivity disorder, conduct disorder (including juvenile delinquency), anxiety disorders of childhood, depressive disorders, several other special symptom disorders, and autism.

Attention-Deficit Hyperactivity Disorder

Attention-deficit hyperactivity disorder (ADHD), often referred to as hyperactivity, is characterized by difficulties that interfere with effective task-oriented behaviour in children, particularly impulsivity, excessive motor activity, and difficulties in sustaining attention. The symptoms of attention-deficit hyperactivity disorder are relatively common among children seen at child guidance centers.

Conduct Disorders

In conduct disorders, aggressive or antisocial behaviour is the focus. Disorder may involve a persistent, repetitive violation of rules and a disregard for the rights of others. These children manifest such characteristics as overt or covert hostility, disobedience, physical and verbal aggressiveness, quarrelsomeness, vengefulness, and destructiveness. Lying, solitary stealing, and temper tantrums are common. Such children tend to be sexually uninhibited and inclined toward sexual aggressiveness. Conduct disorders involve misdeeds that may or may not be against the law; example, *juvenile delinquency.*

Anxiety Disorders of Childhood and Adolescence

These children appear to share many of the following characteristics: over-sensitivity, unrealistic fears, shyness and timidity, pervasive feelings of inadequacy, sleep disturbances, and fear of school. Children diagnosed as suffering from an anxiety disorder typically attempt to cope with their fears by becoming overly dependent on others for support and help.

Separation Anxiety Disorder

It is characterized by unrealistic fears, over-sensitivity, self-consciousness, nightmares, and chronic anxiety. Such Children lack self-confidence, are apprehensive in new situations, and tend to be immature for their age. Such children are described by their parents as shy, sensitive, nervous, submissive, easily discouraged, worried, and frequently moved to tears. Typically, they are overly dependent, particularly on their parents.

Overanxious Disorder

Children with *overanxious disorder* are characterized by excessive worry and persistent fear; however, their fears are usually not specific and are not due to a recent stressful event. Sleeping.problems, especially difficulty in falling asleep, are common. Many children showing overanxious disorder appear to have personality characteristics such as perfectionist ideas and obsessional self-doubt.

Casual Factors in Anxiety Disorders are: An unusual constitutional sensitivity, an easy condition ability by aversive stimuli, and a buildup and generalization of "surplus fear reactions", The undermining of feelings of adequacy and security by early illnesses, accidents, or losses that involved pain and discomfort.

Childhood Depression

Spitz (1946)[10] first described the problem, which he called, as a behaviour pattern, similar to adult depression that occurred in children experiencing prolonged separation from their mothers. This specific childhood depression syndrome included slowed development and such symptomatic behaviour as weepiness, sadness, immobility, and apathy. Depression occurs at about twice the rate for adolescent girls as for adolescent boys.

Other Symptom Disorders

The behaviour disorders are –elimination disorders (enuresis and encopresis), sleepwalking, and tics – typically involve a single outstanding symptom rather than a pervasive maladaptive pattern.

Functional Enuresis

The term *enuresis* refers to the habitual involuntary discharge of urine, usually at night, after the age of expected continence (age five).

A number of possible causal factors: (a) faulty learning, resulting in the failure to acquire a needed adaptive response—that is, inhibition of reflex bladder emptying; (b) personal immaturity, associated with or stemming from emotional problems; (c) disturbed family interactions, particularly those that lead to sustained anxiety, hostility, or both; and (d) stressful events.

Functional Encopresis

The term *encopresis* describes children who have not learned appropriate toileting for bowel movements after age four. This condition is less common than enuresis. Many encopretic children suffer from constipation; thus an important element in the diagnosis of the disorder involves a physical examination to determine whether physiological factors are contributing to the disorder.

Sleepwalking (Somnambulism)

Though the onset of sleepwalking disorder is usually between the ages of 6 and 12. The symptoms of *sleepwalking disorder* involve repeated episodes in which a person leaves his or her bed and walks around without being conscious of the experience or remembering it later. They may walk to another room of the house or even outside, and they may engage in complex activities. Finally, they return to bed and in the morning remember nothing that has taken place.

It appears to be related to some anxiety-arousing situation that has just occurred or is expected to occur in the near future.

Tics: A *tic* is a persistent, intermittent muscle twitch or spasm, usually limited to a localized muscle group. The term is used broadly to include blinking the eye, twitching the mouth, licking the lips, shrugging the shoulders, twisting the neck, clearing the throat, blowing the nose, and grimacing, among other actions.

Pervasive Developmental Disorder: Autism

Autism is a developmental disorder that involves a wide range of problematic behaviours, including deficits in language, perceptual, and motor development; defective reality testing; and an inability to function in social situations.

A cardinal and typical sign is that a child seems apart or aloof from others, even in the earliest stages of life. Typically, autistic children do not show any need for affection or contact with anyone, usually not even seeming to know or care who their parents are. Autistic children do not express emotions. The absence or severely restricted use of speech is characteristic of autistic children. If speech is present, it is almost never used to communicate except in the most rudimentary fashion.

Self-stimulation takes the form of such repetitive movements as head banging, spinning, and rocking. Most of these children seem to be mentally retarded.

Child Abuse

Many abused children show impaired cognitive ability and memory when compared with control children. Abused children are likely to show problems in social adjustment and are likely to feel that the outcomes of events are determined by external factors beyond their own control. They are likely to experience depressive symptoms.

When the abuse involves a sexual component, such as incest or rape, the long-range consequences can be very marked. Individuals who have been sexually abused are more likely to develop substance abuse problems. Jackson and colleagues (1990[11]) found that women who had experienced intra-family sexual abuse had significantly poorer social adjustment, especially in dating relationships. The women also reported significantly lower sexual satisfaction, more sexual dysfunctions and lower self-esteem than control women.

Residual symptoms of sexual abuse are as a type of post-traumatic stress disorder (PTSD) because the symptoms experienced are similar, for example, nightmares, flashbacks, sleep problems, and feelings of estrangement.

Televised Violence

Even if parents do not act aggressively, most children see aggressive models on television.

Aggressive children do watch more television than non-aggressive children, identify more strongly with aggressive characters, and are more likely to believe that aggression on television reflects real life (Eron, 1982). Aggressive acts make a more vivid impression than any punishment the "bad guy" receives. The effects of cartoon violence and violent play are, increases in fighting, kicking, choking, loss of temper, cruelty to animals, and disrespect for others, as well as decreases in sharing, imagination, and school performance.

Conclusion

The study of psychodynamics of Childhood behaviour has undergone a paradigm shift in the recent years and now occupies a central place in human history. Our attempts to understand childhood behaviour is thus critical to a full appreciation of the human condition. The substrates of childhood behaviour are enormously complex and our understanding of them imperfect. Hence we cannot give an accurate or detailed explanation for many behavioural abnormalities.

Induction Techniques

We recommend indirect hypnosis for children. We base the induction on any of the following techniques:

- Story telling, *Panchatantra, Ramayana, Mahabharata* and other epics.
- Travel to the favourite place of choice of the child.
- Alice in wonderland, Anderson Tales, Harry Potter and such other popular themes.
- Only the eye of the bird: Arjuna.
- Television.
- Going for a picnic.
- Deepening: As you play and keep on playing.
- Cricket, balls.
- Companions and peers, Teddy Bear, Dolls.

Family and school are integral part of a child's personality. Before starting hypnotherapy, family situation should be viewed holistically and parents may be involved in therapy too.

Case Studies

1. *Post Traumatic Stress Syndrome: Stealing and Lying: Inability to Study*

A Muslim boy aged 16, studying in VIII class. He was near normal till 2002 when there were riots in and around is small town. On the day of communal violence, his aunty fetched him out of the school. He understood but little, but his aunty says they were very frightened. The boy deteriorated in his studies since then. He started stealing money from home that went upto a large sum at one time. He was sent away to Pune to study with his cousins who were brilliant at studies. He was put an year behind. After an year, when he was brought back, he was again put back one year. Now, he refuses to study; family is reconciled to put him to train in the business. He refuses to do that either. He does not communicate much but most of the time is tuned to computer games.

Goal: Restitution to a functional mode.

Strategy: Age regression, reliving the past, to make friends with supporting forces, applied through story telling inducing indirect hypnosis as:

Very soon we are going to have a period of holy days...the days of *Ramzan*...holy days can be holiday too...you do not have to study on holidays...because on rest of the days you do study...why are some days holy days?...it is because your mummy says so...and, your mummy loves you...so she has brought you to me...to tell you stories about holy days... holy days...when we may not study...but enjoy... play...and while playing we take a deep breath...and we run about... and while playing we take a deep breath...deeper breadth as we take... and we run about faster...and then we enjoy and feel nice, better joy...relax...holy days are holy because on those days we pray God...and you have already learnt how to say *Namaz*...and when we say *Namaz*...seat facing West now...there are holy men in the West...and when we pray to holy men...kind, pious, good people...they love children...they have white beard...and, they love children and like to play with them... protect them...Would you like to meet such a kind protective man? ...he is there for you to ask...you have asked to meet him... he is there...he is putting his hand on your head...he is caressing you...he has a large box of chocolates and sweets...it is all yours for asking...any time you need any thing...this kind man is at your call... the days of *Ramzan*...when he is specially around...we know that there is a God there...up... in the sky...we cannot see Him...but he sent his messenger...his name was the same as your name...he is Ali... you are Ali...and all Alis are good...good boys...they get what they need...and messenger of the God protects all children, all children who are good...provides for them...Ali is a good child...Ali gets what he needs...

Second session was age regression to his age 10 when he was fetched by his aunt from the school. Focusing on the day, it was reinforced that there are protective people all around him…there was his aunt, but there is his mother and so many more.

The boy stopped stealing. He has not lied after four such sessions. The boy refused to study but went to his father's business.

2. Persistent Vomiting without Cause

- *Case 3*

A boy aged 9, brought for repeated bouts of vomiting that occurs particularly during monsoon. Paediatrician has not found any pathology. Establishing rapport with the child who has recently seen a Harry Potter movie:

Little Harry is a magician…and in magic every thing is wonderful…you are also like Harry… you are wonderful…and you can do magic with deep breathing… deep breathing…you do magic… with eyes open…. magic happens with eyes open and… eyes closed…you want to see magic…with deep breathing…with eyes closed…you are seeing Harry… he is my friend too…he has given magic in my hands…I want to give it to your hands…and now you have magic in your hands…and with magic in your hands too… I am snatching away vomiting from your tummy…and you can also stop it when you put your hands on your tummy…there is magic in your hands…that can dry up wet things… that can dry up wet things…wet nappies, wet pants…wet bed…magic can dry your wet things…things get wet in monsoon…with my magical wand, we can ask monsoon to go away…it has stopped raining…you are no more wet…you are dry…completely dry…you are not vomiting any more.

- *Case 4*

A boy of 11 years, vomiting of and on without any organic cause. Fond of playing cricket.

Strategy: You can bowl and bat; field well too…hit straight drives for four…hit a sixer too. Now that you have hit a sixer, thrown your vomiting out of fence…it is out of the game now…you are no more vomiting…

- *Case 5*

With similar strategy, a boy with vomiting stopped doing so for a while. Family stopped therapy. Boy relapsed. He was taken for surgery; duodenojejunostomy was performed. Boy did not improve with surgery.

Notes

1. Inputs by Dr. Radha Mohan, Paediarician, DCAH.
2. Vaillant and Vaillant, Natural History of Male Psychological Health, *Amer. J. Psy.* 147, 31-47, 1990.
3. Kempe C.H. The Battered Child Syndrome, *JAMA*, 181; 17-24, 1962
4. Coster, W.J., Gersten M.S., M. Beeghly, and Cicchetti B., Communicative Functioning in Maltreated Todlers, *Developmental Psychology*, 25; 1020-29, 1989.
5. Oates R.K., Peacock A. and Forrest D., Long Term Effects of Non-Organic Failure to Thrive, *Paediatrics*, 75; 36-40, 1985.
6. G. Stanley Hall, *Adolescent*, New York, 1904.
7. Margaret Mead, *Sex and Temperament in three Primitive Societies*, New York, 1935.
8. Anna Freud, *The Ego and the Mechanism of Defense*, New York, 1946.
9. James Marcia, Identity in Adolescent, in J. Adelson (ed.) *Handbook of Adolescent Psychology*, New York, 1980.
10. Spitz, R.A. *Anaclitic Depression in Psychoanalytic Study of the Child*, Vol. 2. New York (1946).
11. Jackson J.L. *et al.* Yong Adult Women Who Experience Childhood Intrafamilial Sexual Abuse; Subsequent Assessment. *Arch. Sex. Behav.*, 19; 211-221, 1990.

23
Past Life Regression

Past life regression is a fancy with many trainers and hypnotists. As we have said earlier, there are innumerable unproven case studies, which show age regression even to the previous birth. It is impossible to scientifically prove/disprove rebirth and past life. After a life time devotion to research in this area, along with a few collaborators, Ian Stevenson[1,2], (a medical doctor) claims to have scientifically proved past life in a few thousand instances. If we consider this to be true, it requires scientific investigation as to how consciousness can transgress biological limits. Even if Space Time and Consciousness were to converge as a Fifth Dimension[3], biological transmigration is miles away.

A therapist is not concerned with esoteric issues: his concern is to help/cure his client. Regardless of his belief, he is value-neutral when it comes to therapy: he utilizes the currency of country concept. Those subjects who are dysfunctional because of "their unfinished agenda with past life" request–demand past life regression. This we concede in service of clients. Often enough such clients ask before taking therapy: do you believe in rebirth? We answer them by telling them that what we believe is not important; if they believe, we believe in them. When so regressed to past life, they do come back to functional mode. A classic illustration is as follows:

- ***Session 1***

A young lady of 32 years of age, born Aug 3rd 1975, requested past life regression in 2007 March, since she had "unfinished agenda with Lord Krishna" in her past life. She has been dysfunctional since last few years; all her time would go in going to holy places and pious men and gurus in search of a solution to her quest of Krishna.

> 2007 January: went to Allahabad to attend *Ardh-kumbh* and met two illustrious, eminent gurus
> 2006 December: went to Mysore and Ooti
> 2006 November: Went to Varanasi to visit Laheri Baba's house.

2006 July: Served a high priest and attended lectures on *Vedanta*
2006 June: joined an *ashram*
2006 March: Finished course of Kaivalya Dhama Yoga Institute, Lonawala.
2005 November: went to Ranchi at a Centre for Meditation
2005 July: Joined a diploma in yoga at Kaivalya Dhama.
2005 May: Went to Ranchi for 1 month, had a very good experience in meditation as per the Bihar School. Swami convinced her to continue with her yogic studies.
2005 April: Came back home from Rishikesh, disheartened.
1999 December: Read Autobiography of a Yogi for the first time. She has been reading it of and on since then.
1999 October: Read *Ramcharita Manas*
1998 May: Left home for Rishikesh
1998 March: Started listening some shlokas in dreams. Started having some "strong intuitions regarding things which happened in past life".
1997: Started Thakur seva (worship of Lord Krishna installed as an idol)
1996: Went to Vrindavan without informing family. Finished graduation in Fashion Designing.
1995: Decided not to get married, in search of a Guru. Realized that "I have some different meaning to the life."
1994: Finished 12th standard and brother got married.
1993: Started reading Osho.
1992: Completed 10th and sister got married.
1991: Changed the school
1990: Started liking spiritual scriptures and books
1988: Went to Singapore
1985: Visited Vrindavan for the first time with all family members and remembered everything that she saw when again she went back in 1996. It happened in 1996-1997 when she realized that she was connected with Vandravan. She says, a gentle touch on her forearm sometimes helps her to recollect. (A gentle touch assures the subject that therapist is walking—working with her, may have a basis in expression of early activated genes).
(Addressing the name of the subject say, Radha in this session)

Radha, please take a comfortable position in the chair. Slow, leisurely induction with progressive muscular relaxation…Yes very nice. Take a deep breath in and out, wonderful and as you are taking a deep breath in and out…The wave of this energized relaxation is moving upward to make front and back of the entire body relaxed, cool and comfortable…As the coolness enters…You can experience your breathing getting quiet, peaceful and harmonious. The heart is beating regularly and slowly but with great vigor. In expectancy of the experience that you have been waiting for all your life... The fingers of the hand can be moved...when you want to say Yes or No...only...if you like. But due to feeling absolutely free you just enjoy...There are small and fine muscles...When they relax, your whole face relaxes...and you smile...That relaxed, magnificent smile of your face makes you look 10 years younger...That smile of yours is wonderful.

As coolness enters your head...a fine fragrance... a fine fragrance... a fine fragrance..., perhaps of Vrindavan...flowers in Vrindavan... a fine fragrance of flowers in Vrindavan... the mind is enjoying this state of trance...when you are getting your natural due... a fine fragrance of flowers in Vrindavan... and also the whole brain is feeling cool, calm, quiet and heart is happy...Keep enjoying this trance of happiness... your natural due... a fine fragrance of flowers...And, you are now telling me, "I am feeling relaxed, happy, tranquil all over myself, very, very quiet... enjoying this state of natural happiness... this state of being, cool, comfortable and, now I would like to move forward...forward to any place where Krishna is".

So be it...Now you are telling yourself...I am moving out from the room of Ashram and... going out to a place of my choice. going out to a place of my choice...where Krishna is... I am there and it is just before the sun rise. The darkness of night is just disappearing and first ray of light is seen at the horizon on the east...The atmosphere is beautiful...There are big trees and plenty of colourful flower beds...There is fine fragrance of various flowers and it is filling up the whole surrounding... as well as my whole self...The birds are waking up with their biological clock. They are hoping up from one branch to other. They are chirping and also calling their mate... there is a biological clock that ticks and rings too...sings too...That symphony is so nicely tuned.... It really pleases my ears. The cool, fine breeze is passing through the leaves and, also is...spreading fine mixed fragrance all around me. It touches my face and makes me feel very happy. I am enjoying this surrounding with all its contents.

In a short while the east horizon is changing its colour. I see a red streak which gradually rises up and moving forward to become a red ball of fire—The sun. Gradually with the majestic walk it moves upwards into the sky. It gives light all over the place without any discrimination. It enlightens all the people, rich or poor, young or old, healthy or sick! ...How gorgeous! Sun the father...gives like mother' love... Knows only to give without any expectation, any condition...Sun gives for the happiness to others. It gives light, cosmic energy unconditionally...Who ever wants it, they take it. What a virtue! ...It all depends on the individual who takes. But if one surrenders to the Almighty's wish... then you have no exertion, no tension and you can just float like a bird. You have given away the radar in his hand. The almighty...make you float in the right direction... Arjun has given the chariot's control to Lord Krishna...And, Lord Krishna knows which way to go...to take Radha...

The sun is gradually on its journey in the sky, moves higher...and, simultaneously and gradually... from crimson red it has changed its colour to yellow. It is getting hot also. As I turn, I see a nice temple… It has tall, nicely carved various deities, sculptures with pleasant features; it makes me feel very happy…As I enter the temple, it is time for *Arti* (Morning Prayer). I hear the bells ringing and it makes familiar sound… It gives the primordial sound of *AUM*. There are many bells. They all are tuned in a symphony of morning tune… There is one bell as if left for me. I go and ring the bell…a flute joins in this symphony of bells. It fills up myself with immense joy, relaxation, peace, tranquility… a flute joins…I go into trance and become one with the universal consciousness…that is Krishan consciousness… I am in deep trance… This experience of being aware of everything has taken me away to the higher state of consciousness…that is Krishan consciousness… This experience is beyond language… Krishna consciousness… It is Ecstasy!. It is beyond verbal description… It is Ecstasy!. I want to feel it …fill it up …this experience in my heart and head. At any and every time of my need I want this experience to come to me…at the wink of my eyes…only if I wish… wink of my eyes….at the wink of my eyes, when I wish to have it, then I shall wink my eyes…I want this experience to come to me.

Arti is over…I stand in front of the deity. As I stand there in front, I see the expression of welcome in the eyes of the deity. It makes me so happy… There are tears of joy rolling over my cheeks…his cheeks…I am absolutely steady as if I have become a statue…I stand with folded hands… The blessings are being showered… The blessings are being showered…I am being blessed everyday and…today's experience is completely mine…I continue in this state of trance. It makes me feel peaceful from within. Not only that…I am different now… different now than before… in different state of Consciousness. I am Universal Consciousness… I am one with THEE, Krishna! …I feel very, very privileged, special, and happy. I want this experience in my heart…to last for ever. I continue to be in this state till it integrates in me…incorporates within me…(Let subject be in this state for at least few minutes).

Suddenly, I realize that so much of the time has passed. I wake up and birds are flying away for their daily routine leaving their little ones in the nest. I return to the place from where I began my journey and am wide awake.

- ***Session 2***

Age regression for Radha: to previous birth.

Client's detail history is taken and noted from year to year; if need be month wise. Later on it may be ascertained that she did experience. The subject is put into trance by quick induction technique.

Now, you go in to further deep trance. And I want to know Radha, if it is alright for me to carry on our further work… (There is positive signal).

The subject is asked to hold the pen in the right hand. She is asked to sign at each particular junction of life. Later on this is compared with the subject as to how at that age she signed. It is further confirmed later when she is fully awake. As evident, the signature changes with age and also the language like from vernacular to the present state may be English or otherwise whatever way the signature is signed.

Kindly keep watching yourself and, when it is alright, and when it is alright for me to take over; you may please give me your kind consent by signing your name. Very, very nice and, since you have consented, shall we now carry on our work, a bit further forward… a bit further forward or, sometimes further so much backwards (confusion technique)…back is back and back…is sideways back too. But as we make this random movement, I want to know, are you prepared to go back in time…when you were at a place in Tarangini Hall (previous day session). May be, it was evening before yesterday. (Deepening with touch on the arm, pressure between two eyes). Then and then only…when you are wanting to say, 'yes'…Please hold the pen with your hand and, then, and, now… when you are in Tarangini Hall, day before yesterday, now you are in Tarangini Hall… fresh memories…living those memories…of having performed the *pooja*, and meditation…

Now you are boarding a train…You watch the train passing several such stations, as Feb 07…at the station at a glimpse Jan 07… yes, it is a fast moving train… there is Allahabad. There is *Kumbhmela* that is going on…There is Radha, she is a very spiritual person…that she signs her name. You see brilliant, luminating face of Chidanand Saraswati (holy man, a guru that she met, means ecstasy) and… receive his blessings.

Your train is moving fast and we want to go miles and miles at a faster pace, much, much at a faster speed, such that as you reach at a faster speed, you are in July 2006. You are in the spiritual presence of Dayanand Saraswati at Ashram…(name of the place)…You sign in his presence. This place has been familiar to you …you know this place…and we were here only 2 days back.

Radha has a choice…when Radha wants to go slow and it is your choice to go slow…Radha will move any of her fingers of right hand if and it is your choice to go slow… But Radha wants to move miles ahead…she has miles to go…before she wants to go slow…she is now moving fast… she is in Nov 2005, she is in Ranchi……she has miles to go… Radha gives consent to move fast……she has miles to go… and she is already in Ranchi…She sees herself in Ranchi, in Nov. 2005. It is a beautiful place…There are various Ashrams…and temples. She meets many saints, sages, gurus, and, so many…learned people. They are radiating spirituality…… all around you…… all around you, Radha…now…and this spirituality is getting richer and richer…and further rich, by presence of Radha…She feels fine fragrance surrounding her all around…when it is May 2005…we are in Ranchi and you are experiencing aesthetically spiritual experience in meditation…When you feel that spiritual fragrance and, as you are feeling that spiritual fragrance, Radha certifies that by her signature…that spiritual fragrance, Radha is feeling that fragrance…you are being helped to sign…
(Radha signs).

Please Radha, as you have done such an intense work in such a short time... spiritual fragrance. Please hold the pen and sign. Now, please stay at Ranchi. stay at Ranchi for a while to experience the place...It is a serene, quiet, quite peaceful, tranquil place. Please meditate here all by yourself. stay at Ranchi for a while... In that meditation there is silence and stay in that silence for a while...till we decide to go to Rishikesh.

Stay in the state of meditation...you are not hearing my voice any more...till such time that I tell you to hear it once again... nor you hear any other sounds around you...There is only a sound of fine fragrance...a sound of subtle, fine fragrance. My voice has gone further and further far away...it fades into fragrance...

Radha is in deep trance so other participant can ask any question. Even if they do not have, they are made to speak, to ask to confirm later on that she has not listened to the dialogue. This they will share with her to reinforce the experience.

Q. She is not listening to our voice. How will you take her out of Hypnosis?

A. You will see it shortly.

Q. Why do you do age regression and how do you prepare the subject?

A. We get the full history and also there is a dialogue, consent and full information is gathered. The subject writes down in detail with dates the important incidences of life. There will be happy or sad events (like death of near and dear ones or major accidents) which are relevant. The events are written in reverse manner e.g. She writes from 2007 March backwards. Usually, the subject says that he or she does not remember such events.

(At that time she needs to be encouraged as it may be in deep unconscious mind as repressed events.)

When the symptom started; Say may be 1995; she does not remember. We have to age regress till 1993 when she was completely well. Then ask: shall we move forward now? Let us see what happened in 1995, something happened in 1996, 1997; was Radha connected with it? Giving her a gentle touch on forearm sometime helps to recollect.

Once again, Radha, you are with the therapist (Name of the therapist)...once again, it is your natural due to feel...you are in such a wonderful state of meditation; this is the gift of being a spiritual person. We may go to Rishikesh now...may go to Rishikesh? ...If you want to go, please indicate by signing your consent. Sign your consent, please ...

(There is no response)

Take your own time...

(The subject is in deep trance and is taking longer time. Please be patient. Even ask her to move left finger if she does not wish.)

She is taking longer time. So the therapist with the firm tone says: I am asking Radha, a simple question: either go to Rishikesh or think that we had enough of work. Stay where you are and you are to decide.

(As she is not answering, she is in deep trance, the therapist can take own decision. The goal is to go to past life. The therapist once again talks to the subject.)

Radha, it is nice, radiant spiritual glow on your face. Your face is shining with that glow. We have set a goal of going to past birth. And when you are ready, please sign your consent.

(She signs)

Thank you so very much.

You want to go to past life, further and further, to go far, far away. Now, that you have started going, it is fast approaching and is about to approach. We go fast and faster and may be several years backward ...We decide to go with the speed of light...We decide to go with the speed of light...We decide to go with the speed of light and... then, a little slower than the speed of light... you see many *Ashrams*, and you see that you have visited a few of them. You have been there and you are witnessing it. You have put up for few days at Devprayag and few days at Badrinath and Kedarnath (North India). You are moving fast and you are at Baroda (West India) and still faster you are at Rameshwar (South India) and Chitrakut. Here, how nice it is to witness Krishna Leela.

You are at Nasik (These are all holly places of India). But you are so spiritual that you are at the holy river Ganga at Rishikesh. You are at the holiest of all the holy places, where all Hindus (depending on faith, Vatican for Christian, Mecca for Mohammedans etc.) would wish to stay. All the Hindus and such other people who believe in spirituality, Radha, her heart is filled with joy at Varanasi. You are in vast event of *Mahakumbh Mela*. Having had all this spiritual enunciation and initiation with all these holy men, you are going at a high speed and a faster rate. It is year 1996; she is a naughty girl...of 22 years. She decided not to get married...She went to Vrindavan without informing parents...They are worried as to where she has disappeared. But that was to be...as family does not know ...what aim Radha has. She is a different person from the rest of the crowd.

It is year 1994. Radha is very happy for two reasons. Brother is married. She finished her 12th standard.... It is just a simple jump of electron particle...Electron particle has no mass. It also jumps like waves too... She knows all the stuff like electrons and protons and such other particles...It is 10th standard... She passed her 10th standard...and it is the year of sister's marriage...You have a choice now. Either you are in Singapore in a school trip or... at Vrindavan. As you have made the choice...you need not tell me your choice.

May be it is year 1998, or may be 1995, or 1990 or 1985, whatever is your choice, Radha holds the pen and signs her name and certifies once again.

Now, Radha, I am so happy to work with you…I have a great privilege to be associated with you. With one quantum jump of the electron particle, Radha is going to Aug. 3rd, 1975 (Birthday).

The very day, yes, such wonderful day, Aug. 3rd, 1975, and now Radha is traveling at speed of light, in a wink of an eye, Radha sees herself in her mummy's tummy. It is July 1975, June, April, and March, so comfortable in mummy's tummy…The tiny Radha, a tiny dot… Radha, a tiny dot… Radha, a tiny dot…a little beautiful tiny dot…in December 1974, and now Radha goes with the speed of electron or even faster than electron…It is 1974 November, 1973, 1972, 1971, 1970, 1969, 1965, 1960 and as far beyond, as far as you like to go…May be at 10 MB, 20 MB may be 15 MB (confusion technique)… and little less than 100 years…India is in turmoil…1856, the war of independence. It is whole of North India, West India, it is here and there…

Radha is more or less there…She sees what she wants to see, what is she, then and now…In 1986 like speed of light you dart forward 130 years forward and backwards…and it is 1855 and please write…what you want to write.

Yes, you are my friend. We are great friends but I have forgotten your name. "Will you please write your name?" She is under deep trance. She is regressed to past birth. But still she signs her name as Radha. My dear friend, you are a spiritual person and has great spiritual aspiration. You want several phases of past birth, evidently face to face to yourself…it is your doing, I am just walking along you …

You are going so fast. I rather find difficult to travel with you. So I stay behind (ejecting the subject to be independent). You go for further journey, 200 years, 500 years, and 1000 years or years of astronomical figures. All these you are seeing like a flash of light. This was your prerogative. This is your natural due…and you have already met Krishna… had a dance with him…you are having a dance with him…It is a special privilege for Rajni and Bhaskar Vyas to have accompanied you so far, and not any far beyond.

But we have promises to keep and we make the promise that the memory of this sublime spiritual experience will remain fresh and alive with you, whenever, and, every time you want or wish to experience, you will be able to do is in a jiffy.

Let us turn back, fast, faster with a speed of light now from wherever we are in time, space and consciousness, your consciousness is returning back. Now you are returning back to the place where you started (Ashwini Hall) at Nimhans. You are wonderful, great, and supremely spiritual with such a sublime experience now you are pristine pure. Now, you will listen to Rajni. (another therapist).

Radha, now gradually you are waking up, but all that you have experienced is yours to keep. My voice (Dr. Vyas) is going silent. Though I am still sharing spiritual experience with you. We had a long journey back and so we are turning back to the Ashwini Hall with the speed of light. Yes, you are fully relaxed, peaceful, comfortable…

As I count from 10 to 1, you open your eyes, awake, fully awake, all that you have experienced is stored with in you, in your mind, in your brain and, as I am counting backwards 10...9...8...take your time to walk 8...7...6...5...4...3...in to Ashwini Hall, wide awake, alert and fresh in your self and having all the fragrance that you had during the journey... 3——2—— yes Radha, you are feeling light in your eyes, you try and work to open it, and they want to open, allow them to open. Wide awake, and on count of ...5...4...3... 1, 2—1 ...5...4...3...1, 2—1, and Radha, Open your eyes (command). Open your eyes and start breathing normally. Try and move yourself. Alert and wide awake.

Reflections

Usually in age regression, the patient is taken very deep. It takes much longer to go as far as past birth and subject remains hypnoidal, may be even for a day or two. In case of Radha, she remained sleeping for 48 hours: had to be woken up to feed and drink. She was hypnoidal for almost 3 days.

Q. If subject is forcefully woken up, what happens?

A. Psychodynamically her work goes on; she is in trance, in such a situation she has to be made comfortable. Otherwise, there could be severe headache and trance work is left incomplete. She is made to sleep and supervision is kept. Do not ever forcefully wake the subject up. There is dual experience. Therapist is giving such intent session, it is likely that he is also hypnoidal. So always process slowly, deliberately and in a focalized manner.

Q. Why take signature?

A. As one grows in age, the handwriting and the medium of communication changes. So from mother tongue to English and so on.

Post Script to Chapter 19

The following case report illustrates that the belief is the basis: Mind is the slayer, Mind is the healer.

The therapists through their Buddhist leanings became close friends of a Buddhist monk. The monk was the chief lama at the monastery. He will give discourses in the evening and, there will be a gathering of men and women of all ages. The monk in one casual meeting sought the help of therapists. He wondered whether he can be helped with his frozen shoulders and recurrent attacks of migraine. He was sure that some events in his past life are causing these symptoms. Medication has not helped him. He wondered that probably past life regression will help him to identify the *karmic connections*.

Hypnotherapeutic strategies were based on using the currency of the country. Buddhism is routed in the belief of rebirth and reincarnation. Therapist reinforced with absolute concurrence. Immediately he demanded that the therapist must oblige him by past life regression.

The very first session turned out to be stormy. He went into deep trance, did hand levitation without suggestion. At the age past his date of birth he started waving both his arms and burst out sobbing profusely. When the catharsis subsided, the session was terminated. He described his previous life as that of a bird. He saw himself fly in the sky. He found there was a great struggle to remain afloat high in the sky and, there was a great pull to come down. He cancelled his schedule for the rest of the day and, retired to his room.

Next day he told the therapist the following: since few months a young lady is regularly coming to attend his teachings. She keeps staring at him and, he cannot resist reciprocating the same. Some times back the lady has approached him secretly and proposed intimacy. This has rattled him. The therapist suggested that there is a recipe for solution in Buddhism. The monk has accepted vows of celibacy and such other virtues in eight fold path. But Buddha does not enforce any audience. Suffering is real. Its cause can be ascertained and there is a way for liberation from cause.

The monk was very pleased. "This is what I have been teaching but you tell me now as to what should I do?" The therapist advised him, to take refuge in Buddha. There Buddha will guide him to select from two alternatives. If he finds the women irresistible, he may give back his vows to Buddha and, give up monkhood and, become a house holder. Probably he will find a job as a teacher and thus be able to support the family. Alternatively, he has to prohibit the young lady from coming to monastery and delete her from his mind. The lama decided on the second alternative. The therapist continues to meet him to listen to his discourses over last 25 years, during which he occasionally complains of a frozen shoulder.

Notes

1. Ian Stevenson, *Children Who Remember Previous Lives: A Question of Reincarnation*, revised ed., Jefferson, NC, 2001.
2. Bhaskar Vyas and D.V. Nene, *Changing Course of Brahmaputra*, Dalai Lama the Change Initiator, Bombay 1992.
3. Vyas Bhaskar and Vyas Rajni, *Space Time and Consciousness*; The Fifth Dimension New Delhi 2000.

24
Strategies for Spirituality

Spirituality is said to be a pathless land. Meditation is said to happen; it cannot be done. Most we believe otherwise. *Gurus* define a particular method of practice[1] as their own and deny most others. The most famous voyager to the pathless land, J. Krishnamurti, wrote a classic treatise, At the feet of the Masters[2]. He strongly denied any guru, any path or any method. This is often confusing.

Merits and virtues are generated from the generic ground of altered state of consciousness. In order to be better than what we are, we all need to evolve to a better state of consciousness and, no one would want the meditation to happen while driving a car.[3]

Eastern cultures have a vast, varied and magnificent repertoire of strategies. They may be called ways for meditation; but all meditations begin with a *sankalpa* (resolve) that I am now going to meditate. It is, therefore, a beginning with self-hypnosis.

We leave the esoteric aspects of spiritual experience to the sensibilities of the practitioner. Let us straight go to some programmes. At once it should be understood that it is impossible to dwell extensively; *Vajrayana*[4], *Kashmir Shaivism* and Patanjali[5] have several of them. We shall elaborate on just a few.

General Strategy

- ***Person Requesting is Anupama***

There is an *Anupama* (extra ordinary) experience. *Anupama, Anu,* (Atom), The me (3), The *Anupama,* there is no such other person than me that is *Anupama,* no comparable, my highly spiritual motivated self. This is my natural due, I wanted, I aspired. My aspiration is noble... to see God face to face... living... incarnate as... my physical self. As *Anupama* is there, there is no second... there is union with Thee... there is no duality...I have merged into cosmic consciousness.

I The *Anu* (Atom) can become so...small and merge into universe... and also pervade all over the sky...and universe... as universal consciousness. Now

I know… what it is to be with God.… I am with the God… Let there be silence… as I go to highly sublime state… of Tranquility, peace, beauty, and… beautiful by myself. A thing of beauty… is joy for ever… A beautiful state is truly blissful…

- ***Post Hypnotic Suggestion***

I shall be able to experience this any time and every time that I want to. I will listen to the recorded cassette, also it is recorded in my mind… this is a promise to myself that shall be fulfilled.

Buddhist Tradition

Lord Buddha about 2500 years ago sat under the *Bodhi* tree practicing severe penance. After 42 days of fasting and penance, he pondered over the nature of ultimate reality. He attained enlightenment. But this pondering was not dialectical discursive play of thought. Instead, it was in the nature of inner reflection and contemplation. It is the process that begins in the mind and leads one to go beyond mind.

Through this meditative process Buddha came to know the real nature of suffering. The Ultimate Nature of Reality manifested to him as *shunyata* (Void). While the universe has a beginning and end in the very nature of *shunyata,* all the phenomena come to be derived from it. That way, all the occurrences are interconnected and therefore, interdependent. An individual is also a natural phenomenon, therefore, all such occurrences all over the globe-universe, are connected holistically. This deductive logic, though easily understood by ordinarily intelligent persons is not easily realized so that one can derive virtues from it. One has to change the paradigm from the discursive logic to an experience. The experience leads to the gateways of *Vajrayana.*

Vajrayana is full of techniques[6]—*tantra*—that can lead to the attainment of above goals. Its practice generates *Bodhichitta,* a pure state of consciousness. We may reflect on a few *Vajrayana* practices.

For all kinds of initiations, one has to leave one's ego. Interconnectedness and interdependence are appreciated only thorough a realization that no man is an island. So one has to take help from the enlightened ones, from recourse to *dharma,* and by seeking refuge in the collective consciousness/wisdom of the group. Meditating on the deity may be on any one aspect of Buddha such as Vairochana, Ratnasambhava, Amitabha, Amoghasiddhi and Akshobhya. Each one of them signifies a specific aspect in the realm of consciousness.

In *Guhya samaja sadhana*[7], the first step is to take refuge. It is recited as an experience in the inner mind as,

I go for refuge continually to the Buddhas in whose minds abides a mental play (realization of void ness) actualized in stages like the waxing of the stainless moon and infinite methods of pure compassion.

I go for refuge continually to the holy *Dharma* which (as the Noble Truth of the Path) is the basis for total freedom from all misconceptions and the foundation for the excellence of the holy beings, and which (as the Noble Truth of Cessation) is the very nature (of void ness), the single taste of all phenomena.

I go for refuge to the hosts, *Bodhisattvas,* who are masters of discipline, who abide on the stages of progress. The masters are endowed with a glory of *Bodhichitta.* This is incited by supreme compassion. They became freed from the fetters as they progressed.

And following such a surrendering of ones will, there is a resolve that,

I shall generate my mind into a pure *Bodhichitta,* adorned with a pure selfless wish, by application of which the instincts of all the obstacles can be removed.

I arise as *Dveshavajra,* my body dark blue-black in colour, with three faces: black, white and red, and six arms, the right hands holding a *vajra,* wheel and lotus, and the left with a bell, jewel and sword. I embrace *Sparshavajra* who is similar to me. We are both adorned with the eight jewel ornaments. On the upper part of our bodies we are draped with heavenly garments and on the lower parts girded with heavenly silks.

At the crown of my head is Vairochana, at the throat Amitabha, at my heart Akshobhya, at my navel Ratnasambhava and at the energy-channel where my thighs join is Amoghasiddhi. At my navel is Lochana, at my heart Mamaki, at my throat Padnaravasin and at the crown of my head Tara. At my eyes are Kshitigarbhas, at my ears Vajrapanis, at my nose Khagarbha, at my tongue Lokeshvara, at my heart Manjushri, at my secret organ Sarvanivarana-viskambhini, at my joints Samantabhadra and at the crown of my head is Maitreya. At the gateways of my eyes are *Rupavajra,* at the gateways of my ears Shabdavajra, at the gateway of my nose Gandhavajra, at the gateway of my mouth Rasavajra and at the gateway of my *vajra* organ *Sparshavajra.* At my right hand is Yamantakrit, at my left hand *Aparajita,* at my mouth Hayagriva, at my *vajra*-organ Vignantakrit, at the energy-channel of my right shoulder Achala, at the energy-channel of my left shoulder Takkiraja, at my right knee Niladanda, at my left knee Mahabala, at the crown of my head Ushnisha-chakravartin and at the soles of my two feet are Sumbharajas.

From the HUM at my heart, light rays emanate and draw forth from Akanishta the Victorious Ones. JAH HUM BAM HOH! They become non-dual from the symbolic ones. The heads of the Buddha families of each of the deities confer empowerment on each of these deities with a stream of father and mother's *Bodhichitta.*

Om sarva tatha-gata argham, padyam, pushpe, dhupe, aloke, gandhe, naividya, shabda, praticcha hum svaha.

Oh, *Akshobhya* vajra, great pristine awareness, your *vajradhatu* mind is extremely wise, your supreme three *vajras* are three *mandalas.* I prostrate to you, O Melody of Secrets.

Oh Vairochana, great purity, your *vajra*-peace is the greatest joy, your nature is the most supreme Clear Light, I prostrate to you, O Vajra-reveler.

Oh kingly Ratnasambhava, most profound, you are as stainless as *vajra*-space, your nature is pure and without any stain. I prostrate to you, O *vajra*-body.

Oh Vajra Amitabha, greatest king, non-conceptual like space, you are a vajra-holder, you have attained transcendence of longing desire. I prostrate to you, O Vajra-speech.

Oh *Amoghasiddhi-vajra*, complete Enlightened Buddha, you who fulfill every thought, you who have arisen from the very nature of purity, I prostrate to you, O *Vajra*-minded One.

Around the seed-syllable at the heart of the deities of my body *mandala* circles each of their *mantras*.

From the place of union as father and mother, light rays of *Bodhichitta* are emitted, conferring empowerment to all sentient beings, cleansing them of obstacles and transforming them into *HUM's*. These completely fill the expanse of space, and transform to become *Vajradharas* who are brought back by my light rays and dissolve into me. *Om yoga shuddhah sarva dharma yoga shuddho ham.*

By the virtue of this may I swiftly attain the state of *Vajradhara*, the nature of all the Buddhas, and may all beings attain it as well. May I practice both kinds of activities, those actions that are for becoming enlightened, as well as those spoken of by *Bodhivajra* as being those of a fully Enlightened Buddha. May there be no interference to my proper attainment of the completion of this marvelous path. And by spreading and causing it to flourish in all directions and times, may I free all beings by this skillful means.

The deities of my body, Vairochana, Lochana, Kshitigarbha, Rupavajra, Maitreya, Yamantakrit and Achala dissolve in their turn into Clear Light. Then Ratnasambhava, Mamaki, Vajrapani, Shabdavajra, Aparajita and Takkiraja dissolve in their turn into Clear Light. Next Amitabha, Pandaravasin, Khagarbha, Gandhavajra, Hayagriva and Niladanda dissolve in their turn into Clear Light. Then Amoghasiddhi, Tara, Lokeshvara, Rasavajra, Sarvanivarana-viskambhini, Sparshavajra, Samantabhadra, Vighnanta-krit and Mahabala dissolve into Clear Light. Then Ushnisha-chakravartin, then Sumbharaja and then Manjushri dissolve in their turn into Clear Light, and the main figure too dissolves into Clear Light.

The highest initiation in *Vajrayana* is *Kalachakra* which the Dalai Lama offers as a specially privileged and enlightened monk. The meditation here is on a *mandala* where 928 deities are inscribed. While meditating, one extracts an essence of the spiritual qualities of each of the deities and incorporates within as a blessing.

When a transformation is brought about by a ritual and a belief, transformation is there. When we do not understand the psycho-cybernetics, we either call it a myth and discard it or call it a mystery and worship it. The *siddhis* (beneficial values, the nearest inaccurate translation) accrue according to a particular reference.

The classical *mantra* in buddhist meditation, *Om Mani Padme Hum* has a specific meaning for each word of the *mantra* and regardless of the cultural origin of the meditator and his knowledge or ignorance of the meaning of the mantra, it is supposed to be producing beneficial effects.

Om, composed of three letters *a*, *u* and *m* symbolize the impure and pure, body, speech and mind of the meditator and Buddha respectively empty of all its contents: *Mani* literally means jewel, but symbolizes the altruistic intention towards enlightenment, compassion and love. *Padme* stands for wisdom. *Hum* connotes indivisibility of method and wisdom which can lead to a state of nonperturbance by anything.

Other Strategies

It is widely thought that recourse to arousal of *kundalini* leads to inexhaustible reservoir of energy. Zen provides a pathway to wisdom through utter confusion on paradoxes and reflection on apparent utter nonsense. *Vipassyana* meditation may be a reflection on *kayanupassana,* where the flow of the breath and the memory of the body are the objects of contemplation in two different forms called *anapana sati* and *kayagati sati* respectively. *Vedana anupassana* observes the flow of the feelings leading to subtle sharp mind. *Chitta anupassana* passively reflects on the contents of the mind. *Dhammanupassyana,* a contemplation on the philosophical aspects of religious experience like nature, inherent quality, void, merit, and *samadhi* is the final stage of *vipassyana* meditation.

Transcendental meditation begins by an individually assigned specific mantra which is literally meaningless. After practising for a while, when one can get some glimpse of what Maharshi Mahesh Yogi describes as bliss consciousness. Advanced practice is *siddhi* programme. Here, instead of *mantra,* certain words, viz. sutras are given which are to bring about specific effects. The *sutras* are the programmes taken from Patanjali.

As such, meditation is beyond the realm of mind. If we postulate that the happenings during the meditative state may have some connections with mind and through it to the physicality that is brain, we are led to an interesting conclusion. We have seen as to how the thought processes and the secretion of different neurotransmitters are specifically linked. A practice which is thousands of years old and the scientific basis of which we are just about to glimpse, may well have been built on such a perfect understanding of body-mind relationship that the seers evolved specific mantras, sutras, and such other modalities that the meditative "programmes", through the neurolinguistic connections bring about the desired physiological effect.

The utilitarian would ask how much time it is likely to take. At this moment, it is useful once again to remember that the meditative process is not a thought process. How much time the computer takes to go through the kilobytes of memory stored in its chips? The software will discharge functions according to the needs and commands of the practitioner. And of course, the capability of the computer itself will determine its function.

How can a person be free from anxiety, depression, learnt helplessness and such other signs of stress and post-traumatic syndrome? How would compassion, kindness, friendliness, appreciation of other's virtues and ignoring their short comings and most important of all, diminution of ego?

Practice, Practice, Practice is the answer.

Notes

1. Adi Sankaracharya, *Vivekachudamani*. Most easily available is the commentary by Swami Chinmayananad.
2. He was to deny it later: he said to Rohit Mehta that he has not written it. Theosophical Society was made to take off his name as the author.
3. While driving long distance on straight turn pikes, hypnosis does happen. The drivers are warned against it.
4. The Dalai Lama, *The Four Noble Truths*, New Delhi, 1998.
   The Dalai Lama, *Ethics for the New Millenium*, London, 2000.
   Ratanakul P. *The Buddhist Ethics of Metta*, Paper given at the Sion Conference on Ethical Reflections, Netherlands, October 1991.
   The Dalai Lama, *The Four Noble Truths*, New-Delhi 1997, pp. 120-121.
   Ibid., The Way to Freedom. Core Teachings of Tibetan Buddhism, Dharmashala, 2000, p. 133.
   Anil Kumar Sarkar, *The Mysteries of Vajrayana Buddhism from Atisha to Dalai Lama*, New Delhi, 1993, pp. 157-173, 205.
   Geshe Kelsang Gyatso, *Essence of Vajrayana, The Highest Yoga Tantra Practice of Heruka Body Mandala*, London, 1997, p. x-xii.
   Geshe Nyawang Dhargyey, *Kalchakara Tantra*, Dharmashala, 1985.
   Gehse Lhumdub Sopa, Jackson R. and Newman J. *The Wheel of Time: The Kalachakra in Context*, New York, 1991.
   John Blofeld, The Way of Power, *A Practical Guide to the Tantric Mysticism of Tibet*, London, 1970, pp. 190-218.
   The Dalai Lama, *Path to Bliss, A Practical Guide to Stages of Meditation*, New York, 1991, p. 194.
   Lama Thupten Yeshe, *Transference of Consciousness at the Time of Death*, Boston 1991, pp. 1-42.
   Hayward J.W. and Franscisco Varela, Gentle Bridges, *Conversation with the Dalai Lama on the Science of Mind*, Boston, 1992, pp. 106-125.
   Suzuki, D.T. *Essays in Zen Buddhism*, First Series, London, 1980, p. 49.
   Ibid., p. 121.
   Goleman Daniel, *Healing Emotions, Conversations with The Dalai Lama on Mindfulness, Emotions and Health*, Boston, 1997, p. 217.
5. *Viz, Panchstavi*, published by Ramakrishna Ashram at Jammu and Kashmir Shaivism by Jayadeva, Maharshi Mahesh Yogi, Creating an Ideal Society, Seelisberg, 1977.

Wallace Robert Keith, *The Physiological Effects of Transcendental Meditation,* A Proposed Fourth Major State of Consciousness, Los Angeles, 1970.
Orme –Johnson D.W. and Farrow J.T. Scientific Research on the Transcendental Meditation programme: Collected papers. MERU, Switzerland, 1976.
6. Shakti Gowain, *Creative Visualizations,* New York 1987.
7. As taught by the Dalai Lama.

25
Resistance and Failure

Scientific theories and practical applications succeed in statistically significant numbers: one hundred per cent success is a rarity that belongs to the realm of eternal Truth. Induction of hypnosis depends upon the suggestibility of the subject: people have different hypnotic talent. Some will experience a deep trance at the very first session: others will do so after fractionation technique or at subsequent sessions: about two per cent of the population is not hypnotizable. Higher the intellectual level and stronger the motivation, hypnotic suggestibility increases. Expectancy also builds up easier access to the hypnotic state.

Those who challenge are best left alone: therapist is interested in helping his client. He is not in any contest. However, some clients genuinely wish to be helped but are finding it hard to experience altered state of consciousness. Coin technique and the use of pendulum are useful to induce them.

Coin Technique

Several five rupees coins are taken in one hands. The Subject is asked to assess the heaviest coin from the coins in the hand. It is said, "As such all the coins are supposed to be of the same weight but with the fine assessment by you, you will be able to find a very, very fine difference in the weight. You will find one of them to be heaviest".

He shuffles them, evaluates them, and gradually eliminates one by one. He is left with one coin which is heaviest according to him. With the outstretched hand holding the coin on medial aspect of palmer side, he is asked to observe with one eye the coin. The other eye looks at sun and universe and around him self. The coin in right hand is getting heavier and heavier...The coin seems to be a mysterious coin (swallow the saliva, deepening the trance)...Some how the coin seems to be absorbing particles and gaining weight...The coin is so heavy that it is impossible to hold it. And, really it is impossible to hold... it is up to you to hold such heavy weight... carry such load and suffer... You may allow it to fall—It is up to you to hold the heavy weight... so heavy, eyes are closed...sphincters are tight...let the heavy coin... fall down... dropping down... Coin drops...

As soon as the coin drops the right hand also drops in your lap...Heavy weight has fallen down...As soon as it has fallen you are so relaxed, by dropping the heavy weight...no need to hold heavy weight of tension.... As you have dropped the heavy weight, it has fallen down, gone from your hand...your mind...with each deep breath and, weight off your hand, head feels easy. It is profoundly relaxed...deep breath...Enjoy this state of relaxation till I come back to you.

Once the subject is in hypnosis, deepening techniques are applied before therapeutic suggestions are given.

However, even after induction there can be resistance to therapy as described below.

- ***Case 1***

A prematurely retired professor at Medical College was unable to sleep, at times whole of the night since last 11 years. He has been to several psychiatrists and a hypnotherapist before being recommended. He missed his first appointment. He was persuaded so he came for the next without being accompanied, even when he was asked to do so.

He was taken to a medium state of trance before audience of students. He was age regressed to the time of the beginning of his ailment. It was the year when he had let gone a promotion to stay on at the place of his preference. Appropriate ego strengthening and sublimating suggestions were given. The observers were demonstrated hypnotic phenomena. At the end of the session, he refused to have experienced any hypnosis. He did not contact for next appointment. When asked a few days after, he made an excuse and ejected himself.

- ***Case 2***

A highly motivated young brilliant business manager was unable to work because he was getting "vibes". He had several traits of eccentricity. He was ruthlessly honest: so that he would not take a job unless he was himself sure that he can function at his best. He had been to several physicians, other specialists and, was variously diagnosed. He was operated for chronic sinusitis; was not relieved.

Eight sessions of profound, deep hypnosis involving well targeted archetypal symbols did not produce any change. Occupational therapy and cognitive restructuring were also incorporated. There was no change.

- ***Case 3: Session 1***

A medical specialist and hypnotherapist had fatigue, weakness, myalgia, arthalgia, perineal pain, heaviness, heart burn, abdominal pain and tenesmus (proctalgia fugax) of twenty years duration. Symptoms started when he could not take to his chosen specialty. He is super intelligent.

Dr. Siddhartha, the stubborn: **Method of induction**: Pendulum technique

Dr. Siddhartha, do you want to get hypnotized? If yes, let us have the answer from pendulum too. Let us define Yes, No and I do not know answers that can be elucidated from pendulum. Let the pendulum answer. You say yes, keep your eyes closed; and, keep your eyes open (confusion technique,) pendulum will try to find the answer... Pendulum has given the answer.

Pendulum has given the answer, as yes.

If your eyes follow the pendulum, they will go left to right and right to left...you move your eyes as pendulum moves. (Dissociative eye movement technique) and, Dr. Siddhartha is asking the pendulum as the pendulum is moving... It finds his way, as you are asking the question. Pendulum is starting to move left to right and right to left. Dr. Siddhartha, follow the movement of pendulum.... your eyes are following the pendulum left to right and right to left.

If eyes want to close, let them close...as your eyes are closing now ...as you relax.... take a deep...deep breath,... deeper and deeper breath... as you relax...your muscles get loose...muscles of hands and fingers also want to relax (pendulum about to fall, did not fall...patient is in deep trance) And you have under gone, deeper and deeper.... still a state of complete, absolutely complete trance...so well relaxed and so comfortable, your friend is helping you to adjust the chair...a little bit to manage the comfortable position, very nice...., take deep.... deep breath...pendulum falls...

I am letting go your hand, your hand has fallen like a log of wood and you are deeply relaxed... so well relaxed, that for ten long years, you have probably not experienced this profound, absolute, peaceful relaxation...

Hardly ever before, and you have not taken such a deep breath.... A further deep breath. and as you take deeper and deeper breath.... Thank you very much for a perfect understanding, good rapport, absolute trance.

These are, some of the bonds of friendship... and, I am so privileged that, I am your friend and also a friend of your father.

And some of the brightest characteristics of personality, what are the brightest and finest traits of personality, Dr. Siddhartha, you know very well, and he moves and moves forward... and he moves the index finger of right hand to say yes, and he is so well relaxed with harmony, and when you have moved your right finger, there has been so much of peace and joy... not only in your heart but in the heart of all your friends and mine...

We are able to achieve the first goal...you have relaxed...yes... you have relaxed... yes... you have a good experience of hypnosis...yes...you have a good experience of hypnosis... trance... yes...you have a good experience of hypnosis...that is conducive of harmony between your body and mind...between all the systems of your body...yes... you have a good experience of hypnosis... and all most all goals in your therapeutic session will be achieved. That is because it is your natural due. Such highly, specially skilled person...also super intelligent people should know and, you are also aware...that is your natural due...to discover...process of discovery is the natural due for supper intelligent, specially gifted supper intelligent people. And as they take recourse to refined knowledge, we do probing, proving, denying or accepting the inference it offers and they take a path...that may be pathology... that is their natural due...

Deep breath in and out, deeper and deeper and as we have entered into this communion of consciousness, it is your choice to carry on to enjoy as well as at the same time dissociate your self... we don't have to choose Dr. Siddhartha... you don't have to choose Dr. Siddhartha, that is happening in you all the time... let me give you a choice...

And I want to ask you when I give you some thing that is your natural due, your experience, profound sense of relaxation,...... joy and peace... something that has illumined you so far, having a cascading...over whelming cascading effect all over your body...a further deep breath... I want to give you a small gift...would you accept? ...when you want to accept move your yes finger...(moves the finger)... And perceive the fine fragrance of peace...peace coming from all the directions and as this peace also has a fragrance and when you experience this fine fragrance coming from all around, you will move the right index finger (moves the finger), very nice and having got the fine scent of peace, it will give you a certain and sure gift that is your natural due since 2 years, 5 years, 10 years, or many more years. What all excellent accomplishments you have achieved in last 20 years.

You got admission in medical college, you graduated and you overcame the hurdle of career choice... you have made it a success, in choice of your career at the young age of 39. You have a beautiful family... harmonious, love, affection, comfort, joy and at such a age you have access to the finer understanding of body mind relationships...what you understand and I believe can experience also, is seldom available to most people, so shall we make a choice...when you want to accept to take the gift that I am about to give you...you will move the index finger of your right hand. but should you want to wait I will give you some more time as a gift...with out any hesitation. you can certain move index finger of your left hand...your choice very nice you have decided ...as a friend to a friend and...a therapy from therapist to potentially gifted sensible therapist...what you have been denied so far for long...20 years it is my privilege to gift you...this harmony and shall we see before our eyes that what harmony is...I have put the harmony into your being and also I have already put the harmony into the frontal lobe of your brain but it is every where... there in your hypnotherapy...see your hypothalamus in front of your eyes...and, at the top there is thalamus...and around them there is cingulate gyrus...Generating innumerable images of multiple realities as well as generating multiple intelligences, you are seeing them right before your closed eyes.

Super, super intelligent people generate multiple intelligences and this multiplicity of intelligence cause, they do cause enormous kinds of emotionality.

And you see them...all kinds of different emotions, dancing before your eyes in chaotic session... it indeed is a chaos... Now, that you have this splendid gift from a friend to a friend and you have accepted it so willingly and gracefully, splendid gift so much rooted in your prefrontal cortex, as well as in your thalamus, hypothalamus and cingulate gyrus, that you see this chaotic dance and as you intently keep watching it, and as you intently keep watching it...

Like watching enormous length and breadth of breath, endless pains and in that space as you watch this dance that appeared a little while ago a chaotic, unorganized, disorderly dance, you suddenly see the emergence of an order, the things are taking shape. The emotions are crystallizing in character and the dominance is that of peace, order and harmony.

Out of this chaotic state, a harmonious pattern has emerged and there is the face of a scientist that you knew, with whom you met long ago and with whom you have made friends, and as you see his face as a scientist...take a deep breath in and out and further deep breath in and out...we are face to face with Claude Bernard who introduced you with homeostasis.

And you know homeostasis perfect... to the pH of 7.2 to 7.4, you know the perfect balances of sodium, potassium, chloride, sodium bicarbonate, blood urea, blood creatinine, and ...what not... and now you have this master key to so ordain your own homeostasis, so that everyday morning you will set a part 20 minutes time for your own self.

That... Sidddharth, Dr. Siddhartha's gift to himself and no sooner you will sit by your side, close your eyes, see a pendulum in front of your eyes, may be real...may be imagery, your eyes will move...left to right and right to left, left to right and right to left, left to right and right to left...

And you are in wonderful state of deep, deep and deep profound trance, and the chaos your autonomic nervous system is experiencing, will surely, suddenly and certainly get into the rhythmic dance of harmony. Indeed it is my privilege to have worked with you. It is indeed your privilege to accept it because it is your natural due to your heart.

But to accept the harmony and having accepted harmony, how much harmony is all around you, Siddhartha, that you know now.

Every year, winter follows monsoon, it is a good season of rains and, the spring follows the winter... and so does summer follow the spring and then harder the summer...better are the rains...you had hard times so far...

Again there is a harmonious change of day and night, night and day.... day and night, night and day...And disorder and order, chaos and harmony, they are also a harmonious chain of self recovering, self caring, and change that you have perceived rather within you.

This perception of entire harmony, and entire harmony in your body and mind will now set in motion... now set in motion emotions...so that, limbic system in your brain is set to order. It perceives everything, but response appropriately without exaggeration and certainly down to the reality...

Take your own time to wake up from this profound sense of peace and harmony, harmony is peace and only when there is peace and then there is harmony.

- *Session 2*

Strategy: Exploration of the unconscious mind: cognitive restructuring. Induction technique: use of pendulum.

Dr. Siddhartha, pendulum is asking you to relax and when you are fully relaxed let pendulum fall down...pendulum falls...very nice. Dr. Siddhartha you are totally and profoundly relaxed.

You perceive a fine perfume...And as perfume pervades now in your breath, it spreads down in your heart, and there in your blood it circulates all over your body...I just want to tell you that profound reality that you know and you do not know that you know... And, yet so small and so simple a secret. When you want to listen that secret... move the index finger of your right hand... very nice Dr. Siddhartha. It is a secret, it is profound reality, it is really certain... is yet small and simple...I am going to tell you, never mind, various kind of noises around you, noises around within you...you will not listen. You will listen, only my voice...your secret...within you... All other voices are fading far far away. And I in this state of focal awareness, (other subject in the group had catharsis by way of a bout of coughing)... nobody is coughing, nobody is talking, even the birds have stopped chirping. I am telling you a small and simple secret... Believe me, it is your natural due.

The secret.... the secret is that you are a master therapist yourself. You have excess to those mind body linkages. We know that the mind is the cause where symptoms of the disease arise. We have also seen that diseases are metaphors of mind that the body displays. Because of displeasures, discomfort and dislikes of the mind, diseases arise. They are just metaphors and metaphor conveys a message in different words. Dr. Siddhartha has direct, discrete, access to the understanding of this metaphor. The discomfort must go and the disease just gets cured. Displeasure is replaced when radiology translates into pathology. one branch is as much tree as the other...every branch is tree itself...tree unfolds into different branches and yet, it remains tree...a tree is a tree......a tree is a tree......a tree is a tree with different branches.

Some likes and dislikes are a part of life. There is a day and there is a night, there is dusk and there is dawn, finally at the bottom line being so intelligent a person and having been so privileged to understand psycho cybernetics... and what is this psycho cybernetics. It is what you can control in a moment is likely to happen in your mind. You do not have to exercise the control, cybernetics pathways are already triggered, so that from this moment onwards you are profoundly gifted with the faculty of healing your self. You are excelling in your personal healing, so that, you now have a special faculty to heal others and yourself. Enjoy this special gift, gift that is from a friend to a friend, and so he is giving. The giver also is gifted with that faculty. Giver also has gained, and feel yourself, so privileged to have such psycho cybernetic ability…you will like to wake up now…and, you will only wake up after your psycho cybernetic work is done…when you want to wake up, you will wake up, it will not take more than 20 minutes.

- ***Session 3***

Cognitive restructuring through hypnoanalysis

(For hypnoanalysis, a different technique is utilized here. The subject is taken into deep trance. It requires repeated suggestions for deepening. Yes and No signals are defined and through out the session there is permissive cajoling to elucidate the response. The resistance and denial are bypassed by leisurely play for the positive. After the end of the session subject remains hypnoidal for a long time and may require assistance to go home. He may be asked to retire. At times he sleeps it off for a few hours. At such a session, psychodynamic work goes on for few days. He may not be disturbed and should be allowed to work at unconscious level. After some time either he communicates, or he has queries or doubts which he may want to clear or he develops insight and gets cured or relief).

Make your self comfortable, Dr. Siddhartha, you can directly put your self in trance. If you want to start doing *kapala bhati pranayama,* please take a deep breath in and out…smell of your choice is felt around you. It is getting around you. This causes the activation of certain genes in the nasal mucosa…and as you relax, relax even more and when you answer my question by telling me yes, you may move finger of right hand and for no move any finger of left hand.

(Arm levitation is being done as he is showing resistance). Let your self go, thank you, let all the tension go, all disturbing thoughts go, thank you for the trust that you have put in me. (Now, the hand is allowed to fall in the lap) when I let go your hand, it lies on your thighs comfortably, wonderful, great, when we trust. There is so much of relaxation on the face and is so much better to breath, to breath in a space of trust and confidence and you have by this time acquired a tremendous knowledge about final and minute understanding of body mind connection.

Body mind connection…And the various cells, their arrangement, their alignment with each other. And you know Dr. Siddhartha, the structure of a cell which probably very few know. You are privileged to know the structure of cell…those are cells in nasal mucosa that can smell various perfumes… you know this Dr. Siddhartha, don't you? ...that olfactory cells give us the sense of smell.

... would you like to listen the stories of this perfume? 'Yes', it is my privilege to talk with such a talented friend. Only a few will understand and that there are cells in mucosa of nose and in this refined, relaxed, joyful, pleasant, highly creative state...and in this highly creative state...the cells in our body have a nucleus Dr. Siddhartha...

You are seeing a cell under the microscope in your lab. As you increase the power of magnification...you have increased the power of observation...and you can see the chromosomes and when you see the chromosomes, move any of the finger that is the 'yes' finger. You are adjusting the power of magnification. Now, you have isolated the cell and focused on nucleus. They have the wonderful magical dots... You know Dr. Siddhartha that there are genes in these chromosomes.... Wonderful, marvelous.... you are observing.

The story...you are seeing genes and you are now seeing those genes in your nasal mucosa and would you like to count those... 'yes' as you started counting those genes... tell me yes, by movement of your any of the fingers of your right hand...Fine... Fine perfume...genes...your friends... they are 1, 2, 15, 35, 49 may be even more than 100...they are wondering... joyful...and they are sending messages to decode the perfume... body has... particularly a human being has... such wondrous abilities, that not only, we smell through the activation of genes in nasal mucous... yes, is the activation of genes in nasal mucosa, ...you have the ability to arouse cells...all over your...Dr. Siddhartha...body...to make them feel this wonderful perfume, believe me... you have ability to arouse this all over your body as you take a deep breath in and out, you are arousing genes all over your body so that you experience this wonderful perfume...and if and only if you want this perfume to percolate into your cells of esophagus, shall we do that? ...yes...this perfume in your esophagus..., tell me by smelling this perfume and as you are having the feel of this instant perfume... I want you to drink this instant perfume so that your esophagus, which now is loaded with healing and soothing perfume... hold this bottle of water, it is perfume bottle... hold it, even while you remain in trance, drink this perfumed water... you have drank that water easily...this wonderful feeling has gone down in your stomach and all over your body...when you are going to urinate... or any time you will go for toilet...to urinate yes, or no... yes for sure you will go down to urinate...as the urine flows pass your bladder mucosa and the urethra the same fine cooling, soothing effect that you just now have, you will experience that perfume will ones again...your genes will get activated...

Every day you do 20 minutes of this *Yognidra* and arousal of your genes and we may not need to do any other hypnoanalysis. It is all your choice, would you undergo any further hypnoanalysis... when you are cured? The aim is to be well...not hypnoanalysis...You don't need to answer, if you need it, I surely will explore with you.

Take your own your time to immerge your self in this perfume and take your own time to come out from this perfume take your time, soothing in the perfume, you will feel relieved in your bladder and prostate. The relief will stay for ever.

Dr. Siddhartha is a successful hypnotherapist and has helped many to rejuvenate. He denies having been cured. Hypnoanalytic explorations can extend to any depths. The goal is limited to a cure/alleviation to being functional within a certain number of sessions.

Post Script to Chapter 25

Hypnosis is Not the Panacea

- *Case 1*

A high school graduate, an eighteen year old boy residing in a small town nearing a major city belonging to a minority community, he was happy to have quit study to be a small part in family business. He was brought with complaint of persistent vomiting after food since last six months. He has lost weight. His clinical examinations did not reveal any abnormality. The laboratory and radiological investigations were normal. The psychiatrist did not find any apparent psychiatric illness. When the placebo therapy with antacids and gastric sedatives failed, the psychiatrist referred him to hypnotherapist. Hypnotherapist observed that the psychodynamic cause seem to be "residing" in his home town. If he stayed in the city where he came for his hypnotherapeutic sessions his vomiting would cease. It recurred no sooner he was back to his village town.

Further probing revealed one important cue. Before the onset of his symptoms he was engaged to a girl much more affluent and with higher social status compared to his own family. She was living in the same town. The hypnotherapy approach utilized several different modes. The goal was to make him generate insight about the possible conflict in the new relationship and sort out a resolution by himself. This approach continued for about six months with persistent failure.

The psychiatrist took the courage and the charge. He used confrontation therapy with the family and the patient together. He told them straight that the entire team of the therapists is convinced that the boy is bottled up with frustration about the new relationship imposed upon him by the family. That is why he is throwing it out.

The family snapped the tie. The boy was cured of his vomiting.

Hypnosis is not the Panacea so as to cure always by itself:at times, one must hammer the nail where it pinches.

- *Case 2*

A high profile medical professional, well passed his middle age, highly successful, vastly creative and productive, developed aggravation of his diabetic status. On further laboratory investigations he was diagnosed to have triple hormonal autoimmune disorder. Here, thyroid, pancreas and adrenal glands are affected.

Choice of the endocrinologist, obviously, was to correct the dose of anti-diabetic drugs and institute thyroid replacement. Cortisone was thought of but deferred at the request of the patient. High levels of stress were also noticed. So, the patient was referred to hypnotherapist.

At the first interview only, highly perfectionist personality of the patient was obvious. He was late to report at the reception. He apologized simply; but in the process, blamed himself profusely. He was a professional writer; specifically mentioning that he cannot pardon the modern generation for omitting the dots on the Is and forgetting to cross the Ts.

Further lead along these lines made him to assert that he would like to replace capital "I" in modern civilization with small "i": and of course I has to be crossed so that we remember Jesus Christ: this will also remind us that we all have to bear our own cross. He described his philosophy by quoting Romain Rolland, "to strive, to struggle, NOT to find, NOT to yield.

Stress reduced with hypnotherapy. Further sessions focused on insight generation. He was given a strategic programme to delete redundant files; de-fragment the hard disc and, reduce the data. When he said, Yes to whether he would like to increase RAM of his computer, therapy was further enhanced with Ayurvedic[1] drugs. Yoga was incorporated in the daily routine with a teacher in attendance.

The patient meticulously attended for more than an year. He gave up therapy having benefited by what he declared "holistic" approach combined with his own knowledge of modern medicine.

Note

1. *Ashvagandha,* derived from the roots of a plant is proved to rejuvenate; particularly basal areas of brain.

26
Epilogue

Our efforts in compiling the book shall be more than worthwhile when the readers and practitioners find it a helpful guide in their professional pursuit in this less charted route. The book should help many to get over their health problems; it should open up new vistas for personality development and creativity enhancement. If the book succeeds in creating scientific awareness of body-mind being a single entity, we shall consider that as a further reward.

But there is a further goal. Hard core scientists do not divert from their successful careers to other domain in search of mere professionalism. For those who have taken to hypnosis, we hope the book inspires confidence to call it an emerging scientific discipline. Practising hypnotherapists shall hereafter find academic support to call research in different states of consciousness as the cutting edge of biomedical sciences. Let the awareness grow that hypnosis is a quantifiable state of consciousness.

Consciousness still eludes scientific deciphering: but here is a handy tool to probe it with. It is decoding of this all pervading mystery in the universe—that bio-scientists call consciousness and philosophers of science extol as *universal intelligence*[1]—that shall give us a grand unified theory of what the universe is all about. Such a theory will not only explain what is hitherto unexplained in biological sciences; —and we venture to call quantum physics a biological science since consciousness is involved; —but shall bring about the convergence of scientific disciplines that remain artificially compartmentalized as of now.

Hypnosis is an experiment in transpersonal psychology. There is communion in consciousness. Further explorations[2] of this different state consciousness have a potential to take psychology to a distinctly different realm that we call technology of transcendence. Evolution to such an overmind state[3] will bring about the dissolution of doubts about the science of mind and resolution of existential and such other perennial questions concerning the spiritual essence.

We end the book by quoting a voice from Pondicherry

"The promises are given and they shall be fulfilled.[4]"

Notes

1. Lester Smith, Intelligence came first, Wheaton, 1975.
2. Bhaskar Vyas and Rajni Vyas, *Space-time-consciousness, The Fifth Dimension*, Delhi, 2004.
3. Sri Aurobindo, *Life Divine*, Pondicherry, 2001.
4. Mother's Agenda, Pondicherry, 1976.

Appendix

Letters at the Back of the Book

October 17th, 2008

Just as the book is about to go to the press, we are informed by Earnest Rossi that he has finally proved his visionary hypothesis of gene expression during hypnosis. This is a great break through that finally catapults hypnosis into high corridors of science. So, that now we may say, "The promises were given and they are fulfilled."[1]

August 15, 1988
A letter from Dr. David Cheek
Dear Kripa:

I have not forgotten your request for an answer to the notes of doctor vyas and his wife.

Here it is. I hope it makes sense to them. They sound like very thoughtful people.

David b. Cheek,

July 25, 1988
Notes on request from kripa thakur, may, 1988
Dear Doctors Vyas:

I am very much interested in your thoughts and your project. I am sure you are on a very productive path but I am not sure your colleagues in India or mine in America will be open to the facts as you will find them. My reasons for saying this are as follows:

1. Gynecologists working only with infertility patients seem to have a narrow view of the problem. They have a need to be doing something with the tools offered by large teaching centers where the inner mind of the patient is not even considered.

---

1. Ernest Rossi, Salvatore Iannotti, Mauro Cozzolino, Stefano Castiglione, Angela Cicatelli, Kathryn Rossi, A Pilot Study of Positive Expectations and Focused Attention via a New Protocol for Optimizing Therapeutic Hypnosis and Psychotherapy Assessed with DNA Microarrays: The Creative Psychosocial Genomic Healing Experience. *The Journal of Sleep and Hypnosis*. Accepted on 8-8-08.

2. The idea that a woman's mind might be keeping her from having children is a very old one but doing something about it needs methods that cannot be categorized and require methods that are not yet taught in major medical centers.

On the other hand, i know you are right. Aside from the general fact that a subconsciously unwilling woman or a subconsciously frightened one will not have enough of her own endocrine balance to make an egg and nurture it after fertilization. we also have to consider the hormones of a timid, emotionally inadequate male.

Regarding the idea that a woman could develop immune bodies to attack the foreign protein from her husband:

Black in England has demonstrated that the tuberculin reaction of a Manteux test made on people infected with the Koch bacillus can be diminished by using hypnosis.

Esdaile in India in 1846 demonstrated that the three cardinal signs of inflammation—redness, swelling and local heat- disappear when pain is removed with mesmerism.

Delboeuf in France in 1877 (noted by Bernheim) demonstrated that hypnotic analgesia prevents blister formation and speeds healing with second degree burns.

I noticed during my early obstetrical practice that the first indications of hemorrhagic disease and fetal edema of the new born (erythroblastosis as later recognized in 1941) only occurred with women who had had 7 or more children.

After discovery of the relationship between Rh negative mother with positive father and erythroblastosis there was increasing concern by parents whose Rh factor was determined during the prenatal examination. Now, we began to see erythroblastotic babies after the 4th pregnancy, the 3rd pregnancy and even during a first pregnancy. Why?

I practiced in northern California from 1946 to 1954 and delivered 527 babies. I was taking only primigravidas and women who had had problems with earlier pregnancies.

Having learned that abortions are often caused by resentment on the side of the mother toward the husband or his side of the family, it seemed reasonable to me that hypersensitivity to the husband's red blood cells could be on the same basis.

I taught all my pregnant patients to consider their unborn child as an entity separate from themselves and separate from the husband's side of the family. I told them to talk to their baby throughout pregnancy. If they became angry with a husband or members of his family they were to explain to their unborn child that this was anger toward that individual and had no relationship to the baby.

I did not have a single jaundiced or erythroblastotic baby although I was the only specialist in that area and had couples with presumed incompatibility potential referred to me. In other words I had a greater chance than the usual 5X potential for trouble.

In 1954 I came to San Francisco and was talking about this at a meeting that was attended by the chief of the obstetrical staff at the Presideo Army Hospital in San Francisco. He invited me to see a woman who had history of having given birth to one normal child followed by a normal child that was mildly jaundiced. The next 9 pregnancies of this woman ended with fatalities due to hydrops, anemia or failed exchange transfusions with premature infants.

I saw this woman at 34 weeks gestation time and learned of her frustration with the actions of her overbearing, pilot, husband. The origin of her initial reaction against red cells occurred during the second pregnancy when her husband was being expelled from law school for objecting to the way the law was taught there. My work was to teach her to use long periods of self hypnosis during the remaining weeks before labour started. I obtained permission of the chief to let the patient indicate when she felt she should be delivered by caesarean section. She had previously known when she began reacting against her fetus. Her warnings had always been ignored by the military doctors. She was going instantly into hypnosis every time her husband visited her in the hospital where she was to spend the last several weeks of her pregnancy.

She went to 38 weeks and was delivered of an Rh positive male child weighing 6 Ibs. His hemoglobin at delivery was 10 grams. It dropped to 6 grams during the 20 minutes it took to get the exchange transfusion started. He survived after 3 exchanges and grew up a fine young man. To my knowledge this history has never been equaled. That was 25 years ago, long before Rhogam. The mother was totally Rh negative and her husband totally Rh positive.

So much for supportive comments regarding maternal immune reactions that are responsible-for incompatibility that can influence fertility and the products of fertilization.

I am much interested in your work and would very much like a copy of your paper when it is completed.

Sincerely yours, DAVID CHEEK M.D.

Trauma Tapping Technique

Addition by Ulf Sandström

Trauma Tapping Technique (TTT) is a simple First Aid technique for Emotional and Post Traumatic Stress that works by allowing a specific sensory input (touch) to create a depotentiation of an encoded reaction in the amygdala, resulting in resolving the symptoms permanently. It is of great value as an extra tool for combining with hypnotherapy.

The key factor in making it work, is for the client to be in affect, in contact with the emotion they wish to release. For this, hypnosis is an invaluable method. We have been using TTT for treating symptoms of Post Traumatic

Stress in Rwanda and Congo Kinshasa since 2007 for tens of thousands of clients, with documented results.

Allow me to share it with you, try it and evaluate for yourself. See our website: www.peacefulheart.see for more information.

This is how Trauma Tapping is done

1. Have the client connect to the emotion that bothers you, ever so slightly (no need for abreaction or flooding.
2. Tap 15 times using two fingers, firmly but gently on the points in the picture
3. Have the client take two deep breaths, short in and long out
4. Repeat the tapping procedure
5. Have the client take two deep breaths, short in and long out
6. Have the client relax and breathe normally

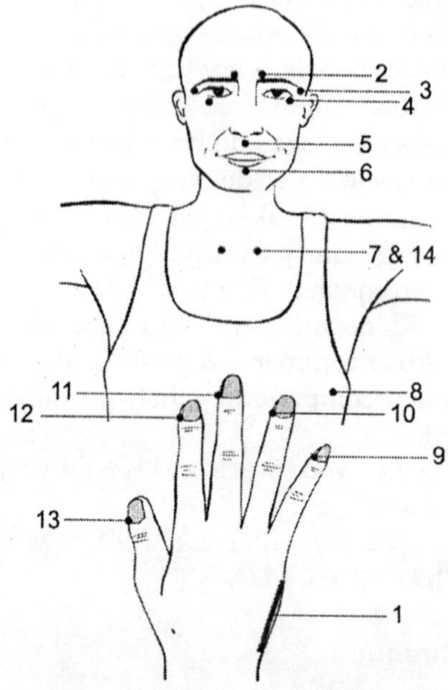

Fig. Trauma Tapping Technique

Points

1. Side of the hand/Karate Point
2. Beginning of the eyebrow
3. Outside eye on the bone
4. Under the eye
5. Under the nose
6. Under the mouth
7. Under the collarbone on the chest
8. Under the arm
9. The inside tip of the little finger
10. The inside tip of the ring finger
11. The inside tip of the middle finger
12. The inside tip of the index finger
13. The outside tip of the thumb
14. Under the collarbone and on the whole chest, like drumming...

Background

The Trauma Tapping Technique belongs to a field Psychosensory treatments for post traumatic stress symptoms and other emotional imbalances which includes for example Eye Movement Desensitization and Reprocessing (EMDR) which is being used successfully for symptoms of traumatic stress and Havening. TTT is also related to Emotional Freedom Technique (EFT) and Thought Field Therapy (TFT) in respect to the tapping of body points, but has been simplified to be content free, language independent and simple enough to be transferable "peer to peer" to make it ideal for areas of post-conflict with a challenged infrastructure.

AXIOMS

Certain statements can be taken for granted. Therapeutic strategy can then be derived from those axioms.

Hypnosis and Hypnotherapy

- Hypnosis is altered state of consciousness. It is distinctly different from other three ordinarily well known three states *viz.* awake, sleep and dream.
- Hypnosis is easy to induce. Anyone can learn to induce hypnosis.
- Most humans can be hypnotized. Those who resist and challenge should be avoided.
- Hypnotherapy is strategic. Such applications of hypnosis require scientific understanding of physiology and psychology. Training and practice that evolves over a number of years are a must for therapist.
- For strategic application of hypnotherapy, diagnosis of the condition being treated is necessary; so is the understanding of pathogenesis.
- Goals as well as intermediate aims in therapy need to be defined at the onset of treatment.
- Familiarity and ability to elicit various phenomena is a must for the therapist.
- The deft application of the above facilitates the treatment. The therapist decides which phenomenon to be invoked.
- Hypnotic state is a state characterized by heightened suggestibility. There is uncritical acceptance of the suggestion.
- The suggestions work like a surgeon's knife.
- It is the duty of the therapist to look after the physical comfort of a hypnotized subject as much as an anesthetist looks after the anesthetized patient.
- In hypnosis there is innate preference for the natural state of well being as well as towards positive aspect.

- Rapport is basic to all forms of psychotherapy. Minimum effort is necessary in hypnotherapy. Rapid and intense rapport is fundamental to the success.

Mind

- There is no substance to the mind; never mind, as long as we mind our mind to manipulate the mind of the subject carefully.
- There is no specific location of mind in the brain. Different centers perceive sensorial inputs at specific locations. Summation of sensorial inputs generates perception. Out of numerous and variable perceptions concepts are generated. *Manah shashti indriyani.* Mind is sixth sense organ. Concepts are basic to intelligence.
- Concepts are the guidelines for function. Valid concepts provide smooth functioning at societal and personal level. Corruption of the conceptualization is basic to psychopathology. *Manah eva manushyanam karanam bandha mokshabhyoho.* Mind alone is the cause of bondage and freedom for the human beings.
- There is no duality between mind and body. One is not separate from the other. There is a mind body continuum; one influences the other continuously and simultaneously.
- French philosopher Descartes was wrong in considering mind as separate from the body but his philosophy still pervades in propagating wrong notion.
- However, Descartes was absolutely correct to say that body mechanisms function as interconnected wheels so that motion in any system sets up a dynamic movement all over.
- Unconscious mind (This collates with the *chitta* in Indian Psychology) constitutes about 90 per cent the psychic contents.
- Subconscious mind is the portion of psyche that can be brought into awareness with some effort.
- Conscious mind, that is ordinary aware, constitutes about 1 per cent of psyche.

Physiology and Pathogenesis

- Homeostasis, i.e. a continuous maintenance of equilibrium of all the parameters at molecular and systemic levels is fundamental to life.
- An aberration in any of the parameters causes a disorder or a disease.
- An infection in the body produces a particular disease. A perpetual conceptual corruption causes psychic disturbance so as to produce stress. This is basic to psychosomatic diseases.
- Psychic disturbances can be behavioural, cognitive or both.

- Corrupt conceptualization is like a virus in software system of a computer. It can crash all the data and even erase the hard disc.
- Psychological disorders and organic diseases are understood at molecular level; however these levels by themselves do not constitute a disorder or a disease. Mere biochemical correction does not reverse the disease process.
- Psychodynamic discreativity either creates the disease or contributes to its propagation. *Pragyaparadha jayate sarve rogan* (All diseases arise from the faulty functioning of discriminative wisdom. This quote from Charak summarizes the etiopathology of all diseases).
- Diseases are the metaphors that body creates to express its discomfort because of a traumatized mind.
- Thoughts and emotions equate with floating particles in blood stream.
- Emotions are further identified with numerous biochemical substances such as hormones, neurotransmitters and other information substances.
- Symptoms arise when events are inadequately processed so that there is repression into unconscious mind.
- Unconscious mind is the hidden dynamo that drives the body functions at all the times.

Therapeutic Process

- Belief is fundamental to therapeutic cure. *Samshayatma Vinashyati.* One who doubts perishes.
- Hypnotherapy is the therapy of new millennium.
- Hypnotherapy is drugless therapy: however drugs do have a justified use and should not be excluded when indicated.
- Hypnotherapist cannot lie. However, he puts bitter truths in sugarcoated form. *Satyam bruyat, priyam bruyat* (You will speak the truth; but speak it in pleasant, acceptable way).
- The therapist should be focalized during the session.
- Wonder and continuous building up of that is one of the most important ingredients in therapy.
- Therapy aims at relief or cure: there is no judgment of the patient/client.
- Values of the client, personal or cultural are his/her property. They have to be respected and so honoured. Use the currency of the country you are in during the proceedings.
- During hypnosis, an event may be relived; so that the memory can be erased or modified. Reliving a happy event can provide substitution for the traumatic one.

Dynamics of Change

- Suggestions work, since in hypnosis, surreal is identified as real. This is reinforced by the therapist. Metaphors are surreal symbols.
- Language, semantically as well as through syntax, is understood by brain. Word is a symbol. During hypnosis, symbol can change its meaning.
- Arousal of emotions potentiates therapy. *Yad bhava, tad bhavana; yad bhavana, tad bhavatu.* As is the experience, so, are the feelings As you feel, so it happens.
- Overall therapeutic stress reduction leads to easier maintenance of homeostasis.
- Therapeutic reversal of aberrant psychodynamics by elimination/ modification of faulty perception.
- Insight generation. A moment sees what the ages toil to express.

Dynamics of Transformation: Plausible Hypotheses

- Creativity is geared to a higher order and may be, to a radically different mode.
- Neurones do not regenerate; however, brain undergoes plasticity through development of new synapses; this may be facilitated by hypnotic process.
- Changes in the conditioned/stereotype pathways in the brain.
- Opening of different functional areas of brain, such as prefrontal cortex and down grading of function of other areas. fMRI studies by us will prove.
- Different gene expression. Gene expression studies by us will prove.

Index